SMOKING

AND

TOBACCO

CONTROL

MONOGRAPH 5

Tobacco and the Clinician

Interventions for Medical and Dental Practice

U.S. DEPARTMENT OF HEALTH
AND HUMAN SERVICES
Public Health Service
National Institutes of Health

NIH Publication No. 94-3693
January 1994

Foreword

As we approach the end of the 20th century, smoking continues to decline in the United States, with fewer than 1 in 4 adults reporting they use cigarettes on a regular basis. Per capita cigarette consumption currently stands at a level not seen since the early 1940s, and total consumption of cigarettes declined by 140 billion units in the past decade alone.

This stands in sharp contrast to the midpoint of the century when smoking rates were increasing, especially among women, and per capita cigarette consumption did not reach its peak until 1963, the year preceding publication of the first Surgeon General's report. Like America in 1950, cigarette manufacturers were enjoying unparalleled success and showing no sign of weakening. Then the cigarettes of choice were not the Marlboro, Winston, and Salems of today, but unfiltered Camels, Lucky Strike, Chesterfield, and Philip Morris. These four brands accounted for more than 75 percent of all brands sold in the United States. Camels, which had battled with Luckies for the top spot in the U.S. market for decades, had regained that position in 1949 and in 1950 had a 27-percent market share, leading Lucky Strike's 23 percent. Marlboro, the top-selling cigarette brand among the current generation of smokers with a 25 percent market share, had less than one-half of one percent.

At the beginning of the 1950s, the practice of cigarette smoking enjoyed nearly universal acceptance and widespread social appeal, not only in this country but also in many other parts of the world. Cigarette smoking was practiced by a substantial majority of adult males, with some age groups experiencing 70 to 75 percent smoking rates. Regular use of pipes and cigars was also common among men. The prevalence of smoking among physicians and dentists was equal to and even exceeded that seen in the general male population, whereas today less than 10 percent of physicians or dentists report themselves as cigarette smokers.

Smoking among women still lagged behind that of men, but by the mid-1950s nearly 3 of every 10 women reported they smoked cigarettes regularly. Just a few decades earlier women had been openly criticized for smoking, especially in public. However, by the end of the second world war, major social and environmental change that affected women's lifestyle choices, including smoking, had already begun. These changes, fueled by aggressive cigarette advertising and marketing, led to a rapid rise in the number of women smoking. By the end of the 1950s, smoking by women became not only socially acceptable but the expected norm among some strata of women.

It is useful to examine some of the processes by which the cigarette manufacturers were able to produce this widespread social acceptance and high level of cigarette use, and particularly for the purposes of this monograph, it is enlightening to examine how the credibility of physicians, dentists, and other health personnel was used to create a positive image for cigarette smoking. The reassuring image of physicians and other health care practioners was used extensively to convince the public that cigarette smoking was safe, acceptable, and without risk.

The growing public recognition of scientific methods was used to convince the consumer that smoking was healthy and to create confusion about the scientific certainty with which smoking had been established as a cause of disease. Both the health care and scientific communities were slow to recognize and respond to the cigarette manufacturers' use of their credibility to aid in the sale of cigarettes, and we therefore carry a special burden of responsibility in dealing with what is currently our largest preventible cause of death and disability.

The same authority and credibility that was used by cigarette manufacturers to sell cigarettes must now be applied by the health care community to reduce and eliminate the damage caused by tobacco in our society. This monograph is intended to present a comprehensive picture of what physicians, dentists, and other health care providers can do for their patients and communities to eliminate the needless disease and suffering produced by tobacco use. It is also a call to arms so that they can understand and combat the misuse of science and health imagery in the promotion of tobacco.

USE OF HEALTH THEMES AND MEDICAL PERSONNEL IN CIGARETTE ADVERTISING

The first modern blended U.S. cigarette—Camels—was introduced in 1913. Accompanying this change in manufacturing technique was the application of newly developed mass marketing approaches and advertising campaigns that relied heavily on health themes to promote cigarette consumption. During the period from the mid-1920s through the end of the 1950s, all the major cigarette manufacturers in the United States used health-based themes in their advertising. These themes usually consisted of one or more of the following concepts:

- direct health claims—wherein a particular brand of cigarettes was promoted as having a "desirable" health benefit compared with competitors;
- images of health professionals—using models of physicians, dentists, or nurses, they were often used in conjunction with ads purporting a health benefit; and
- medical statements and testimonials—usually quoting scientists or doctors or citing information from surveys of health professionals or Government reports in an effort to minimize the perceived health risks of smoking or to imply that smoking a specific brand of cigarettes was safe or safer than other brands.

WHEN HEALTH BECAME AN ISSUE

During the late 1920s and early 1930s, health themes began to appear increasingly in cigarette advertisements. As early as 1927, Lucky Strike was claiming that dangerous irritants in tobacco should be removed through heating. "It's toasted" was a slogan used for years in all Lucky Strike ads. "Toasting," according to these ads, removed "tobacco's harmful corrosive ACRIDS." One ad in this series even asserted that the dangerous irritants removed from Lucky Strike tobaccos were sold to chemical companies.

Camels stressed how they "increase your flow of energy," and famous athletes affirmed that Camels "don't get your wind . . . you can smoke all you want!" Old Gold cigarettes promised "not a cough in a carload," and Philip Morris instructed the smoker, "Sure you inhale, so play safe with your throat . . . scientifically proved less irritating . . . ."

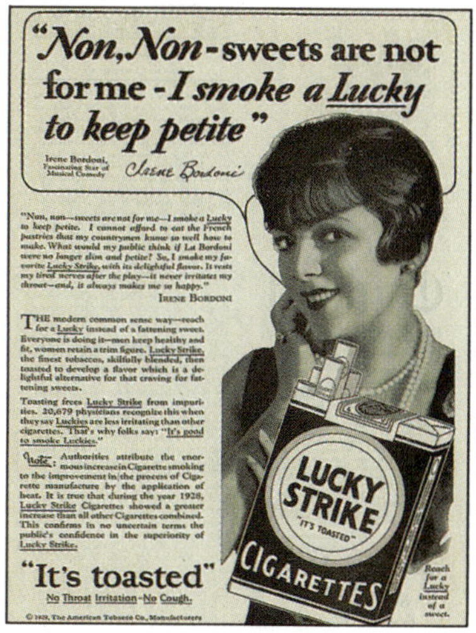

Perhaps one of the most notorious cigarette ad campaigns ever began in 1928 with Lucky Strike's "Reach for a Lucky Instead of a Sweet." Designed especially to entice women into the smoking ranks, this ad theme and its variations ran for several years and often featured well-known entertainers or sports figures attesting to the fact that Luckies kept them slim and petite. Even today, many cigarette ads promote the concept that smoking helps control weight—thus implying a health benefit. Brands such as "Virginia Slims" and "Superslims" directly foster this concept and are marketed exclusively as female brands.

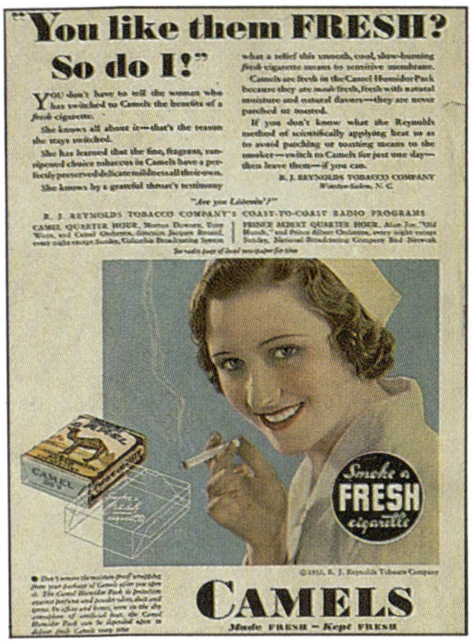

Some ads were obviously intended to convince both smokers and would-be smokers that not only was smoking safe, it was possibly even good for you. In many such advertisements, models portraying physicians, nurses, or scientists were prominently displayed.

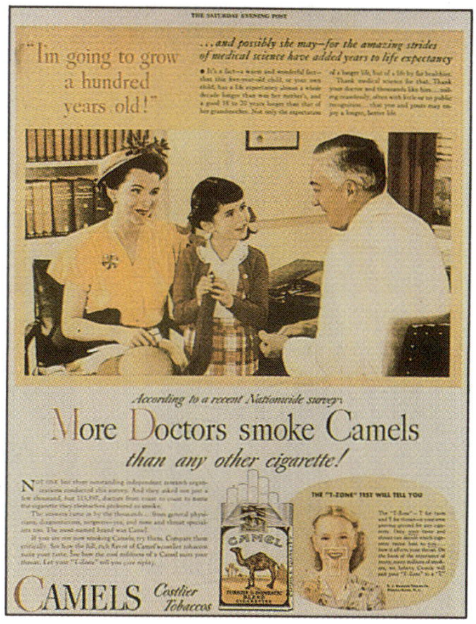

We know today that such health claims were not grounded in science but were fabricated by Madison Avenue in a direct attempt to calm people's growing fears about the dangers of smoking.

The Filtered Fifties The publication in the early 1950s of the first retrospective and prospective studies to conclusively link smoking with lung

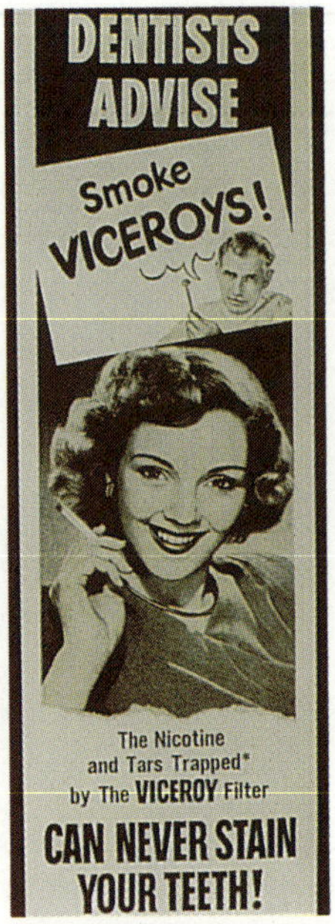
DENTISTS ADVISE
Smoke VICEROYS!
The Nicotine and Tars Trapped* by The VICEROY Filter
CAN NEVER STAIN YOUR TEETH!

cancer led to a new barrage of health claims and medical "testimonials" based on the cigarette industry's newest technological "breakthrough"—the filtered cigarette.

Filter cigarettes were not entirely new, however, but merely a variation of an existing concept, the "tipped" or "mouthpiece" cigarette. Even prior to 1900 filter cigarettes such as Obak and Imperiale were marketed in this country from Europe, but the first major U.S. development in this field occurred in 1931 when Benson and Hedges introduced Parliament filter cigarettes. Viceroy brand cigarettes, marketed 5 years later, originally contained a hollow cotton tube and changed to a cellulose acetate filter in 1954. As the first such company to use cellulose, Brown and Williamson made the point of promoting the "20,000 individual filters in every Viceroy tip." Cellulose acetate became the industry standard for filter cigarettes and is used to this day. Kool cigarettes came with a cork-tipped mouthpiece, whereas Marlboro, initially promoted as a cigarette for women, came with a choice of ivory tips and beauty tips (in red) in addition to their "plain end." Until health became an issue, however, no brand of tipped or filtered cigarettes ever enjoyed much popular or commercial success.

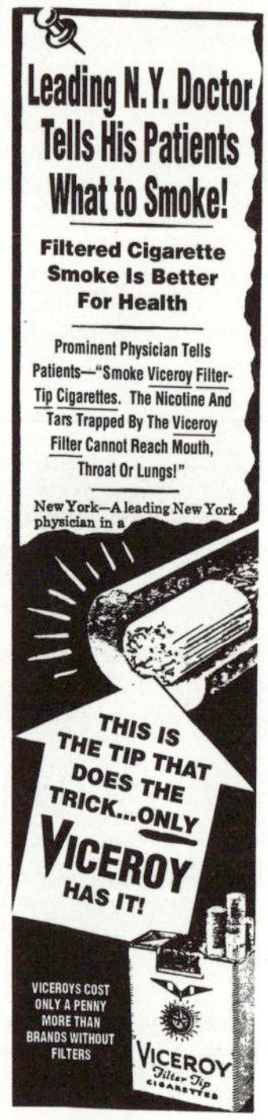

Filter cigarettes soon became the "new" technology that the manufacturers exploited to reassure smokers that regardless of any bad things in cigarettes, "science" now had a solution. At the same time that medical science was increasingly implicating smoking as a health threat, cigarette advertising extolled filter cigarettes as the scientific answer to the health "question." In addition to print advertising, the companies increasingly used the new medium of television to promote these new cigarette product lines as safe. Even popular television shows such as the "Ben Casey, M.D." and "Dr. Kildare" medical dramas were brought into millions of homes each week via cigarette sponsorship—and health protection was a commonly implied theme.

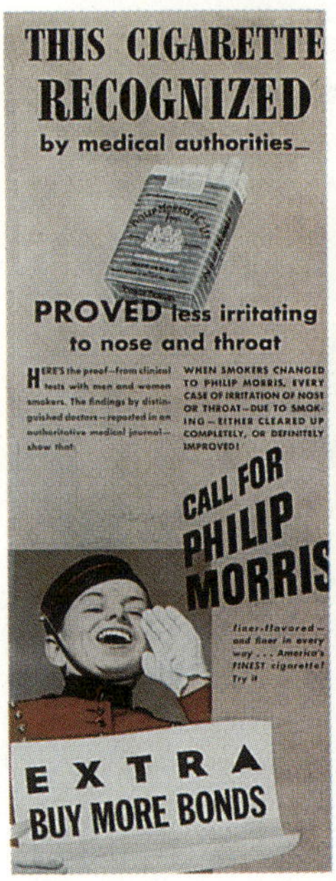

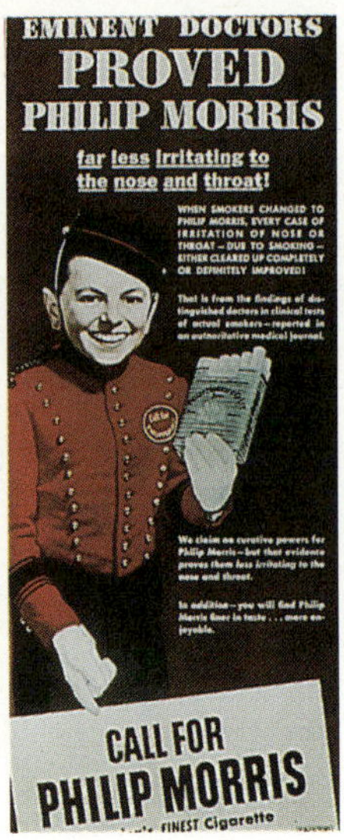
EMINENT DOCTORS PROVED PHILIP MORRIS
far less irritating to the nose and throat!
CALL FOR PHILIP MORRIS

What can be labeled the greatest health fraud in cigarette history occurred in March 1952, when Lorillard Tobacco Company introduced Kent cigarettes with its new

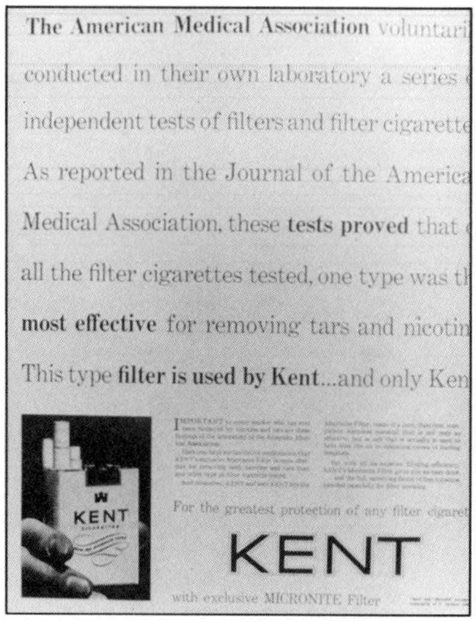
The American Medical Association voluntari
conducted in their own laboratory a series
independent tests of filters and filter cigarette
As reported in the Journal of the Americ
Medical Association, these tests proved that
all the filter cigarettes tested, one type was t
most effective for removing tars and nicotin
This type filter is used by Kent...and only Ke
KENT
For the greatest protection of any filter cigare
KENT
with exclusive MICRONITE Filter

"Micronite filter" that was "developed by researchers in atomic energy plants." Lorillard ad copy stressed that the new filter removed seven times more tar and nicotine than any other brand. To bolster its claim, Lorillard cited none other than the *Journal of the American Medical Association* as its source.

After strenuous objections from the AMA, Kent discontinued any direct reference to that organization but continued to picture health professionals and used the "health protection" theme in both print and television ads for years, sometimes citing pseudoscientific test results in an effort to lend a degree of medical credibility to their claims.

Ironically, the substance in the Kent micronite filter that allegedly provided "health protection" turned out to be asbestos—one of the more dangerous occupational lung carcinogens known. Without any public disclosure whatsoever, the company quietly replaced the asbestos with cellulose in 1957. Millions of smokers who had switched to Kents were never informed either that the filter had contained asbestos or that the asbestos had been replaced.

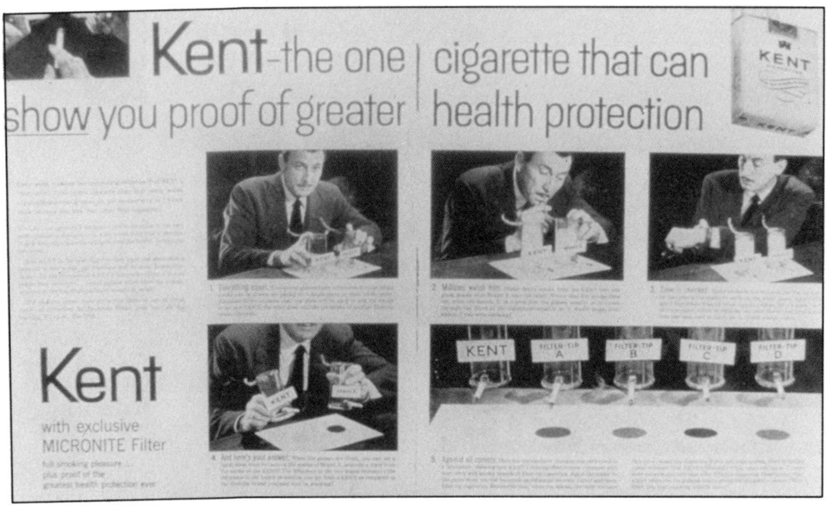
Kent-the one cigarette that can
show you proof of greater health protection
KENT
Kent
with exclusive
MICRONITE Filter
KENT
FILTER-TIP A
FILTER-TIP B
FILTER-TIP C
FILTER-TIP D

As the decade of the fifties drew to a close, filter cigarettes, virtually nonexistent at the beginning of the decade, had captured 50 percent of the U.S. market. This dramatic change in brand market share provides indisputable evidence that cigarette advertising can alter consumer demand. A survey conducted by the Memorial Sloan-Kettering Cancer Center showed that 70 percent of smokers who switched from regular to filter-tipped cigarettes did so for reasons of health. Today, nearly 98 percent of all cigarettes sold in the United States are filtered.

Some Health Themes in Contemporary Advertising

Health claims in advertising did not end with the 1950s but continued well after the Surgeon General issued his now-famous 1964 report. By the beginning of the 1960s, the scientific consensus on the health consequences of smoking was overwhelming, and use of health professionals in cigarette ads could no longer be justified. Nonetheless, health themes are evident even in today's cigarette advertisements.

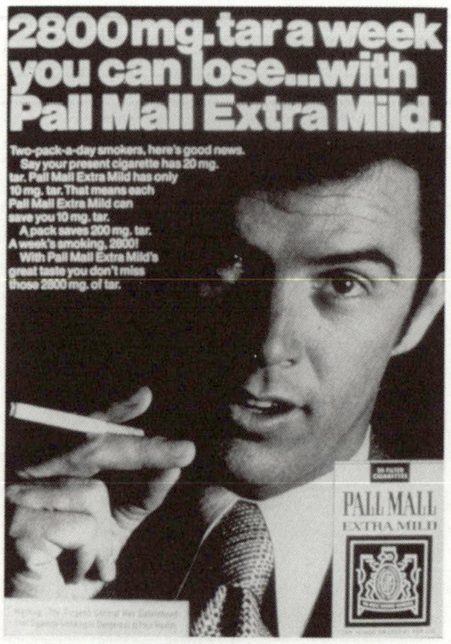
2800 mg. tar a week you can lose...with Pall Mall Extra Mild.
Two-pack-a-day smokers, here's good news.
Say your present cigarette has 20 mg. tar. Pall Mall Extra Mild has only 10 mg. tar. That means each Pall Mall Extra Mild can save you 10 mg. tar.
A pack saves 200 mg. tar. A week's smoking, 2800!
With Pall Mall Extra Mild's great taste you don't miss those 2800 mg. of tar.
PALL MALL
EXTRA MILD

After the 1964 Surgeon General's report, the cigarette companies began citing official Government sources and statistics to promote some brands that were reportedly lower in tar and nicotine. Carlton cigarettes for years used Federal Trade Commission (FTC) test results to proclaim, "Latest U.S. Gov't Report Confirms Carlton is Lowest" or "U.S. Gov't Report: A whole carton of Carlton has less tar than a single pack of . . . ." Now cigarette ads stated, "Now is Lowest" in tar; Pall Mall Extra Mild used FTC data to compare its cigarette brand to others with "2800 mg tar a week you can lose . . . with Pall Mall Extra Mild." Later, it would be found that many cigarette brands had been purposefully engineered to test low in tar/nicotine content based on machine measurement but that they generated much higher yields when smoked by people.

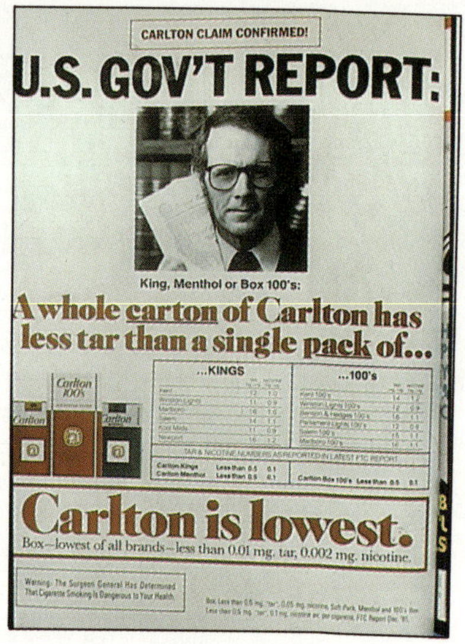
CARLTON CLAIM CONFIRMED!
U.S. GOV'T REPORT:
King, Menthol or Box 100's:
A whole carton of Carlton has less tar than a single pack of...
...KINGS
...100's
Carlton is lowest.
Box—lowest of all brands—less than 0.01 mg. tar, 0.002 mg. nicotine.

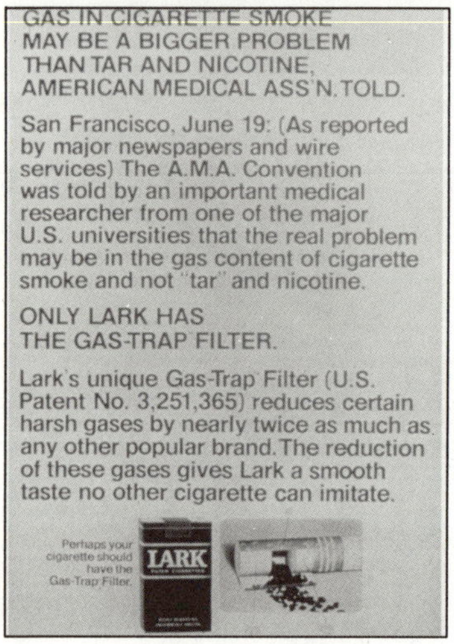
GAS IN CIGARETTE SMOKE MAY BE A BIGGER PROBLEM THAN TAR AND NICOTINE, AMERICAN MEDICAL ASS'N. TOLD.
San Francisco, June 19: (As reported by major newspapers and wire services) The A.M.A. Convention was told by an important medical researcher from one of the major U.S. universities that the real problem may be in the gas content of cigarette smoke and not "tar" and nicotine.
ONLY LARK HAS THE GAS-TRAP FILTER.
Lark's unique Gas-Trap Filter (U.S. Patent No. 3,251,365) reduces certain harsh gases by nearly twice as much as any other popular brand. The reduction of these gases gives Lark a smooth taste no other cigarette can imitate.
Perhaps your cigarette should have the Gas-Trap Filter.
LARK

Direct Attack On Smoking Health Risk Information

Earlier cigarette advertising was intended to create doubt among smokers and would-be smokers regarding the "alleged" association between smoking and health, but a series of R.J. Reynolds ads in 1984 took a more direct approach. Published in national news magazines, Reynolds emphatically stated that "studies which conclude that smoking causes disease have regularly ignored significant evidence to the contrary." This statement was made 30 years after the publication of numerous studies linking smoking to lung cancer and other diseases and 20 years after the Surgeon General's report provided a clear scientific

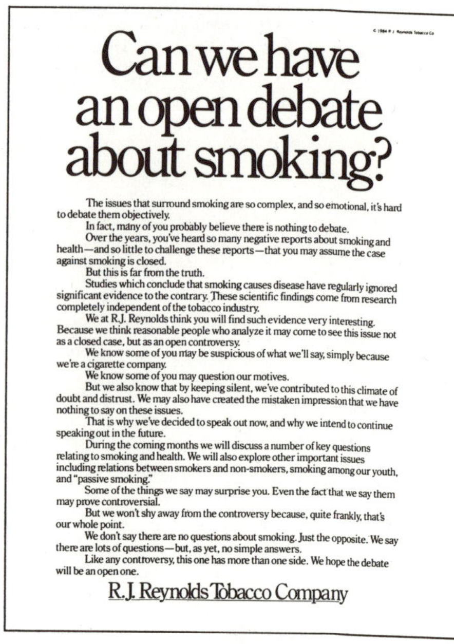

consensus that "Cigarette smoking is a health hazard of sufficient importance in the United States to warrant appropriate remedial action."

In a followup ad, Reynolds even boasts, "We believe in science. That is why we continue to provide funding for independent research into smoking and health."

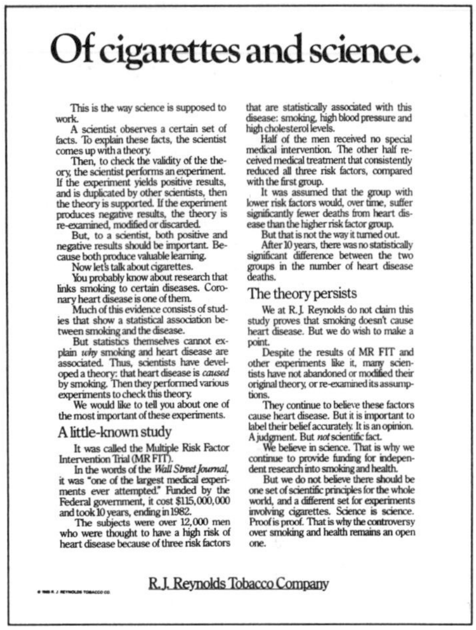

Of cigarettes and science.

This is the way science is supposed to work.

A scientist observes a certain set of facts. To explain these facts, the scientist comes up with a theory.

Then, to check the validity of the theory, the scientist performs an experiment. If the experiment yields positive results, and is duplicated by other scientists, then the theory is supported. If the experiment produces negative results, the theory is re-examined, modified or discarded.

But, to a scientist, both positive and negative results should be important. Because both produce valuable learning.

Now let's talk about cigarettes.

You probably know about research that links smoking to certain diseases. Coronary heart disease is one of them.

Much of this evidence consists of studies that show a statistical association between smoking and the disease.

But statistics themselves cannot explain *why* smoking and heart disease are associated. Thus, scientists have developed a theory: that heart disease is *caused* by smoking. Then they performed various experiments to check this theory.

We would like to tell you about one of the most important of these experiments.

A little-known study

It was called the Multiple Risk Factor Intervention Trial (MR FIT).

In the words of the *Wall Street Journal*, it was "one of the largest medical experiments ever attempted." Funded by the Federal government, it cost $115,000,000 and took 10 years, ending in 1982.

The subjects were over 12,000 men who were thought to have a high risk of heart disease because of three risk factors that are statistically associated with this disease: smoking, high blood pressure and high cholesterol levels.

Half of the men received no special medical intervention. The other half received medical treatment that consistently reduced all three risk factors, compared with the first group.

It was assumed that the group with lower risk factors would, over time, suffer significantly fewer deaths from heart disease than the higher risk factor group.

But that is not the way it turned out.

After 10 years, there was no statistically significant difference between the two groups in the number of heart disease deaths.

The theory persists

We at R.J. Reynolds do not claim this study proves that smoking doesn't cause heart disease. But we do wish to make a point.

Despite the results of MR FIT and other experiments like it, many scientists have not abandoned or modified their original theory, or re-examined its assumptions.

They continue to believe these factors cause heart disease. But it is important to label their belief accurately. It is an opinion. A judgment. But *not* scientific fact.

We believe in science. That is why we continue to provide funding for independent research into smoking and health.

But we do not believe there should be one set of scientific principles for the whole world, and a different set for experiments involving cigarettes. Science is science. Proof is proof. That is why the controversy over smoking and health remains an open one.

R.J. Reynolds Tobacco Company

It is difficult to determine exactly what effect such ads have on the public. At the very least, they serve to create doubt in some smokers' mind about whether the link between smoking and health is real, especially among those individuals who are considering quitting and who may delay taking action that could benefit their health. However, there is no question that these ads are a deliberate misrepresentation of the scientific knowledge of the disease risks associated with cigarette smoking.

Tobacco and The Clinician

This monograph provides important information on how health care professionals can contribute to the national effort to reduce smoking both among individual patients and in our communities. Health professionals have a responsibility to ensure that the 50 million people who continue to smoke fully understand the true health consequences of their behavior, and where appropriate, the health professional should provide direct assistance to help them become nonsmokers.

Equally important, we need to become smoking experts within our communities to counter tobacco industry-sponsored misrepresentation of scientific fact. Whether it is providing justification for policies protecting nonsmokers from the harm caused by passive smoking, preventing underage youth from having easy access to tobacco, or restricting certain types of cigarette promotions, health professionals need to acquire the skills necessary to effectively address these issues. After all, if we don't, who will?

Philip R. Lee, M.D.
Assistant Secretary for Health

Preface

This monograph, the fifth in the NCI Smoking and Tobacco Control series, provides important information for clinicians interested in reducing the tremendous burden of disease caused by cigarettes and other tobacco products. As health professionals we can and must contribute to this effort, both by assisting individual patient cessation and by contributing to broader tobacco control activities in our communities.

Cigarette smoking is still this Nation's largest cause of premature death and disability and remains the only product that, when used as intended by the manufacturer, will kill the consumer. Every physician and dentist can and should become a smoking expert to counter the pervasive attempts by the tobacco industry to convince smokers and would-be smokers that smoking is desirable, sexy, or fun.

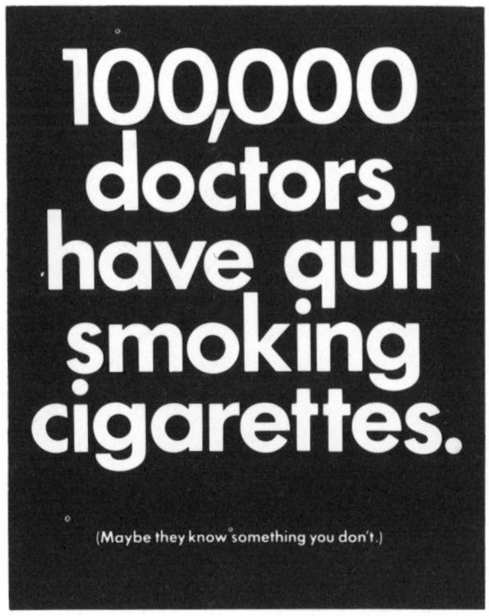
100,000
doctors
have quit
smoking
cigarettes.
(Maybe they know something you don't.)

We need to remind ourselves that for decades the cigarette industry blatantly used the medical profession in cigarette advertising and enticed entire generations into believing that smoking was safe. Even today, 30 years after it became known with overwhelming scientific certainty that smoking was a major health threat, cigarette advertisers still portray smoking as free from any significant health risk.

Health professionals have been an integral part of the national effort to reduce smoking in the United States, and in fact, the first major smoking information campaign launched by the U.S. Public Health Service was based on changes in physicians' smoking behavior.[1] However, we must do more.

TOBACCO AND THE CLINICIANS' RESPONSIBILITY

Today more than 400,000 of our citizens die needlessly each year because they smoke cigarettes. Additional thousands more will die or experience a diminished quality of life because of diseases that result from use of other tobacco products. As health professionals, we have the responsibility to stem this tide of needless suffering by providing assistance to those patients who want to stop smoking and by becoming more active in our communities, supporting policies that can reduce smoking among all segments of society, especially the young.

---

[1] The campaign, consisting of a series of office posters and public service print ads placed on all U.S. Postal Service delivery trucks, was short-lived because the cigarette industry aggressively attacked both the validity of the survey and the campaign, forcing the postal service to withdraw its support.

Assisting patients to quit adds to the number of nonsmokers and facilitates the growing social unacceptability of smoking in general. Although the percentage of physicians who routinely counsel smokers to quit has doubled in the past 15 years, it is disheartening that only about 50 percent of current smokers report they have ever received such advice from a physician. However, on a cost-benefit basis advice about smoking cessation is more cost-effective than many other valuable medical interventions, including preventive measures for hypertension and hypercholesterolemia. The cost was estimated at $748 per year of life saved. It would be unthinkable for a physician not to routinely monitor patients for high blood pressure, yet many physicians and dentists do not have an office system for even identifying patients who smoke.

Involvement in community-based smoking control activities poses a different, but no less important, challenge. Medical professionals' responsibility for the health of patients cannot be limited solely to those procedures performed in an office practice. Indeed, we need to recognize that the tobacco industry views the community as "a vector" to help spread the disease of tobacco addiction, and it is our responsibility to prevent it from doing so. As this monograph points out, the promotion of tobacco in our communities is still widespread. All kinds of events—from auto races to rock concerts to athletic contests and even community charity fundraisers—are often sponsored with tobacco industry money. Sponsorship of these events is intended to buy social acceptance and legitimacy, and health professionals must take the lead in discouraging such tobacco-promotion activities to the extent possible.

THE NCI NATIONAL HEALTH PROFESSIONAL TRAINING PROGRAM

In 1984 the National Cancer Institute began funding a series of 12 clinical trials in an effort to develop more effective intervention methods for use by physicians, dentists, and other health care professionals with their patients who smoke. More than 100,000 patients and 6,100 physicians and dentists were involved in these trials.

Brief Physician and Dentist Protocol for Patient Smoking Cessation

1. **ASK** about smoking at every opportunity.
2. **ADVISE** all smokers to stop.
3. **ASSIST** patients with stopping by setting a quit date, providing self-help materials, and prescribing nicotine replacement therapy as appropriate.
4. **ARRANGE** followup visits to foster maintenance and prevent relapse.

This monograph distills from these and other related studies a clear picture of not only what interventions work but also how to recruit and motivate clinicians to provide assistance and how to institutionalize the provision of cessation assistance within the health care delivery system. The monograph also provides many practical tips for involvement in community-based smoking control activities.

Recognizing that health practitioners committed to cessation assistance require training and skills to successfully deliver such services, the National Cancer Institute initiated a national training program for clinicians with the goal of training 100,000 primary care physicians and 50,000 oral health professionals.

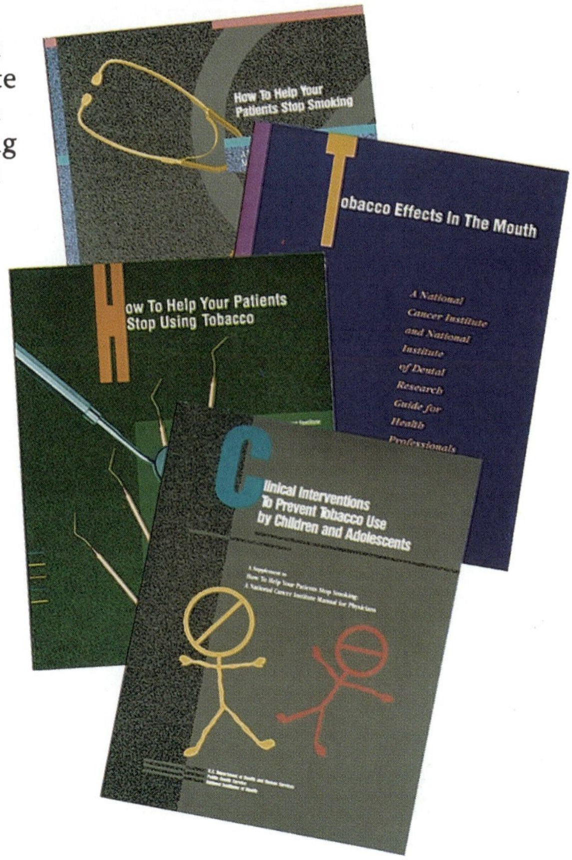

When these goals are realized, the program will produce between 1 and 2 million additional former smokers each year. And last year, in cooperation with the American Academy of Pediatrics, NCI expanded its training protocol to include primary prevention of smoking for those primary care providers who routinely see children and adolescents in their practices. Results from this national training program will have a substantial impact on the health and well-being of the Nation and will ultimately save billions of health care dollars as well.

Samuel Broder, M.D.
Director, National Cancer Institute

Acknowledgments

Tobacco and the Clinician: Interventions for Medical and Dental Practice was developed under the general editorship of the Smoking and Tobacco Control Program (STCP), **Donald R. Shopland**, Coordinator, National Cancer Institute, Bethesda, Maryland. The senior scientific editor was **David M. Burns, M.D.**, Professor of Medicine, University of California, San Diego; Dr. Burns also served as scientific editor for Chapters 1 and 5. The scientific editors for Chapters 2, 3, and 4, respectively, were

Stuart J. Cohen, Ed.D., M.A.
Director of Primary Care Research
AMC Cancer Research Center
Denver, Colorado

Thomas E. Kottke, M.D., M.S.P.H.
Section of Clinical Epidemiology
Department of Health Sciences Research
Mayo Clinic
Rochester, Minnesota

Ellen R. Gritz, Ph.D.
Professor in Residence, Department of Surgery
Director, Division of Cancer Control
Jonsson Comprehensive Cancer Center
University of California, Los Angeles
Los Angeles, California

The STCP staff gratefully acknowledges the authors who made this monograph possible. Attributions for each chapter, in alphabetical order, are as follows:

Chapter 1	**Strategies for Office-Based Smoking Cessation Assistance**	Alan Blum, M.D. Department of Family Medicine Baylor College of Medicine Houston, Texas David M. Burns, M.D. University of California, San Diego San Diego, California Elizabeth Gilpin, M.S. Department of Cancer Prevention and Control Cancer Center University of California, San Diego La Jolla, California

Chapter 1 (continued)

Thomas P. Houston, M.D.
Department of Preventive Medicine
American Medical Association
Chicago, Illinois

John P. Pierce, Ph.D.
Department of Cancer Prevention and Control
Cancer Center
University of California, San Diego
La Jolla, California

John W. Richards, Jr., M.D.
Department of Family Medicine
Medical College of Georgia
Augusta, Georgia

Chapter 2 **Recruitment and Training of Practicing Physicians, Dentists, And Their Office Staffs**

Anthony Biglan, Ph.D.
Oregon Research Institute
Eugene, Oregon

Mark J. Brekke, M.A.
Brekke Associates
Minneapolis, Minnesota

Milo L. Brekke, Ph.D.
Brekke Associates
Minneapolis, Minnesota

Thomas J. Coates, Ph.D.
University of California, San Francisco
San Francisco, California

Stuart J. Cohen, Ed.D., M.A.
AMC Cancer Research Center
Denver, Colorado

Shirley A. Conn, R.N., M.S., M.S.N.
Blue Plus, Blue Cross/Blue Shield of Minnesota
St. Paul, Minnesota

Steven R. Cummings, M.D.
University of California, San Francisco
San Francisco, California

Jack F. Hollis, Ph.D.
Kaiser Permanente Center for Health Research
Portland, Oregon

Chapter 2 (continued)

John R. Hughes, M.D.
University of Vermont
Burlington, Vermont

Sue A. Kelly, C.D.A.
Oral Health Research Institute
Indiana University School of Dentistry
Indianapolis, Indiana

Thomas E. Kottke, M.D., M.S.P.H.
Section of Clinical Epidemiolgy
Department of Health Sciences Research
Mayo Clinic
Rochester, Minnesota

Edward Lichtenstein, Ph.D.
Oregon Research Institute
Eugene, Oregon

Elizabeth A. Lindsay, Ph.D.
COMMIT, Waterloo Smoking Projects
University of Waterloo
Waterloo, Ontario, Canada

Patricia Maxwell, R.N.
Pacific Medical Clinic
Bellevue, Washington

Roger H. Secker-Walker, M.B., F.R.C.P.
College of Medicine
University of Vermont
Burlington, Vermont

Herbert Severson, Ph.D.
Oregon Research Institute
Eugene, Oregon

Leif I. Solberg, M.D.
Minneapolis, Minnesota

Mort J. Stein, M.D.
Kaiser Permanente
San Francisco, California

Victor Stevens, Ph.D.
Northwest Kaiser Permanente
Portland, Oregon

George K. Stookey, Ph.D.
Oral Health Research Institute
Indiana University School of Dentistry
Indianapolis, Indiana

Chapter 2 (continued)

Neil D. Swan
R.O.W. Sciences, Inc.
Rockville, Maryland

Thomas M. Vogt, M.D.
Kaiser Permanente Center for
Health Research
Portland, Oregon

William C. Wadland, M.D.
College of Human Medicine
Michigan State University
East Lansing, Michigan

Douglas M. Wilson, M.D.
McMaster University Health
Sciences Centre
Hamilton, Ontario, Canada

Chapter 3 Training of Physicians In Training

Elizabeth E. Campbell, M.D.
Department of Medicine
University of North Carolina
Chapel Hill, North Carolina

Suzanne W. Fletcher, M.D.
Annals of Internal Medicine
Philadelphia, Pennsylvania

Robert Goldberg, Ph.D.
University of Massachusetts
Medical School
Worcester, Massachusetts

Jorge J. Gonzalez, M.D.
Internal Medicine Teaching Program
New Hanover Memorial Hospital
Wilmington, North Carolina

Thomas G. Irons, M.D.
East Carolina University
School of Medicine and Medical Center
Greenville, North Carolina

Katherine Kalan
University of Massachusetts
Medical School
Worcester, Massachusetts

Richard D. Kenney, M.D.
Director of Pediatrics
Scottish Rite Children's Med. Ctr.
Atlanta, Georgia

Chapter 3 (continued)

Thomas E. Kottke, M.D., M.S.P.H.
Section of Clinical Epidemiology
Department of Health Sciences Research
Mayo Clinic
Rochester, Minnesota

Jean Kristeller, Ph.D.
Department of Psychology
Indiana State University
Terre Haute, Indiana

Mary F. Lyles, M.D.
Department of Medicine
Bowman Gray School of Medicine
Winston-Salem, North Carolina

Judith K. Ockene, Ph.D.
University of Massachusetts
Worcester, Massachusetts

Michael S. O'Malley, M.D.
School of Public Health
University of North Carolina
Chapel Hill, North Carolina

C. Stewart Rogers, M.D.
Internal Medicine Teaching Service
Moses Cone Memorial Hospital
Greensboro, North Carolina

Clare J. Sanchez, M.D.
Department of Medicine and Psychiatry
Dorothea Dix Hospital
Raleigh, North Carolina

Victor J. Strecher, Ph.D.
School of Public Health
University of North Carolina
Chapel Hill, North Carolina

Frank T. Stritter, Ph.D.
University of North Carolina
School of Medicine
Chapel Hill, North Carolina

Robert C. Turner, M.D.
Department of Medicine
East Carolina University
School of Medicine
Greenville, North Carolina

Chapter 3 (continued)

Victor G. Villagra, M.D.
Department of General Internal Medicine
Geisinger Medical Center
Danville, Pennsylvania

Susanne T. White, M.D.
Louisiana State University
School of Medicine and Medical Center
New Orleans, Louisiana

Chapter 4 Special Practice Settings

John Beumer, D.D.S., M.S.
University of California, Los Angeles,
School of Dentistry
Los Angeles, California

Steven Cahill, M.P.H.
Department of Epidemiology
and Family Medicine
University of Maryland
Baltimore, Maryland

Clifford R. Carr, Ed.D.
Jonsson Comprehensive Cancer Center
University of California, Los Angeles
Los Angeles, California

Cindy Chang, M.S.
Jonsson Comprehensive Cancer Center
University of California, Los Angeles
Los Angeles, California

Timothy R. Cline, Ph.D.
University of Mississippi
Jackson, Mississippi

Barbara L. Frankowski, M.D., M.P.H.
College of Medicine
University of Vermont
Burlington, Vermont

Ellen R. Gritz, Ph.D.
Jonsson Comprehensive Cancer Center
University of California, Los Angeles
Los Angeles, California

Laura C. Leviton, Ph.D.
Health Services Administration
University of Pittsburgh
Pittsburgh, Pennsylvania

Chapter 4 (continued)

David A. Rapkin, Ph.D.
Jonsson Comprehensive Cancer Center
University of California, Los Angeles
Los Angeles, California

Roger H. Secker-Walker, M.B., F.R.C.P.
College of Medicine
University of Vermont
Burlington, Vermont

Mary Sexton, Ph.D., M.P.H.
Department of Epidemiology
and Family Medicine
University of Maryland
School of Medicine
Baltimore, Maryland

Saul Shiffman, Ph.D.
Department of Psychology
University of Pittsburgh
Pittsburgh, Pennsylvania

Joan Stine, M.H.S., M.S., C.H.E.S.
Department of Epidemiology
and Family Medicine
University of Maryland
School of Medicine
Baltimore, Maryland

Paul H. Ward, M.D.
University of California, Los Angeles
Los Angeles, California

Chapter 5 Dissemination, Facilitation, and Maintenance of Office-Based Cessation Advice

Larry Berger, M.D.
Health Services Division
Lovelace Medical Foundation
Albuquerque, New Mexico

Joyce Adair Bird, Ph.D.
Division of General Internal Medicine
University of California, San Francisco
San Francisco, California

David M. Burns, M.D.
University of California, San Diego
San Diego, California

Catherine Dubé, Ed.D.
Brown University School of Medicine and
the Miriam Hospital
Providence, Rhode Island

Chapter 5 (continued)

Roselyn P. Epps, M.D., M.P.H.
Public Health Applications Research Branch
National Cancer Institute
Bethesda, Maryland

Don Fordham, M.D., M.P.H.
Division of General Internal Medicine
University of California, San Francisco
San Francisco, California

Michael G. Goldstein, M.D.
Brown University School of Medicine and the Miriam Hospital
Providence, Rhode Island

Corinne Husten, M.D., M.P.H.
Public Health Applications Research Branch
National Cancer Institute
Bethesda, Maryland

Norman Hymowitz, Ph.D.
Department of Psychiatry and Mental Health Sciences
University of Medicine and Dentistry of New Jersey
Newark, New Jersey

Elizabeth A. Lindsay, Ph.D.
COMMIT, Waterloo Smoking Projects
University of Waterloo
Waterloo, Ontario, Canada

Nancy A. MacDonald, M.P.H., C.H.E.S.
Brown University and the Miriam Hospital
Providence, Rhode Island

Marc Manley, M.D.
Public Health Applications Research Branch
National Cancer Institute
Bethesda, Maryland

Stephen J. McPhee, M.D.
Division of General Internal Medicine
University of California, San Francisco
San Francisco, California

Robert Mecklenburg, D.D.S., M.P.H.
R.O.W. Sciences, Inc.
Rockville, Maryland

Chapter 5 (continued)

Raymond Niaura, Ph.D.
Brown University School of Medicine and the Miriam Hospital
Providence, Rhode Island

Judith K. Ockene, Ph.D.
University of Massachusetts
Worcester, Massachusetts

Emilie H. Osborn, M.D., M.P.H.
Division of General Internal Medicine
University of California, San Francisco
San Francisco, California

Paul Pomrehn, M.D., M.S.
Department of Family Medicine
University of Iowa
Iowa City, Iowa

Jonathan E. Rodnick, M.D., M.P.H.
Division of General Internal Medicine
University of California, San Francisco
San Francisco, California

Leif I. Solberg, M.D.
Minneapolis, Minnesota

Douglas M. Wilson, M.D.
McMaster University
Health Sciences Centre
Hamilton, Ontario, Canada

The editors gratefully acknowledge also the following distinguished scientists, researchers, and others, both in and outside government, who contributed critical reviews:

John J. Ambre, M.D., Ph.D.
Department of Toxicology and Drug Abuse
American Medical Association
Chicago, Illinois

Frederick Bass, M.D.
Stop Smoking Program
British Columbia Medical Association
Vancouver, B.C., Canada

Renaldo N. Battista, M.D., Sc.D.
Montreal General Hospital
Montreal, Quebec, Canada

David S. Brody, M.D.
Mercy Catholic Medical Center
Darby, Pennsylvania

Steven Brunton, M.D.
Long Beach Memorial Medical Center
Long Beach, California

Arden G. Christen, D.D.S., M.S.D., M.A.
Indiana University School of Dentistry
Indianapolis, Indiana

Michael P. Eriksen, Sc.D.
Office on Smoking and Health
Center for Chronic Disease Prevention and Health Promotion
Centers for Disease Control and Prevention
Atlanta, Georgia

Paul M. Fischer, M.D.
Medical College of Georgia
Augusta, Georgia

Gary Giovino, Ph.D.
Office on Smoking and Health
Center for Chronic Disease Prevention and Health Promotion
Centers for Disease Control and Prevention
Atlanta, Georgia

Dorothy Hatsukami, M.D.
Department of Psychiatry
University of Minnesota
Minneapolis, Minnesota

Shirley B. Lansky, M.D.
Illinois Cancer Center
Chicago, Illinois

J. Michael McGinnis, M.D.
Office of Disease Prevention and Health Promotion
Office of the Assistant Secretary for Health
Department of Health and Human Services
Washington, D.C.

Robert Mecklenburg, D.D.S., M.P.H.
R.O.W. Sciences, Inc.
Rockville, Maryland

Clifford H. Miller, D.D.S.
Division of Education
American Dental Association
Chicago, Illinois

Karen Monaco
American Lung Association
Chapel Hill, North Carolina

Walter W. Rosser, M.D.
Department of Family and Community Medicine
University of Toronto
Toronto, Ontario, Canada

Dr. Carlo Senore
Montreal General Hospital
Montreal, Quebec, Canada

J. Christopher Shank, M.D.
Hassler Center for Family Medicine
Fairview General Hospital
Cleveland, Ohio

Susan Sullivan, Ph.D., M.P.H.
Cancer Control Research Program
Duke Comprehensive Cancer Center
Duke University Medical Center
Durham, North Carolina

Richard B. Warnecke, Ph.D.
Survey Research Laboratory
University of Illinois at Chicago
Chicago, Illinois

Richard A. Windsor, Ph.D., M.P.H.
National Heart, Lung, and Blood Institute
Bethesda, Maryland

The editor acknowledges the contributions of the following staff members of R.O.W. Sciences, Inc., Rockville, Maryland, who provided technical and editorial assistance in the preparation of this monograph:

Richard H. Amacher, Project Manager

Douglas Bishop, Art Director

Jean Brady, Research Assistant

Karen Bray, Technical Assistant

Rebecca Charton, Librarian

Catherine Godfrey, Word Processing Specialist

Faye A. Grant, Administrative Secretary

Susan E. Jones, Administrative Secretary

James R. Libbey, Coordinator, Proofreader

Janet Mullaney, Copy Editor

Frances Nebesky, Copy Editor

Theodora Radcliffe, Copy Editor, Indexer

Donna Selig, Proofreader

Barbara Shine, Managing Editor

Keith W. Stanger, Graphics Specialist

Sonia Van Putten, Word Processing Specialist

William Ward, Copy Editor

Debra Waugh, Copy Editor

Ronald W. Wolf, Senior Copy Editor.

Contents

		Page
	Foreword	iii
	Preface	xi
	Acknowledgments	xv
Chapter 1.	**Strategies for Office-Based Smoking Cessation Assistance**	1
	Overview of Office-Based Smoking Cessation Assistance David M. Burns	3
	Trends in Physicians' Smoking Behavior and Patterns of Advice To Quit John P. Pierce and Elizabeth Gilpin	12
	The Health Professional's Responsibility in Smoking Cessation: Strategies for Office and Community John W. Richards, Jr., Thomas P. Houston, and Alan Blum	24
	Appendix A. Magazines Without Tobacco Advertising	38
Chapter 2.	**Recruitment and Training of Practicing Physicians, Dentists, and Their Office Staffs**	41
	Introduction Stuart J. Cohen	45
	Effects of Training Family Physicians in a Comprehensive Smoking Cessation Intervention Elizabeth A. Lindsay and Douglas M. Wilson	48
	Doctors Helping Smokers: Development of a Clinic-Based Smoking Intervention System Thomas E. Kottke, Leif I. Solberg, Milo L. Brekke, Shirley A. Conn, Patricia Maxwell, and Mark J. Brekke	69
	Prompting Smoking Cessation in Family Practice William C. Wadland, John R. Hughes, and Roger H. Secker-Walker	92
	Smoking Cessation in Primary Care Practice: Summary of Results From the Quit for Life Project Steven R. Cummings, Thomas J. Coates, Mort J. Stein, Neil D. Swan, and the Quit for Life Research Group	102

Physician and Dentist Interventions
For Smoking Cessation 113
Stuart J. Cohen, George K. Stookey, and Sue A. Kelly

The Tobacco Reduction and Cancer Control
(TRACC) Program: Team Approaches to
Counseling in Medical and Dental Settings 143
Jack F. Hollis, Thomas M. Vogt, Victor Stevens,
Anthony Biglan, Herbert Severson, and Edward Lichtenstein

Appendixes
A. Screening Form for Study on
Assessing Patient's Health Risks 169
B. Study on Physician Advice for
Smoking Cessation 170
C. Entry Questionnaire 171
D. Medical Screening Form 174
E. Generic Reminder Sheet 175
F. Reminder Sheet for Gum Group 176
G. Reminder Sheet for No-Gum Group 177
H. Physician Data: Initial Visit 178
I. Exit Questionnaire #1 (All Patients) 179
J. Exit Questionnaire #2 (No-Gum Group) 181
K. Exit Questionnaire #3 (Nicotine Gum Group) 182
L. One- to Two-Week Followup for
Smoking Cessation Study 183
M. Six-Month Followup for
Smoking Cessation Study 184
N. Followup Questionnaire on the
Use of Nicotine Gum 185

Chapter 3. Training of Physicians in Training 187

Introduction 189
Thomas E. Kottke

Interventions for Smoking Prevention and Cessation 191
Robert Goldberg, Judith K. Ockene,
Katherine Kalan, and Jean Kristeller

Effects of Two Realistic Interventions To Teach
Smoking Cessation Counseling to
Primary Care Residents: A Randomized Trial 207
Victor J. Strecher, Michael S. O'Malley, Victor G. Villagra,
Elizabeth E. Campbell, Jorge J. Gonzalez, Thomas G. Irons,
Richard D. Kenney, Robert C. Turner, C. Stewart Rogers,
Mary F. Lyles, Susanne T. White, Clare J. Sanchez,
Frank T. Stritter, and Suzanne W. Fletcher

Appendixes
A. Smoking Intervention Communication Grid ... 223
B. Outline of the Advice and Counseling Smoking Intervention Approaches ... 224
C. Physician Responses to Patients' Concerns ... 226

Chapter 4. Special Practice Settings ... 227

Introduction ... 229
Ellen R. Gritz

Pediatricians' Role in Smoking Prevention and Cessation ... 232
Barbara L. Frankowski and Roger H. Secker-Walker

Smoking Intervention by Providers of Health Care for Women ... 246
Mary Sexton, Joan Stine, and Steven Cahill

A Physician- and Dentist-Delivered Smoking Cessation Intervention for Head and Neck Cancer Patients ... 259
Ellen R. Gritz, Clifford R. Carr, David A. Rapkin, Cindy Chang, John Beumer, and Paul H. Ward

Medical Advice as a Communication About Risks of Smoking and Benefits of Quitting ... 272
Laura C. Leviton, Timothy R. Cline, and Saul Shiffman

Appendixes
A. Smoking Materials for Pediatricians ... 287
B. Algorithms for Delivery of Smoking Cessation Advice ... 288
C. Protocol Developed by University of North Carolina Faculty Development Program ... 292
D. Self-Efficacy Intervention ... 293
E. Transcript From a Self-Efficacy Counseling Session ... 295

Chapter 5. Dissemination, Facilitation, and Maintenance Of Office-Based Cessation Assistance ... 299

Introduction ... 301
David M. Burns

Smoking Cessation as a Clinic Quality Improvement Project ... 303
Leif I. Solberg

Computerized Reminder System To Aid Physicians in Assessment and Counseling of Patients Who Smoke ... 321
Stephen J. McPhee, Joyce Adair Bird, Don Fordham, Jonathan E. Rodnick, and Emilie H. Osborn

Physicians' and Dentists' Roles in COMMIT—
The Community Intervention Trial for
Smoking Cessation 334
Elizabeth A. Lindsay, Judith K. Ockene, Larry Berger,
Norman Hymowitz, Paul Pomrehn, and Douglas M. Wilson

Dissemination of Physician-Based
Smoking Cessation Interventions 342
Michael G. Goldstein, Nancy A. MacDonald,
Raymond Niaura, and Catherine Dubé

Clinical Interventions in Tobacco Control:
A National Cancer Institute Training Program
For Health Care Providers 356
Marc Manley, Roselyn P. Epps,
Robert Mecklenburg, and Corinne Husten

Appendix A. Case Studies 369

Index 375

Chapter 1

Strategies for Office-Based Smoking Cessation Assistance

CONTENTS

Overview of Office-Based Smoking Cessation Assistance
David M. Burns 3
Introduction 3
Comprehensive Tobacco Control Strategies 4
Development and Maintenance of Office-Based Assistance 7
References 11

Trends in Physicians' Smoking Behavior and Patterns of Advice To Quit
John P. Pierce and Elizabeth Gilpin 12
Introduction 12
How Smoking Fits Into a Generalist's Practice 12
Smoking Behavior of Physicians 15
Physicians' Advice, as Reported by Patients 17
Summary 21
References 22

The Health Professional's Responsibility in Smoking Cessation: Strategies for Office and Community
John W. Richards, Jr., Thomas P. Houston, and Alan Blum 24
Introduction 24
In the Practitioner's Office 27
Individualizing Interventions 29
Strategies for Counseling 30
Community Awareness and Action 33
References 36

Appendix A. Magazines Without Tobacco Advertising 38

Overview of Office-Based Smoking Cessation Assistance

David M. Burns

INTRODUCTION The burden of premature death and avoidable disability caused by tobacco use in the United States (US DHHS, 1989) and the benefits of cessation (US DHHS, 1990) are well documented. Despite the widespread acceptance of this information by the public and the high frequency with which physicians report that they advise their patients to quit smoking, almost one-half of smokers report never having been told to quit by their physician. Patients do report that they would be likely to try to quit if told by their physician to quit. Because 70 percent of smokers see a physician each year and 60 percent visit a dentist, the potential for the health care community to affect smoking prevalence in the United States is both large and substantially underutilized.

To increase the effectiveness of the health care community in promoting smoking cessation, the National Cancer Institute has funded research efforts to develop more effective intervention methods for use by physicians and dentists and to facilitate the adoption of these methods. This monograph distills from those projects a clear picture of what interventions work, how to recruit and motivate clinicians to provide advice, and how to institutionalize the delivery of smoking cessation assistance within the health care delivery system.

The outcome results of the studies in this report have been published in the peer-reviewed literature. The purpose of this monograph goes beyond a review of the cessation outcome literature to include detailed descriptions of the program content and strategies. In addition, the investigators who drafted the descriptions of their programs were asked to assess which approaches were effective, which were ineffective, and what they would do differently if they could repeat their projects. This departure from the traditional scientific and data-based approach is intentional. It was the experience with what worked and did not work at the program level that formed the core of the interventions tested in the trials described here. It should therefore be no surprise that current concepts of effective approaches to clinician-provided smoking cessation assistance have evolved beyond those that were used to design these research trials, which were funded in the early 1980's. The long delay from the design of a trial and request for funding to publication of the results in the peer-reviewed literature means that the current knowledge of how to implement practice-based smoking cessation assistance frequently has advanced beyond that documented in the literature. This monograph presents the current best judgment of how to implement and sustain an effective office-based cessation effort, by combining the knowledge from both controlled scientific investigation and trial-and-error experience.

COMPREHENSIVE TOBACCO CONTROL STRATEGIES

The current state of the art in comprehensive tobacco control strategies combines multiple environmental changes with multiple programs directed at individuals in different stages of the initiation and cessation processes (US DHHS, 1991). No single approach is best for all smokers, and different smokers are most attracted to and most affected by different programs. Perhaps more importantly, no single channel reaches all smokers and no single time is best for all smokers to make a quit attempt. Persistent and inescapable messages to quit, or to not start, coupled with continuous support for individual cessation efforts provided through multiple channels reinforced by environmental incentives to be a nonsmoker currently characterize comprehensive tobacco control strategies.

An essential corollary of this understanding of tobacco control is that smoking cessation assistance provided by physicians and dentists represents only one channel in a multichannel effort and that cessation efforts supported by clinicians are likely to be most effective when they draw on and are integrated with other forces promoting smoking cessation. The traditional therapeutic model, in which treatment is designed to be effective regardless of the factors in the patient's environment, is unlikely to be successful in stopping cigarette smoking when environmental factors determine both the personal, psychological, and sociological utility of smoking and the motivation for cessation. Rather than perceiving the clinician as the provider of a clinically proven "magic bullet" that will cure a patient forever, it may be more realistic to see the physician's or dentist's function as that of focusing and magnifying the forces promoting cessation. This change in perspective may help to reduce the frustration and futility that many practitioners have when working with their smoking patients.

To understand the role of the physician or dentist in smoking cessation, it is useful to have an understanding of the processes of smoking initiation and cessation and of the interventions that can influence the stages in that process. One formulation of the influences involved in cigarette initiation and cessation is presented in Figure 1. Exploration and initiation of regular use of cigarettes are largely confined to adolescence, with regular use and dependence occurring during late adolescence and early adulthood. Experimentation with cigarettes and initial cigarette use are influenced by the factors that affect adolescent development, whereas dependency develops when the psychological and sociological utility of smoking is incorporated into the approaches used by the smoker to function in and cope with the adult world. Many adolescents experiment with tobacco use but never become regular smokers; some adolescent regular smokers stop before they develop dependence on cigarette use.

The process of stopping smoking is often a cyclical one, with the smoker making a number of attempts to quit before finally succeeding. Nationally, the vast majority of smokers would like to quit and approximately one-third of current smokers attempt to quit each year. Ninety percent or more of

Figure 1
The processes of smoking initiation and cessation

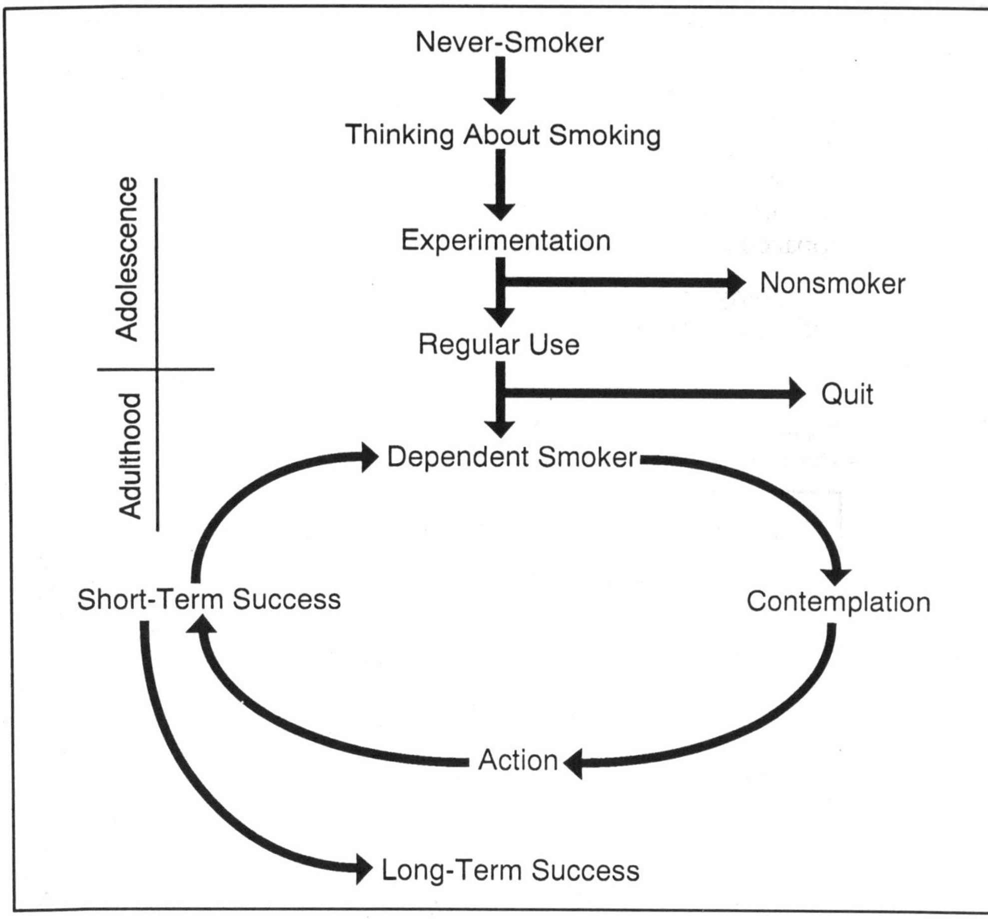

Source: US DHHS, 1991.

those quit attempts fail (Pierce and Hatziandreu, 1989). Smokers have been categorized into three groups:

- Those who are not thinking about quitting (in precontemplation);
- Those who are thinking about quitting (in contemplation); and
- Those who are in the act of quitting.

Clearly those who have attempted to quit and failed need motivation to make another attempt, and the cessation process is one in which smokers cycle through the stages of cessation, with a few more smokers succeeding in their cessation efforts each time. One goal of practice-based smoking interventions is moving smokers from one position in the cessation cycle to the next, rather than using long-term cessation as the only goal.

The cyclical pattern of precontemplation, contemplation, and attempting to quit generates a new set of nonsmokers each time a group of smokers passes around the cycle (Prochaska and DiClemente, 1986). One formulation of the process of cessation and the points at which the multiple channels of a comprehensive tobacco control effort can influence cessation is presented in Figure 2. This figure simplifies the effects of these tobacco control efforts but provides an overview of the possible interactions in a comprehensive tobacco control program.

Many of the environmental influences and tobacco control programs influence smokers at different points in this cycle. Public information

Figure 2
The process of cessation

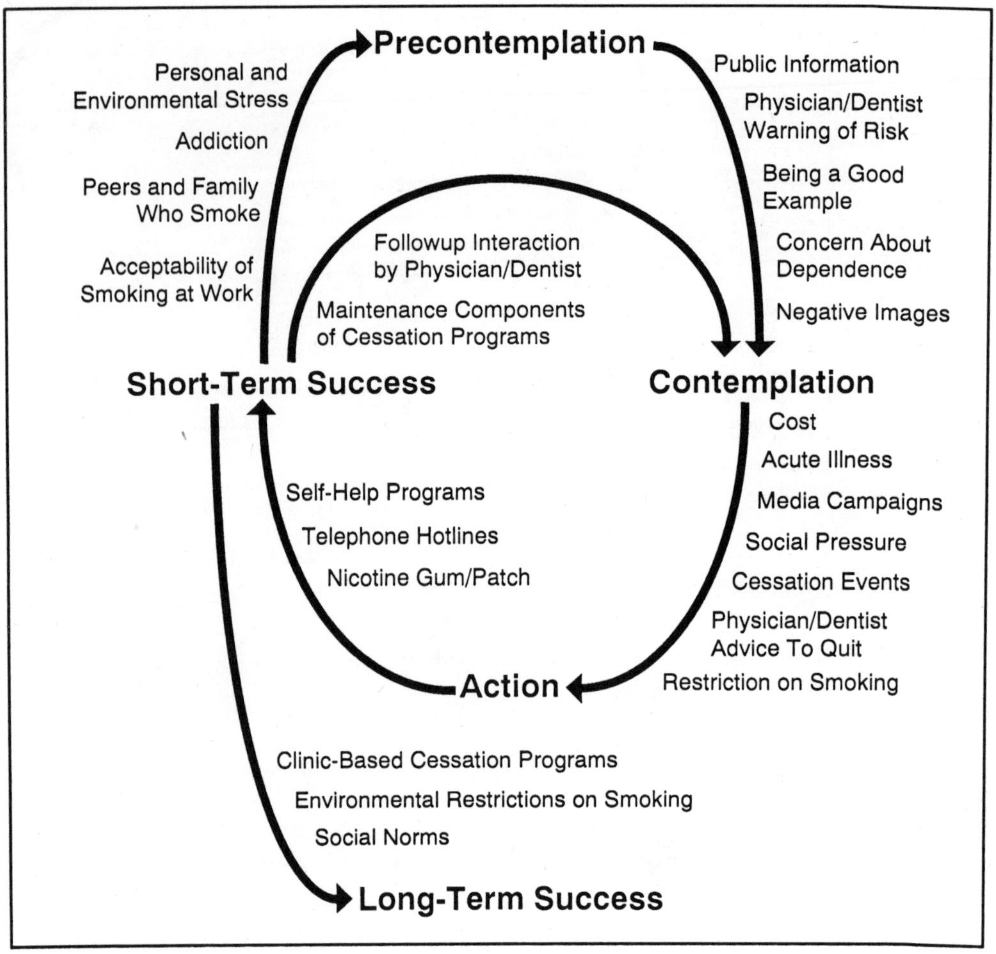

Source: US DHHS, 1991.

campaigns and physician or dentist warnings about the risks associated with smoking move smokers from the precontemplation to the contemplation stage. However, there are other reasons why smokers think about quitting, including concerns about dependency and interest in setting a good example for others. Recently the negative image of the smoker and the social unacceptability of smoking have also provided strong reasons why smokers think about quitting. Individual tobacco control programs have been targeted at altering the frequency and intensity with which these motivational issues are presented to the smoker.

The move from thinking about quitting to trying to quit is often triggered by environmental stimuli. The cost of cigarettes can be a powerful trigger for cessation attempts. Physician advice to quit, particularly at the time of an acute illness, is also a powerful trigger for cessation activity, with up to half of the patients who are advised to quit making a cessation effort. Media campaigns, especially when coupled with cessation events such as the Great American Smokeout, are also able to trigger a large number of cessation attempts (Gunby, 1984). Changes in rules to restrict smoking in the workplace have been associated with quit attempts by substantial numbers of workers.

Triggering cessation efforts is an important tobacco control strategy because each round of cessation activity results in a few more nonsmokers. The large number of smokers who attempt to quit each year attests to the success of those components of the tobacco control effort that move smokers from precontemplation to contemplation and from contemplation to action. The major gap in current tobacco control efforts is in converting a cessation attempt into a long-term success.

Self-help programs, telephone hotlines, and nicotine replacement therapy enhance short-term cessation success, and clinic-based cessation programs have a substantial benefit for long-term cessation for those who participate (Schwartz, 1987). The recruitment of smokers into clinic-based cessation programs is one of the areas in which office-based effort can be particularly effective. However, the major barriers to long-term success remain difficult to alter and are, for the most part, in the smoker's environment. Barriers include social norms and workplace rules that promote smoking and facilitate relapse, the continued smoking behavior of peers and family members, tobacco advertising, and unusual episodes of personal or environmental stress that lead the smoker to fall back on old coping strategies, including smoking. Recognizing these influences and customizing advice for the smoker is one way that physicians and dentists can integrate their cessation assistance into a comprehensive tobacco control effort.

DEVELOPMENT AND MAINTENANCE OF OFFICE-BASED ASSISTANCE

Just as the process of smoking initiation and cessation can be thought of as a series of stages, so too the process of developing and sustaining an office-based smoking cessation program can be divided into stages with different forces acting at the different stages. Figure 3 diagrams this process and divides the factors acting at each stage into those components that act on a single clinician or within a practice and those that are part of the health care delivery environment.

Figure 3
Development and maintenance of office-based smoking cessation assistance

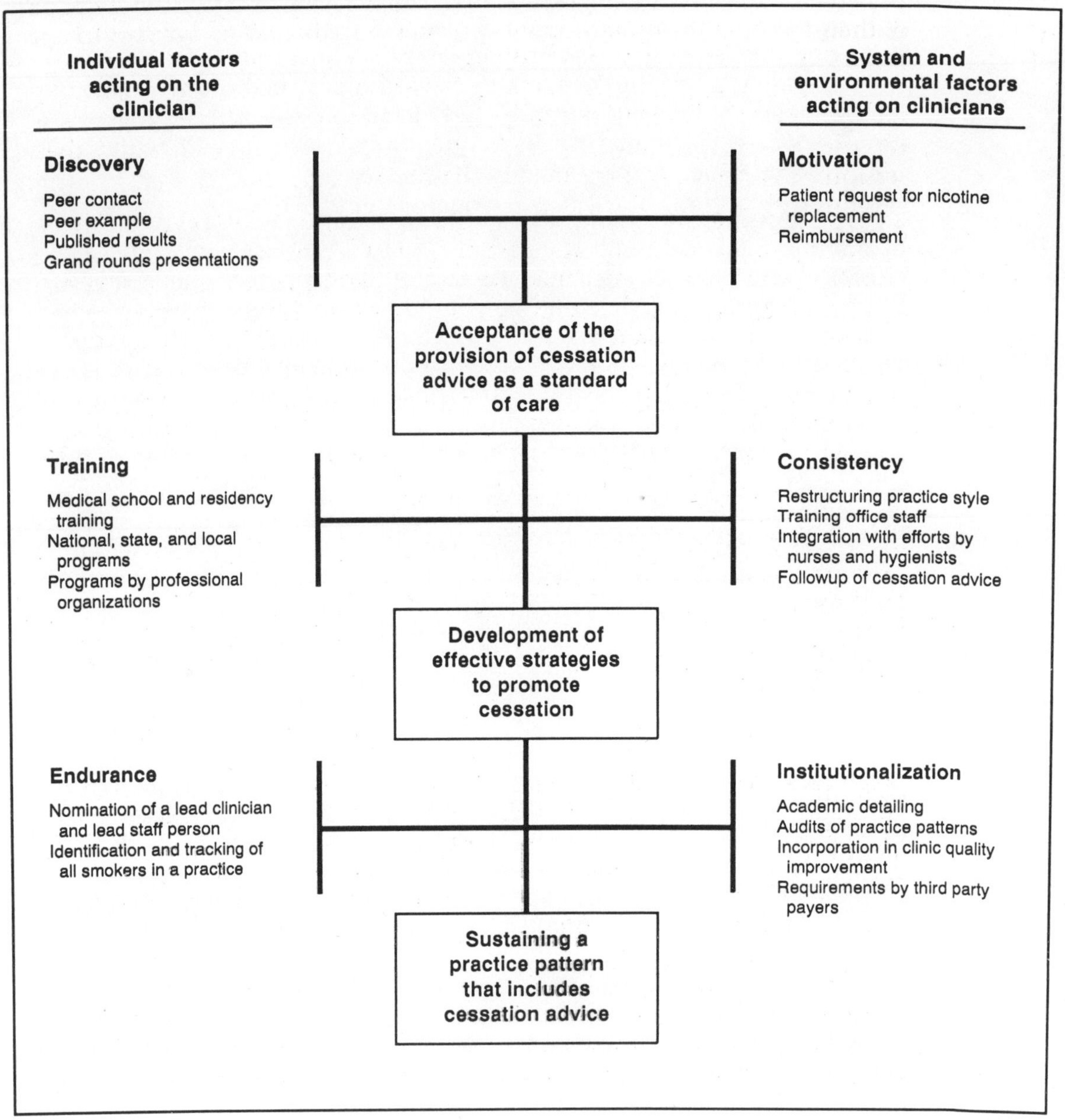

Because individual clinicians may be at different points on this continuum, the strategies to change behavior and the behavioral changes expected will differ. For clinicians who do not perceive cessation advice as part of their practice, the offer of training in the skills to counsel smokers to quit may be less effective than a grand rounds that defines the importance and success rates of clinician-based cessation programs. Conversely, it is unlikely that clinicians interested in improving the effectiveness of cessation advice can get the skills training needed in a single 45-minute grand-rounds-type session. The need to devote time and energy to both short and long training sessions can be confusing unless one recognizes that they are directed at different practitioners with different levels of interest and experience.

The first change needed in clinicians is the recognition that they have a responsibility to every patient who smokes to present the risks associated with smoking and to urge them to quit at an appropriate point in their care. This responsibility goes beyond providing advice to quit to those who have smoking-related disease processes, where cessation may be of therapeutic importance; it includes that larger segment of the smoking population for whom cessation advice is provided exclusively for preventive benefits. Interactions with peers and the example of peers are a major part of the process by which clinicians define standards of care and evaluate their performance relative to those standards. As more physicians and dentists deliver routine cessation assistance, the standards shift and performance pressure mounts on those practitioners who lag behind. One of the tools used to define and advance practice standards is publication of the results of studies and consensus positions. This tool can be effective, albeit slowly, in influencing that vast majority of clinicians who are committed to high-quality care.

Physicians and dentists are in a service delivery profession and are, therefore, influenced by patient expectations and demands. The introduction of nicotine gum, and now the transdermal nicotine patch, both of which require physician or dentist prescriptions, mandates physician and dentist involvement with patients' efforts to quit smoking. The wide recognition of these products by the general public has led to patients' requesting prescriptions from their physicians or dentists. Such requests have led some practitioners to incorporate cessation assistance into their practice; without the need to write a prescription, they might not have done so.

Reimbursement is a significant motivator in health care delivery, and many health care structures now include preventive services in their contracts with physicians. As the standards of care shift to include cessation as a mandatory component of preventive services, and as payers reimburse clinicians on the basis of documentation of the delivery of these services, practitioners who had not considered smoking assistance as part of their role will be obligated to reconsider.

Those practitioners who are committed to cessation assistance will need the training and skills to deliver cessation advice. Many medical school, dental school, and residency curricula are beginning to provide this training (see Chapter 3). Efforts to provide training to those practitioners who have already completed their training are described in Chapter 2, and it is likely that these training efforts are, at least in part, responsible for the increase in the proportion of smokers who report having received advice to quit from their physician or dentist.

Training of the practitioner has a limited effect on the actual office practice. Almost universally, the programs described in this monograph stress the importance of changing the patient intake process and information flow in the office and the training and participation of the office staff. Similarly, the integration of physician or dentist advice with cessation advice and assistance provided by nurses, hygienists, or other office staff facilitates the effectiveness of the advice and the likelihood that it will be offered consistently. The identification and tracking of smokers also are critical to the consistent delivery of advice and, perhaps more importantly, to followup of that advice on subsequent visits.

The most difficult barrier to the successful long-term change in an office practice is the maintenance of that change once the initial enthusiasm of instituting change dissipates. Changes in the office personnel and members of the practice, alterations in the volume of patient visits, and time available for counseling can lead to the failure to sustain a change in office practice, even without a conscious decision to go back to prior procedures. The need to orient new professional and administrative staff members to the smoking cessation assistance approaches used in the practice can create an educational burden that the practice cannot sustain. The identification of individuals in the office who accept the responsibility for the continuity of the cessation approach and the availability of "academic detail" personnel who can come into the office periodically to provide and upgrade training are two of the approaches discussed in Chapter 5.

Building smoking cessation assistance into the continuous quality improvement or audit mechanisms that are a part of the quality assurance programs both within the practice setting and by those agencies responsible for reimbursement is a powerful tool to promote cessation advice in health care. A computer-based system for tracking smokers in a practice and for generating the summary data needed to incorporate cessation assistance in a quality assurance program is also described in Chapter 5.

The remainder of this first chapter discusses the roles that practitioners can play in a tobacco control effort and the actual smoking behavior and counseling practices of physicians and dentists. Subsequent chapters present detailed descriptions of what works in physician and dental practices (Chapter 2), in residency training programs (Chapter 3), and in special practice settings (Chapter 4). Chapter 5 describes the efforts to disseminate and maintain office-based smoking cessation assistance.

REFERENCES

Gunby, P. Smokeout could preface "smoke-free society." *Journal of the American Medical Association* 252: 2803-2804, 1984.

Pierce, J., Hatziandreu, E. *Report of the 1986 Adult Use of Tobacco Survey.* U.S. Department of Health and Human Services, Public Health Service, Centers for Disease Control, Office on Smoking and Health. Publication No. 10491, 1989.

Prochaska, J.O., DiClemente, C.C. Toward a comprehensive model of change. In: *Treating Addictive Behaviors: Processes of Change,* W.R. Miller and N. Heather (Editors). New York: Plenum Press, 1986, pp. 3-27.

Schwartz, J.L. *Review and Evaluation of Smoking Cessation Methods: The United States and Canada, 1978-1985.* U.S. Department of Health and Human Services, Public Health Service, National Institutes of Health, National Cancer Institute, Division of Cancer Prevention and Control. NIH Publication No. 87-2940, 1987.

U.S. Department of Health and Human Services. *The Health Benefits of Smoking Cessation: A Report of the Surgeon General.* U.S. Department of Health and Human Services, Public Health Service, Centers for Disease Control, Center for Chronic Disease Prevention and Health Promotion, Office on Smoking and Health. DHHS Publication No. (CDC) 90-8416, 1990.

U.S. Department of Health and Human Services. *Reducing the Health Consequences of Smoking: 25 Years of Progress. A Report of the Surgeon General.* U.S. Department of Health and Human Services, Public Health Service, Centers for Disease Control, Center for Chronic Disease Prevention and Health Promotion, Office on Smoking and Health. DHHS Publication No. (CDC) 89-8411, 1989.

U.S. Department of Health and Human Services. *Strategies To Control Tobacco Use in the United States: A Blueprint for Public Health Action in the 1990's.* U.S. Department of Health and Human Services, Public Health Service, National Institutes of Health, National Cancer Institute. NIH Publication No. 92-3316, 1991.

Trends in Physicians' Smoking Behavior and Patterns of Advice To Quit

John P. Pierce and Elizabeth Gilpin

INTRODUCTION

In this section, we first discuss the smoking profile of patients in a medical practice. How many patients are smokers, and what do we know about them? How much work is involved for a physician to implement the National Cancer Institute guidelines? Next, we look at the prevalence of smoking among physicians and medical students. We address the issue of physicians advising smokers to quit, from the patient's perspective. Is there any evidence that physicians are advising more patients to quit? How many and what type of smokers perceive that they have been so advised?

HOW SMOKING FITS INTO A GENERALIST'S PRACTICE

Who Are The Smokers?

In two separate samples (rounds I and III) of Kottke and associates' Doctors Helping Smokers studies, approximately 20 percent of those who visited the general practice were smokers (Kottke et al., 1989, and Chapter 2, this volume). This result is identical to that from the 1990 California Tobacco Survey, which identified 20 percent of all patients who had seen a physician in the last year as smokers (Burns and Pierce, 1992). Also, in the California Tobacco Survey, 20 percent of all patient visits in the year prior to the survey had been made by smokers.

The California Tobacco Survey also provides a demographic analysis of smokers who report visiting a physician in the last year (Table 1). Altogether 25.8 percent of the population who had not visited a physician in the previous 12 months were smokers, compared with 20.0 percent who visited a physician.

Among the population who visit a physician, the proportion of men who are smokers is slightly higher than the proportion of women (22.1 vs. 18.2 percent). Indeed, the proportion of smokers visiting a physician in most subgroups is about 20 percent, with the following exceptions: those over the age of 65 years (10.9 percent), Hispanics (16.5 percent), blacks (27.4 percent), Asians (15.5 percent), and those with a college degree (11.8 percent) (Burns and Pierce, 1992).

The self-reported level of health for those who visited a physician varied according to whether or not the patient was a smoker (Table 2). Nonsmokers are more likely to consider themselves to be in excellent health, whereas smokers are more likely to rate their health as poor, fair, or good. Approximately two-thirds of nonsmokers who visited a physician in the last year considered themselves to be in either excellent or very good health compared

Table 1
Demographics of smokers, by visit to physician in last 12 months, California, 1990

	Visited Physician in Last Year Percentage		
	Yes	No	Ratio
Total	20.0%	25.8%	0.76
Sex			
Male	22.1	28.8	0.77
Female	18.2	21.0	0.86
Age			
18 to 24 yr	20.9	35.5	0.82
25 to 44	22.5	26.7	0.84
45 to 64	20.3	25.9	0.78
65+	10.9	20.2	0.54
Ethnicity			
Hispanic	16.5	20.4	0.81
Non-Hispanic	20.7	28.6	0.72
Race			
White	19.8	25.8	0.76
Black	27.9	34.0	0.81
Asian/Pacific Islander	12.0	19.7	0.61
Education			
< 12 yr	24.5	28.5	0.86
12	23.1	29.2	0.79
13 to 15	19.8	25.1	0.79
16+	11.8	15.5	0.76

Source: 1990 California Tobacco Survey, as cited in Burns and Pierce, 1992.

with about 53 percent of smokers. About 18 percent of smokers indicated that they were in fair or poor health, compared with about 13 percent of nonsmokers. Nevertheless, the majority of smokers who visit a general practice will feel that they are in good health (Burns and Pierce, 1992).

Whom Can Physicians And Dentists Help?

The four principles for physician and dentist intervention outlined by NCI are *ask*, *advise*, *assist*, and *arrange*. From the studies reported in this monograph, we can estimate the likely percentages of smokers with whom a physician or dentist will be able to undertake each of these activities successfully.

Ask

If an effective smoking-advice system is to be achieved in a general practice, each patient's smoking status must be known and the medical or dental charts must be flagged to prompt the physician or dentist to discuss smoking with the appropriate patients. As described earlier, this system

Table 2
Health status of patients who visited a physician in the last year, California, 1990

	Percentage of Smokers	Percentage of Nonsmokers
Self-Reported Status		
Excellent health	19.6%	30.4%
Very good health	33.2	33.4
Good health	29.3	23.3
Fair health	14.6	10.6
Poor health	3.3	2.3

Source: 1990 California Tobacco Survey, as cited in Burns and Pierce, 1992.

should result in flags on about 20 percent of all charts from any particular day. Two methods have been popular for determining whether a patient is a smoker: (1) the receptionist obtains the information at the front desk or (2) the nurse or dental hygienist asks the patient while recording vital signs. With either approach, determination of smoking status requires a slight change in the practice's system. Elsewhere in this monograph, researchers discuss various methods to implement this change.

Advise

Anecdotal experience from physician and dentist trials suggests that, if a comprehensive program is used, nearly all smokers who visit a physician or dentist can be counseled to quit (T. Kottke, personal communication; A. Christen, personal communication). Generally, there are two situations in which patients are not counseled to quit: when the patient is too distraught to concentrate and when the clinician is too far behind schedule to be completely in control of the patient encounter. Experience in the Nokomis Clinic in Minnesota suggests that these situations arise in about 15 percent of all physician visits (T. Kottke, personal communication).

Assist

The level of assistance that the health care provider can offer varies considerably, including assessing whether the smoker is ready to quit, discussing quitting, eliciting barriers and fears about making a quit attempt, helping to set a quit date, and in some cases prescribing a nicotine substitute. With an aggressive approach, physicians, dentists, or their smoking cessation coordinators can get many of their smoking patients to set a quit date (see Cummings et al., Chapter 2, this volume). Prescribing of a nicotine supplement as an aid to quitting has been studied extensively.

The most successful systems for smoking advice include designation of a smoking advice coordinator who first discusses smoking with the patient. Then, the physician or dentist gives 1 to 2 minutes of strong advice to encourage the patient to quit. Because this system involves minimum physician or dentist time to urge the patient to set a quit date, approximately 90 percent of clinicians are comfortable complying with this smoking advice strategy. More than 80 percent of patients seem prepared to discuss their smoking further with the designated smoking coordinator, and about 30 percent are prepared to negotiate a quit date (see Hollis et al., Chapter 2, this volume).

Arrange

The majority of smoking cessation attempts are not successful. Nationally, approximately 30 percent of smokers reported that they had tried to quit in any given year (Hatziandreu et al., 1990), but very few of those smokers sought any external aid to help them succeed (Fiore et al., 1990). In the Nokomis Clinic in Minnesota, researchers estimate that approximately 1 in 1,000 smokers actively seek information on programs to help them quit.

Arranging for help to quit and for followup has been the most difficult step in the comprehensive smoking-advice system. As described in Chapter 2 (Hollis et al.), only 10 percent of smokers attended a scheduled followup visit to review their progress.

SMOKING BEHAVIOR OF PHYSICIANS

The smoking behavior of U.S. physicians has been surveyed regularly since 1949. In that year, some 60 percent of physicians smoked. This percentage declined, and by 1964, at the time of the first Surgeon General's report detailing the health consequences of smoking (US DHEW, 1964), the percentage of physicians who smoked had decreased to around 30 percent (Garfinkel and Stellman, 1976). Smoking prevalence among physicians continued to decline, and by the early 1980's, only 5 to 10 percent of physicians were smoking (Buechner et al., 1986; Sachs, 1983). The most recent data come from an anonymous, self-report survey conducted in 1989 to 1990, involving responses from 5,426 physicians (Hughes et al., 1992). In this survey, 51.1 percent of respondents reported ever using tobacco, 13.7 percent reported tobacco use in the last year, 10.6 percent reported use in the last month, and 6.3 percent labeled themselves daily consumers. The reduction in smoking prevalence among physicians resulted from a decrease in smoking uptake among new physicians and by the successful quitting of experienced physicians (US DHHS, 1989).

As the negative health consequences of smoking become widely known, we would expect smoking uptake rates to change much more rapidly than quitting behavior because it is easier not to start than to quit an addictive behavior. In the United States, taking up smoking generally has occurred between the ages of 12 and 25 (Pierce et al., 1991; US DHHS, 1989). Therefore, studies of smoking prevalence among medical students should indicate quite accurately the proportion of new physicians who will smoke. The Johns Hopkins Precursors Study and the Preventive Cardiology studies provide data on smoking uptake among medical students.

From 1948 through 1964 at the Johns Hopkins Medical School (Baltimore, Maryland), the behavior of medical students was analyzed by annual surveys, now known as the "Precursors Study" (M. Klag, personal communication). Members of each admitted class were surveyed on several categories of behavior, including current cigarette use. The average smoking prevalence among medical students at Johns Hopkins Medical School was 65.4 percent for the years 1948 through 1951 (Figure 4), a rate only slightly higher than the prevalence of smoking among physicians during these years. However, by 1965 the prevalence for the medical students had dropped below 40 percent. Presumably, if surveyed later as practicing physicians, some would be found to have quit.

Throughout the 1980's, the National Heart, Lung, and Blood Institute provided a series of preventive cardiology awards to several investigators at medical schools (Stone et al., 1990). As part of these awards, investigators undertook cardiovascular risk surveys of medical school students. Dr. Tom Pearson of Bassett Hospital (Cooperstown, New York) combined and computerized data from eight medical schools (Johns Hopkins University, Case Western Reserve University, Mt. Sinai, St. Louis University, State University of New York at Rochester, University of Utah, George Washington University, and the University of California at Irvine) (T. Pearson, personal

Figure 4
Smoking prevalence among medical students

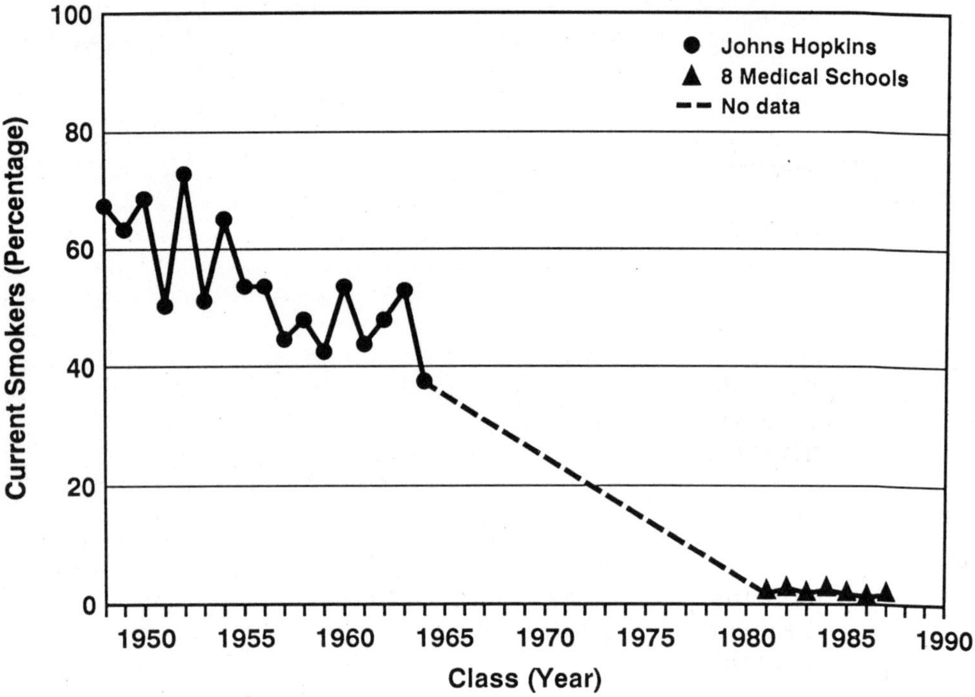

Sources: Derived from unpublished data, Precursors Study and Preventive Cardiology Series.

communication). In general, first- and fourth-year medical students from the graduating classes of 1981 through 1987 were surveyed. In these medical schools, from 1981 through 1987, the maximum prevalence was less than 3 percent in any year. These data seem to indicate that medical students in the United States had become almost smoke-free by the early 1980's.

Smoking prevalence among medical students can be put in context by comparison with the smoking prevalence in 22- to 26-year-old individuals in the population with 16 or more years of education, as determined from the National Health Interview Surveys. In 1965, an estimated 40 percent of the NHIS population in the age and education ranges given above were current smokers, about the same percentages observed for the Johns Hopkins medical students in that year. Prevalence declined steadily in the general population over time, and by 1987 it was down to 14 percent (which is at least 10 percentage points higher than smoking prevalence among medical students in the Preventive Cardiology series). One explanation for the difference between the change in the smoking behavior of medical students and that of their peers is the radical change in social norms among aspiring physicians with respect to the acceptability of smoking after publication of the 1964 Surgeon General's report.

PHYSICIANS' ADVICE, AS REPORTED BY PATIENTS

Gritz (1988) has estimated that some 70 percent of the population visit a physician each year. In California in 1990 (Burns and Pierce, 1992), 72.4 percent of the total population visited a physician in the year prior to the survey. This included 66.8 percent of all current smokers. Indeed, 40.2 percent of current smokers visited their physician on more than one occasion during that 12-month period. Physicians have both the mandate and the opportunity to advise smoking patients to quit; they are in the position to provide that advice at low cost on a one-to-one basis to the majority of smokers each year.

Data Sources and Measures

Information on whether physicians had advised individual patients to quit smoking was obtained from three National Health Interview Surveys (1974, 1976, and the 1987 Cancer Risk Factor Supplement) and the 1986 Adult Use of Tobacco Survey (AUTS). The three NHIS studies were household in-person interview surveys with questions related to smoking asked directly of the respondent (response rate more than 85 percent). Details of the survey methodology were reported previously (NCHS, 1985 and 1987). The 1986 AUTS survey was a random-digit-dialing telephone survey; within an identified household, eligible respondents answered the questions themselves (US DHHS, 1986b). The response rate was 74 percent. Rates of physicians' advice from the surveys, reported previously (Gilpin et al., 1992), are summarized below.

In each survey year, ever-smokers were defined as those who had smoked more than 100 cigarettes in their lifetime. Current smokers were defined by the question, "Do you smoke cigarettes now?" Ever-smokers who answered no to the question about current smoking were labeled "former smokers."

In the 1974 and 1976 surveys, respondents were asked, "Have you ever been advised by a doctor to quit smoking?" In the 1986 survey, respondents were asked, "Did any doctor ever advise you to quit smoking?" Finally, in the 1987 survey the question was, "Has a doctor ever advised you to quit smoking?" For this discussion, the sample of respondents analyzed included current and former smokers, aged 20 or older at the time of interview, who indicated whether or not they had received advice to quit from a physician. When respondents were asked whether they had ever received advice to quit smoking from a physician, no time interval was mentioned.

Increase in Reported Advice

Three separate analyses of changes in reported advice with time were performed. The first analysis considered former smokers, the second focused on current smokers, and the third included both current and former smokers and used information on the date of smoking cessation. The analysis of current smokers alone should give a better picture of recent advice patterns. Finally, in the third analysis, respondents who had been former smokers the longest would generally have been more likely to be advised at an earlier date than those who quit more recently or who are current smokers, thus providing another indication of changes in physicians' advice patterns.

Advice rates over time or over time since former smokers smoked were compared with the χ^2 test for trend. Figure 5 presents the overall percentages of current and former smokers who had been advised to quit smoking, as reported in each survey year. These percentages have increased steadily over the years ($p < 10^{-8}$), especially in the last two survey years compared with the first two. In 1974, only 26.4 percent of current smokers reported receiving advice, and by 1987 the percentage had reached 50.9 percent. Furthermore, the percentages of former smokers (by interval since they smoked) and current smokers advised to quit smoking in the combined 1986 and 1987 surveys also show the trend for increased advice to quit with time ($p < 10^{-8}$) (Figure 6).

The trend to increased reporting of advice with time has been noted previously within these same surveys and those for earlier years (US DHHS, 1990). For the 1964 AUTS survey, 15 percent of current smokers reported receiving advice. By the 1966 AUTS survey, the percentage of smokers reporting they received advice had reached 16.9 percent, and by the 1970 AUTS survey, it climbed to 21.8 percent (US DHHS, 1990).

Demographic Subgroups

To examine the relationship of demographic factors to the reported rates of advice among current smokers, the earlier 2 years, 1974 and 1976 (from NHIS), and the later 2 years, 1986 and 1987 (from AUTS and NHIS, respectively), were combined. There are some important demographic differences in who is likely to have received advice to quit smoking (Table 3). In both periods, more female smokers than male smokers reported having been advised to quit smoking (28.9 vs. 25.8 percent in the 1970's, and 53.3 vs. 45.6 percent in the 1980's).

Figure 5
Physician advice, as reported by current and former smokers

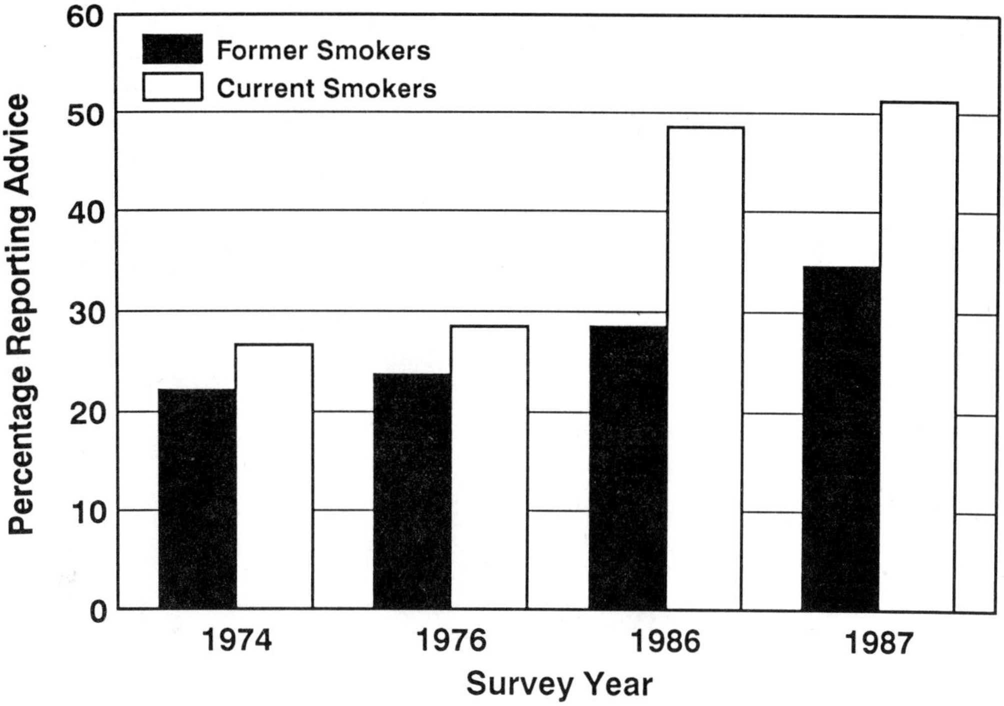

Sources: 1974, 1976, 1987 National Health Interview Surveys; 1986 Adult Use of Tobacco Survey.

In both survey periods, a clear trend for age was seen: More advice is reported with advancing age of the patient. However, in the later period (1986 and 1987) this trend was less pronounced. This finding could result from more frequent visits to the physician by older people, from an aging of the population, or both (US DHHS, 1986a).

In both survey periods, white respondents reported receiving advice more than did blacks (28.5 vs. 18.4 percent in the 1970's, and 51.5 vs. 39.4 percent in the 1980's). This indicates that physicians may not be advising blacks to quit smoking as often or as strongly as they are advising whites.

Smokers with more than a high school education reported receiving advice more often than did those with less education, and all educational levels showed the same increase with time. While the average age of the population has been advancing in recent years, so has its level of education. These changes may tend to offset one another and probably account for the absence of a more substantial trend in reported advice relative to education level.

Figure 6
Physician advice, by interval since patient last smoked

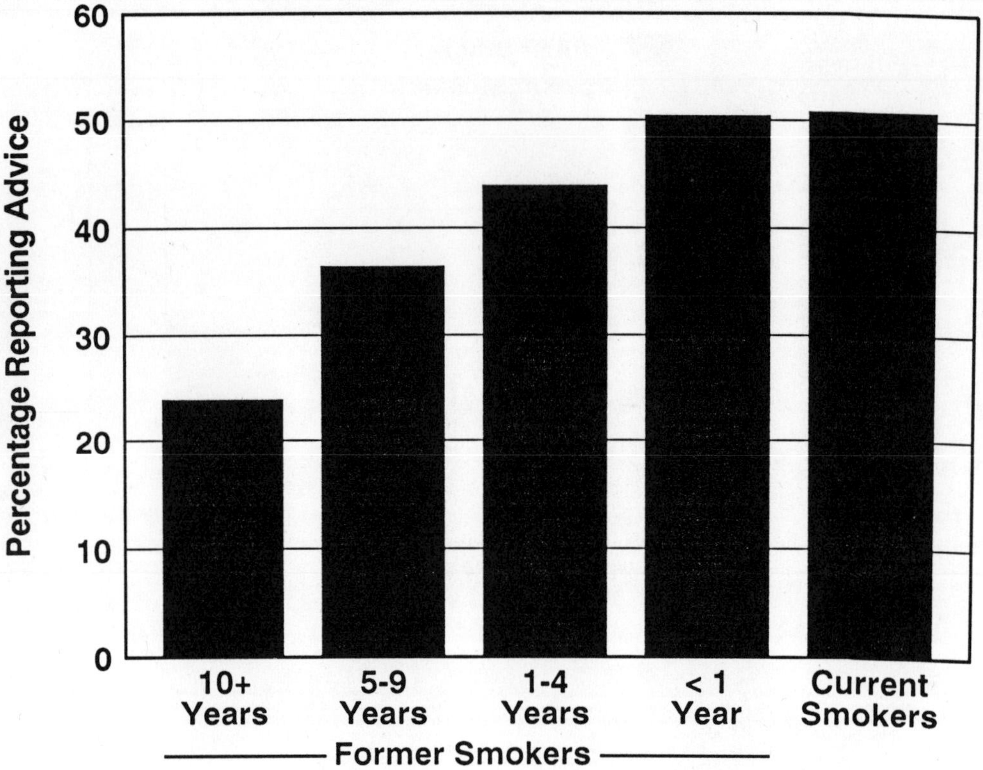

Sources: 1986 Adult Use of Tobacco Survey, 1987 National Health Interview Survey.

Differences in Physicians' And Patients' Reports

In 1986 and 1987, half of all current smokers reported that they had been advised to quit smoking by a physician. In seven studies that relied on physician self-report (including two national surveys of family practitioners), the proportion of physicians reporting regularly advising their smoking patients to quit ranged from 52 to 97 percent (Fortmann et al., 1985; Ockene et al., 1986; Orleans et al., 1985; Rimer et al., 1986; Rosen et al., 1984; Valente et al., 1986; Wechsler et al., 1983; Wells et al., 1986).

Several factors may account for the discrepancy in the advice rates reported by patients and those reported by physicians. First, physicians who do not respond to voluntary surveys about their practices for advising patients to quit smoking may not routinely give such advice. Second, the physicians seen most often by smokers may not be cardiopulmonary specialists and may not be as aware of the importance of advising patients to quit, and therefore do not give their patients as much advice (Wells et al., 1986). Third, physicians may be more likely to advise patients who have smoking-related illnesses (Cummings et al., 1987; Ockene et al., 1987). Results from

Table 3
Current smokers advised to quit, by time period and demographic characteristics

	1974 to 1976 (n=16,033)	1986 to 1987 (n=10,403)	Ratio
	Percentage (Standard Error)		
Overall	27.3% (0.4)	49.7% (0.5)	1.8
Sex			
Male	25.8 (0.5)	45.8 (0.7)	1.8
Female	28.9 (0.5)	53.3 (0.7)	1.8
Age			
20 to 29 yr	19.4 (0.7)	41.9 (1.1)	2.2
30 to 44	26.7 (0.6)	49.6 (0.8)	1.9
45 to 64	33.0 (0.9)	55.1 (1.1)	1.7
≥ 65	33.4 (1.2)	54.5 (1.4)	1.6
Race			
White	28.5 (0.4)	51.5 (0.5)	1.8
Black	18.4 (0.9)	39.4 (1.3)	2.1
Other	15.9 (3.1)	44.1 (3.0)	2.8
Education			
< 12 yr	27.2 (0.6)	47.9 (1.0)	1.8
12	25.2 (0.6)	48.5 (0.8)	1.9
13 to 15	28.5 (0.6)	52.1 (0.9)	1.8
≥ 16	30.8 (1.3)	53.4 (1.5)	1.7

Sources: 1976, 1984, 1987 National Health Interview Surveys, 1986 Adult Use of Tobacco Survey.

a national survey of internists indicated that, although 82 percent of the group reported counseling more than 75 percent of smokers with heart disease, only 52 percent reported counseling more than 75 percent of all patients who smoke (Wells et al., 1986). Finally, physicians may have given advice that patients do not remember. A physician's simple statement to a patient, "You should quit smoking," may not have the same impact as active counseling or multiple messages (Kottke et al., 1988; Schwartz, 1987).

SUMMARY Although more smokers in recent years are receiving health professionals' advice to quit smoking, many still are not being reached by this important avenue. Physicians and dentists may hesitate to advise smoking patients to quit because they perceive that such advice has little impact compared with standard therapies for other ailments. Physicians and dentists need to understand that the success of their efforts is not measured in how many patients become ex-smokers in the year after advice is given. On that scale, only about a 5-percent quit rate is to be expected (Cummings et al., 1987; U.S. Preventive Services Task Force, 1989). Rather, advice will lead the patient along a cyclical path to quitting. Smokers generally move through stages of not thinking about quitting, then thinking about it, making a quit attempt followed by relapse, and another period of no interest (Prochaska and DiClemente, 1983). However, repeated advice to quit, together with messages from other sources, will help reinforce the process so that eventually the smoker will make a successful attempt and become one of the 5 percent who quit.

REFERENCES

Buechner, J.S., Perry, D.K., Scott, H.D., et al. Cigarette smoking behavior among Rhode Island physicians, 1963-83. *American Journal of Public Health* 76: 285-286, 1986.

Burns, D., Pierce, J.P. *Tobacco Use in California 1990-1991.* Sacramento: California Department of Health Services, 1992.

Cummings, K.M., Giovino, G., Sciandra, R., Koenigsberg, M., Emont, S.L. Physician advice to quit smoking: Who gets it and who doesn't. *American Journal of Preventive Medicine* 3: 69-74, 1987.

Fiore, M.C., Novotny, T.E., Pierce, J.P., Giovino, G.A., Hatziandreu, E.J., Newcomb, P.A., Surawicz, T.S., Davis, R.M. Methods used to quit smoking in the United States. *Journal of the American Medical Association* 253: 2760-2765, 1990.

Fortmann, S.P., Sallis, J.F., Magnus, P.M., Farquhar, J.W. Attitudes and practices of physicians regarding hypertension and smoking: The Stanford Five-City Project. *Preventive Medicine* 14: 70-80, 1985.

Garfinkel, L., Stellman, S.D. Cigarette smoking among physicians, dentists and other health professionals, 1959-1972. *CA—A Cancer Journal for Clinicians* 26: 373-375, 1976.

Gilpin, E., Pierce, J., Goodman, J., Giovino, G., Berry, C., Burns, D. Trends in physicians' giving advice to stop smoking, United States, 1974-87. *Tobacco Control* 1: 1-36, 1992.

Gritz, E.R. Cigarette smoking: The need for action by health professionals. *CA—A Cancer Journal for Clinicians* 38: 194-212, 1988.

Hatziandreu, E.J., Pierce, J.P., Lefkopoulou, M., Fiore, M.C., Mills, S., Novotny, T.E., Giovino, G., Davis, R.M. Quitting smoking in the United States: Who tries and who succeeds. *Journal of the National Cancer Institute* 82: 1402-1406, 1990.

Hughes, P.H., Brandenberg, N., Baldwin, D.C., Storr, C.L., Williams, K.M., Anthony, J.C., Sheehan, D.W. Prevalence of substance use among U.S. physicians. *Journal of the American Medical Association* 267: 2333-2339, 1992.

Kottke, T.E., Battista, R.N., DeFriese, G.H., Brekke, M.L. Attributes of successful smoking cessation interventions in medical practice: A meta-analysis of 39 controlled trials. *Journal of the American Medical Association* 259: 2882-2889, 1988.

Kottke, T.E., Brekke, M.L., Solberg, L.I., Hughes, J.R. A randomized trial to increase smoking intervention by physicians: Doctors Helping Smokers, round I. *Journal of the American Medical Association* 261: 2101-2106, 1989.

National Center for Health Statistics. *Current Estimates from the Health Interview Survey.* U.S. Department of Health and Human Services, Ser. 10, No. 166, 1987.

National Center for Health Statistics. *The National Health Interview Survey Design, 1973-84, and Procedures 1975-1983.* U.S. Department of Health and Human Services. DHHS Publication No. (PHS) 85-1320, 1985.

Ockene, J.K., Hosmer, D.W., Williams, J.W., Goldberg, R.J., Ockene, I.S., Biliouris, T., Dalen, J.E. The relationship of patient characteristics to physician delivery of advice to stop smoking. *Journal of General Internal Medicine* 2: 337-340, 1987.

Ockene, J.K., Williams, J., Hosmer, D., Goldberg, R.J., Raia, T.J. A survey of physicians' smoking intervention practices. Presented at the Annual Meeting of the Society for Behavioral Medicine, San Francisco, California, March 1986.

Orleans, C.T., George, L.K., Houpt, J.L., Brodie, K.H. Health promotion in primary care: A survey of U.S. family practitioners. *Preventive Medicine* 14: 636-647, 1985.

Pierce, J.P., Naquin, M., Gilpin, E., Giovino, G., Mills, S., Marcus, S. Smoking initiation in the United States: A role for worksite and college smoking bans. *Journal of the National Cancer Institute* 83: 1009-1013, 1991.

Prochaska, J.O., DiClemente, C.C. Stages and processes of self-change of smoking: Toward an integrative model of change. *Journal of Consulting and Clinical Psychology* 51(3): 390-395, 1983.

Rimer, B.K., Strecher, V.J., Keintz, M.K., Engstrom, P.F. A survey of physicians' views and practices of patient education for smoking cessation. *Preventive Medicine* 15: 92-98, 1986.

Rosen, M.A., Logsdon, D.N., Demak, M.M. Prevention and health promotion in primary care: Baseline results on physicians from the Insure project on life-cycle preventive health services. *Preventive Medicine* 13: 535-548, 1984.

Sachs, D.P.L. Smoking habits of pulmonary physicians. *New England Journal of Medicine* 309: 799, 1983.

Schwartz, J.L. *Review and Evaluation of Smoking Cessation Methods: The United States and Canada, 1978-1985.* U.S. Department of Health and Human Services, Public Health Service, National Institutes of Health, National Cancer Institute, Division of Cancer Prevention and Control. NIH Publication No. 87-2940, 1987.

Stone, E.J., Van Citters, R.L., Pearson, T.A. (Editors). Preventive cardiology: Perspectives in physician education. *American Journal of Preventive Medicine* 6(Suppl.): 1-100, 1990.

U.S. Department of Health and Human Services. *The Health Benefits of Smoking Cessation: A Report of the Surgeon General.* U.S. Department of Health and Human Services, Public Health Service, Centers for Disease Control, Center for Chronic Disease Prevention and Health Promotion, Office on Smoking and Health. DHHS Publication No. (CDC) 90-8416, 1990.

U.S. Department of Health and Human Services. *Health United States 1986 and Prevention Profile.* U.S. Department of Health and Human Services. DHHS Publication No. (PHS) 87-1232, 1986a.

U.S. Department of Health and Human Services. *Reducing the Health Consequences of Smoking: 25 Years of Progress. A Report of the Surgeon General.* U.S. Department of Health and Human Services, Public Health Service, Centers for Disease Control, Center for Chronic Disease Prevention and Health Promotion, Office on Smoking and Health. DHHS Publication No. (CDC) 89-8411, 1989.

U.S. Department of Health and Human Services. *Tobacco Use in 1986: Methods and Basic Tabulations from Adult Use of Tobacco Survey.* U.S. Department of Health and Human Services, Public Health Service, Centers for Disease Control, 1986b.

U.S. Department of Health, Education, and Welfare. *Smoking and Health: A Report of the Advisory Committee to the Surgeon General of the Public Health Service.* U.S. Department of Health, Education, and Welfare; Public Health Service. PHS Publication No. 1103, 1964.

U.S. Preventive Services Task Force. *Guidelines to Clinical Preventive Service: An Assessment of the Effectiveness of 169 Interventions. Report of the U.S. Preventive Services Task Force.* Baltimore: Williams and Wilkins, 1989.

Valente, C.M., Sobal, J., Muncie, H.L., Levine, D.M., Antlitz, A.M. Health promotion: Physicians' beliefs, attitudes and practices. *American Journal of Preventive Medicine* 2: 82-88, 1986.

Wechsler, H., Levine, S., Idelson, R.K., Rohman, M., Taylor, J.O. The physician's role in health promotion: A survey of primary care practitioners. *New England Journal of Medicine* 308: 97-100, 1983.

Wells, K.B., Lewis, C.E., Leuke, B., Schleiter, M.K., Brook, P.H. The practices of general and subspecialty internists in counseling about smoking and exercise. *American Journal of Public Health* 76: 1009-1013, 1986.

The Health Professional's Responsibility in Smoking Cessation: Strategies for Office and Community

John W. Richards, Jr., Thomas P. Houston, and Alan Blum

INTRODUCTION Achieving behavior change among individuals exposed to risks is a complex task. The field of risk communication is an evolving science, often poorly understood by both its practitioners and those who should be. It seems evident, however, that providing information about a potential risk is only the first of several steps in affecting behavior. Information, motivation, and sometimes legislation are needed to reduce personal and societal risks. Seat belt campaigns that have culminated in automobile safety laws for adults and children are a case in point.

The personal and professional role and responsibility of health professionals go beyond merely giving relevant information about smoking. Needed are office-based and community efforts that can help motivate patients and activate other health professionals to address more effectively the single largest cause of illness and death in our society, smoking.

In reviewing categories of behavior change, Green and colleagues (1988) identified three types of behavioral influence that apply to clinicians: predisposing, enabling, and reinforcing factors. Knowledge and attitudes toward health promotion and disease prevention, the health behavior of the professional, confidence in counseling skills, and belief about their patients' interest in such advice are the predisposing factors that can be both positive and negative cues toward health promotion behavior. Factors that promote or enable health promotion activities include a feeling of confidence about performing preventive care services, reimbursement for these activities, and an organized practice setting that facilitates preventive medicine. Reinforcing factors include positive feedback from patients, evidence of intermediate results, peer support, and a perception that health promotion activities add to the role of healer.

Many of these characteristics are not easily fulfilled in the case of smoking cessation. Although many health professionals have adequate knowledge about the pathophysiology of tobacco use and its adverse consequences on health, most are not adequately trained in medical or dental school, or during residency, to counsel patients about smoking cessation (Horton, 1986). Likewise, although many patients desire health promotion advice from their physicians, the physicians often do not fulfill the patients' expectations. In a study by Owen and Davies (1990), 67 percent of smokers preferred receiving advice from a health professional over other means of assistance with smoking cessation. Physicians and dentists, however, are notoriously lax about advising patients to stop smoking. Only about 45 percent of smokers report that a physician has ever advised them to stop smoking (Anda et al., 1987; Davis, 1988).

Good news about physician counseling behavior comes from a survey in which 98 percent of recently trained family physicians reported that they counsel patients about smoking, even when no smoking-related disease is present. Thirty percent of that group also said they believed they were influential in their patients' smoking cessation (Goldstein et al., 1987).

Many health professionals do not feel empowered to engage in smoking cessation efforts because of reimbursement issues and the perception that smoking cessation requires inordinate amounts of time. Green and coworkers' identified reinforcing factors (Green et al., 1988) also may be perceived as blockers when physicians' partners and peers do not support their beliefs about smoking cessation, when feedback from patients is not as readily apparent as with self-limiting or easily treated illnesses, or when there is discouragement because of failure to achieve a 100-percent cure among patients who smoke.

On the other hand, most physicians have adopted health behaviors that are conducive to smoking cessation in practice. A 1987 study conducted by the American Medical Association showed that only 9 percent of randomly selected physicians were smokers (Harvey and Shubat, 1987). Because health professionals have frequent contact with patients who smoke, there is opportunity for intervention. More than 70 percent of Americans see a physician at least annually, and more than 60 percent see a dentist each year. Smokers average 4.3 physician visits each year (Wetzler and Cruess, 1985), and even a brief intervention by physicians can be successful in doubling the spontaneous quit rate of 2 to 4 percent (Ockene, 1987; Schwartz, 1987).

At this point, a brief review of the hazards of smoking and the benefits of cessation is in order. Smoking's effects on health constitute the single largest cause of preventable disease and death in American society. The Office on Smoking and Health has estimated that more than 430,000 Americans die each year from diseases related to smoking (Centers for Disease Control, 1991). Nearly one of every five deaths in the United States is caused by smoking; this represents more deaths than the combined total of deaths each year from AIDS, automobile accidents, homicide, suicide, and illegal drugs.

The 1990 Surgeon General's report (US DHHS, 1990) points out that smoking is the leading cause of lung cancer among both men and women; the risk of lung cancer is 22 times higher among male smokers and 12 times higher among female smokers than nonsmokers. After smoking cessation, the risk of lung cancer declines, so after about 10 years of abstinence, the risk of lung cancer for the ex-smoker is between 30 and 50 percent of the risk for those who have continued to smoke.

Smokers have about two times the risk of nonsmokers of dying from heart disease. Cessation reduces the excess risk by about 50 percent after only 1 year. After 15 years of cessation, the risk is similar to that for persons who have never smoked.

Stroke is the third leading cause of death in the United States. Stroke prior to age 55 is twice as common among smokers as it is among non-smokers. It is less clear how quickly stroke risks return to baseline for persons who have stopped smoking—probably between 5 and 15 years.

Smoking is the major cause of chronic obstructive lung disease, the fifth leading cause of death in the United States. Again, we see benefits in cessation because the progression of chronic obstructive pulmonary disease is reduced with abstinence from smoking. Cigarette smoking is one of the major causes of peripheral artery disease and increases the mortality from abdominal aortic aneurysm between two and five times.

Women have special risks from smoking besides lung cancer, now the leading cancer killer among women. These include an increased risk of cervical cancer and several complications of pregnancy, including bleeding during pregnancy, premature rupture of membranes, preterm delivery, placenta previa, abruptio placenta, and producing a baby with low birth weight. Women who stop smoking before becoming pregnant or stop smoking during the first trimester of pregnancy apparently reverse the risk of low birth weight for the baby as well as reducing the other pregnancy-associated risks.

Recent data show also that smoking during pregnancy affects the growth and development of young children, in both the physical and cognitive areas. Stopping smoking early in pregnancy prevents these effects, just as the in utero risks are reduced by smoking cessation (Sexton et al., 1990a and 1990b).

Both smoked and smokeless forms of tobacco have deleterious effects on the soft and hard tissues of the oral cavity.

Because the facts about smoking and the benefits of cessation are known, and 80 to 90 percent of patients want to stop smoking, it is incumbent on physicians and dentists as community members to participate in smoking cessation counseling. Clinicians are bestowed with an enormous mantle of authority: Most smokers who express a preference want information about smoking cessation from physicians in preference to other sources; and one-half of smokers say they would try to quit if their dentist advised them to quit. Physicians and dentists also have an ethical duty to prevent illness and reduce the burden of disease and suffering.

Our patients do not wake up one morning and suddenly decide to become smokers; rather, they are bombarded from an early age with messages and role models that encourage tobacco use. A health professional's approach to smoking cessation should therefore be a longitudinal strategy involving a multitiered approach that includes the office, hospitals, schools, civic organizations, and the mass media, in addition to the more traditional individual patient encounter. What follows reflects trial and error by physicians and research efforts by members of Doctors Ought to Care, a physician-led group advocating smoking cessation strategies as an essential part of every practice (Blum, 1980 and 1982). Moreover, there is growing evidence that these techniques are effective.

IN THE PRACTITIONER'S OFFICE

Most physicians' and dentists' offices are remarkably underused for smoking cessation, especially in light of the above-described devastation of health by tobacco use. The entire office staff must work to create an environment conducive to nonsmoking behavior among patients. The first step is to assume a patient's perspective and tour the office with the objective of creating an atmosphere that clearly conveys the message that nonsmoking is the norm. Because the amount of time the patient spends registering and waiting may be as long as the health care encounter itself, every opportunity to encourage and support nonsmoking behavior must be used throughout the office environment. The following details what can be done in different office areas.

The Reception Area

As part of the professional office, the reception area automatically grants credibility and implies endorsement to whatever editorial or commercial material it may contain. Health professionals are the target, therefore, of publishers who are trying to get their magazines displayed in patient care facilities. In fact, many magazines such as *Better Homes and Gardens, Working Woman, Family Circle, Woman's Day,* and *People* offer very low "professional rates." Each of these magazines contains an average of 10 cigarette advertisements per issue. These are often juxtaposed with health articles, most of which are unrelated to the subject of tobacco (Houston, 1984). Indeed, *Time, Newsweek, Sports Illustrated, Better Homes and Gardens, U.S. News and World Report, Ladies Home Journal,* and *People*—the most frequently purchased magazines for doctor's offices (Fischer, 1985)—have many advertisements encouraging and glamorizing tobacco use. In addition, most of them have deliberately avoided the subject of tobacco's effects on health (Richards, 1991).

It is absurd to display glamorous models in highly desirable settings to promote cigarettes in a physician's or dentist's waiting room. Health care professionals can send a message to patients and publishers alike by canceling subscriptions to these publications and subscribing to publications that do not promote tobacco (Richards, 1983; also see Appendix A). An alternative technique is to call attention to the harmful and often untruthful nature of these advertisements by stamping or pasting stickers on the advertisements with comments such as, "This ad is a rip-off" or "Your doctor does not approve of this ad" (Figure 7). Moreover, a sign might be placed in the reception area alerting patients to the reason specific reading material has been provided. Of course, a sign should be displayed that informs patients that the office is a smoke-free zone. Other signs in the office can invite patients to inquire about smoking cessation and inform them that smoking cessation activities are available.

Figure 7
Sticker for waiting room magazines

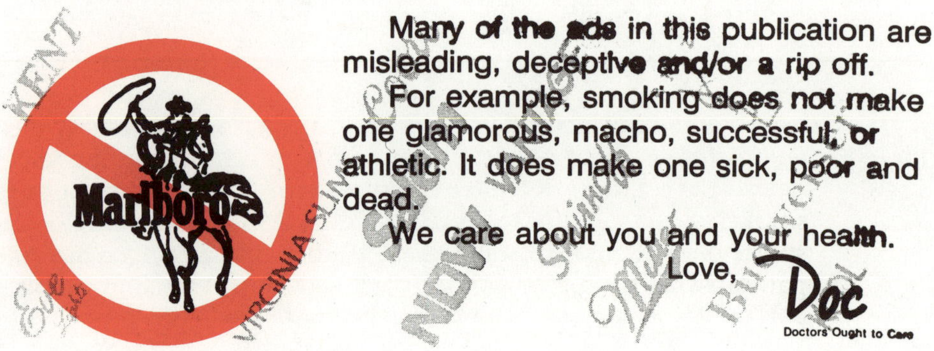

Source: Doctors Ought to Care; copyright 1987; used with permission.

Other areas of the office, such as the restrooms, can be provided with eye-catching posters and reading material that promote healthful behavior. Even the ceilings of exam rooms are open for attention-getting posters or messages. These would be supplements to the traditional use of time spent in the exam room, when patients can read carefully selected materials.

Vital Signs In almost all practices, vital signs are noted prior to the patient-physician encounter. Because tobacco use is the principal cause of premature morbidity and mortality in this country, a column should be added to the vital signs record and headed "tobacco" (Richards, 1991). A simple question—"Do you use tobacco?"—should be asked as a part of checking vital signs. The utility of this simple screening test is far greater than most screening used in practice. When the response is positive, the physician or dentist has information that is a powerful predictor of both acute and chronic disease in the patient and his family. Moreover, it signifies to nonsmokers as well as to smoking patients that tobacco use is a very important factor in health and that the health care provider is concerned about smoking.

The Examination Whether the presenting complaint is acute or chronic, smoking cessation can and should be a part of each visit. Tobacco use, once identified, should be placed on the problem list as a permanent problem. Just as a physician routinely takes blood pressure readings for formerly hypertensive individuals, the physician should continue to inquire about tobacco use even after cessation is achieved. This reinforces patient efforts because physician concern is often cited by patients as an important influence on smoking behavior.

Identifying and using "teachable moments," such as during or just after an illness, can significantly increase chances for a successful intervention by providing new motivating factors on which to build (Brunton, 1984).

However, it is not sufficient to wait for teachable moments: Experienced physicians can and should create them.

To the alert physician or dentist, the presenting complaint will often lead to smoking cessation opportunities. For example, a child with an ear infection or even a cold offers a teachable moment to talk with parents about their cigarette smoking. Prenatal visits, the intrapartum hospital stay, and well-child visits provide the opportunity to discuss protecting children from environmental tobacco smoke as well as to remind parents about their own health risks. Routine dental appointments can become opportunities for smokeless tobacco education, especially among adolescent boys. The school sports physical, the camp physical, routine checkups for diabetic or asthmatic patients—all should be used as teaching encounters about tobacco use.

During the examination itself, opportunities abound. Instead of a spot on the wall for a patient to look at during the funduscopic exam, substitute an attention-getting poster to make productive use of 30 seconds of direct concentration. Casual comments while examining the mouth ("Still smoking, I see") or while listening to the lungs ("Still smoking, I hear") plant seeds for change. However, asking the traditional question, "How much do you smoke?," may lead the patient to interpret that there is a safe level of consumption, so the physician must be prepared with an appropriate disclaimer to follow the patient's response.

INDIVIDUALIZING INTERVENTIONS

To increase effectiveness, physicians and dentists should examine closely the basic reasons for patients' smoking, keeping in mind the techniques used to sell cigarettes and encourage consumption. Most people, especially teenagers, choose cigarettes that advertisers promise will make them look macho, mature, sexy, successful, or more acceptable to their peers. Because cigarettes, if used, actually cause the *opposite* appearance, the very same Madison Avenue images that promote buying and using cigarettes can also be employed successfully by physicians to promote *un*buying or *non*smoking.

Smoking cessation is really no different from many other medical interventions. However, with smoking cessation the average person who stops smoking has tried several times over a prolonged period—sometimes years—before becoming a successful nonsmoker. This can be frustrating for the physician who is accustomed to achieving success with measurable results in a matter of days.

For example, consider the urinary tract infection. The patient complains of frequency, urgency, and dysuria. A culture is taken. Antibiotics are selected and prescribed. The sensitivity confirms the correct choice. The patient generally gets better quickly and is well in a week. If the patient with a urinary tract infection were to come back in a week with continued symptoms, no physician would say, "I'm sorry, but we tried an antibiotic; unfortunately, it did not work. I guess you'll have to suffer with this until you figure out a way to get better. However, you might get pyelonephritis and septicemia and die."

With smoking cessation, the practitioner does a "culture" by performing a general assessment of the patient's situation; determines the "sensitivity" by asking the question, "What brand do you smoke?"; and then selects the verbal "antibiotic" according to a combination of the above. If the first verbal antibiotic for smoking cessation does not work, the clinician should try another and then another, until success is achieved.

Just as a medical student is uncomfortable and apprehensive when using antibiotics to treat his or her first patient with a urinary tract infection, the same feelings are to be expected when first using various smoking cessation techniques. With practice, however, using smoking interventions will become as routine as treating a urinary tract infection.

One must remember that smoking cessation efforts, like other therapy, must be individualized through consideration of agent (strategies that have the best efficacy for a given situation), absorption and elimination (factors that enhance or detract), dose (enough to be therapeutic, yet not toxic), and timing (frequency and relation to other agents). Rather than a source of frustration, each intervention should be considered a learning experience for both the clinician and the patient. Realistic expectations are a must. Achieving a smoking cessation rate of 25 percent of patients at 1 year might seem disappointing for the physician accustomed to a 100-percent success rate for treating urinary tract infections. However, one must keep in mind that 25 percent would be an incredible success rate when contrasted with a reported baseline rate of 2 to 4 percent per year. Clinicians would jump at the chance to prescribe an antibiotic that is 100 percent more effective than competing products. Practiced, thoughtful smoking cessation efforts can be 1,000 percent better than no intervention.

STRATEGIES FOR COUNSELING

Words

Selecting the proper words to discuss smoking with a patient is every bit as important as selecting the proper pharmacologic agents for other health problems. Unfortunately, little time in training is devoted to developing this skill. Selecting the verbal "drug of choice" is not difficult, however, once a proper culture and sensitivity have been established.

In a recent article, Richards (1992) discussed 5 of the most important questions for the physician to ask and 20 of the excuses most commonly given by patients. Practice in these anticipated dialogues will better equip the health care provider to deal with one-on-one smoking intervention opportunities.

Money

Money is a powerful motivator. A high school freshman might respond to information that money saved by not buying cigarettes could be used to purchase a stereo at the end of a year or a car after the junior year of school. The young executive might be persuaded to give up a two-pack-per-day habit if told that the same money placed in an 8-percent annuity might be worth more than $1 million at retirement. In a similar fashion, a reward can be paid for not smoking by taking the money one would have spent each day on cigarettes and putting it in a "nonsmoking piggy bank." This money can be deposited in the bank, put into an account for children, used to pay for holidays or vacations, or, in a more immediate way, spent at the end of each nonsmoking month on a gift for the new nonsmoker or the family. At current prices, one pack per day comes to more than $50 per month, which requires a pretax income of $70 to $100. A patient who quits smoking in celebration of the birth of a child will have saved enough money over 18 years of abstinence to pay for the child's college education.

Demarketing Turning the tables on Madison Avenue can be an easy and effective strategy. A 15-year-old girl who smokes Virginia Slims (or another fashion-image brand) to appear sexy and independent might listen to information about how smoking causes "zoo breath" and yellow teeth, and that kissing a smoker is like "licking an ashtray." It is unlikely that teenagers will listen to statistics about possible deaths or disease in 30 or 40 years.

A 35- or 40-year-old woman might respond to the knowledge that premature wrinkling of the face is a cosmetic side effect of smoking. Both teenaged and young adult women might have second thoughts when reminded that Philip Morris is exploiting women by making them think that they have "come a long way," when actually the company is mocking women's independence by telling them what to do and getting them addicted to cigarettes.

The smoker of Now, True, Carlton, or other "low-tar" brands is concerned about health. Would the same person buy bread marketed as the "lowest in poison" or a soup that has "only 3 milligrams arsenic"? Appealing to health concerns and reinforcing the health benefits of cessation may be most effective for this subcategory of smokers (Blum, 1979).

Another way to point out the illogic of smoking is to ask the patient who refuses to stop smoking to switch to a brand inconsistent with the patient's desired image. For example, for the Marlboro-smoking truck driver, suggest Virginia Slims or Eve. This often leads the smoker to smile and realize the absurdity of smoking, which seems to break the ice and resistance to further efforts. For the patient for whom no technique seems to work, despite many attempts, a tactic to prolong the amount of time the patient considers the doctor's suggestions after leaving the office might be beneficial (for example, giving pamphlets or handouts to enhance the patient's absorption of the message).

In all the above techniques and strategies, the physician or dentist must take care to create an alliance with the patient against an enemy, that is, the companies selling tobacco products. By pointing out the deceitful marketing and unethical business practices of the cigarette industry and the manufacturer of their brand in particular, patients, especially teens, may become angry enough to stop purchasing their products. We must never lose sight of the fact that our patients, the smokers, are victims of an industry that has addicted them to nicotine. We must never look on the smoker as the enemy or take sides against smokers in our efforts. Even though many of our patients may not be able to stop smoking, we must continue to treat them with compassion and kindness.

The Quit Date Much has been written about establishing a quit date. Although beneficial to most patients, if it appears so hard to quit that the patient has to spend excessive time and effort getting ready, some may assume that it is just too difficult to stop smoking and will never even try.

Asking, "Have you set a quit date?" is really a way of determining the patient's readiness to stop smoking. If the answer is "yes," then follow with, "When?" and "What is it about that date that makes it a good one?" This will gather important additional motivating information for use in selecting the verbal drug of choice. This may also rapidly identify blockers to be dealt with or myths to be debunked.

If the patient has not already set a quit date, suggest setting one immediately. For patients who have tried to stop several times in the past, or for those who have relapsed after significant periods of cessation, "Why not today?" should be the next question. These patients may merely need a new boost for their previous success, and a lengthy period of contemplation before the stop date may actually allow them to put off the decision.

If the patient will not set a quit date, then explore the rationale with a statement such as, "You're an intelligent person. With all you know about what smoking is doing to you and the fact that you will die about 18 years earlier because of it, help me understand how you came to this decision." The patient's answer will offer an enormous insight into his or her thinking and motivation and will provide information for advising other patients as well. More often than not, the patient's rationale is based on inaccurate information. Thus, it provides an opportunity to correct the myth, educate the patient, and further encourage the smoker along the path toward becoming a nonsmoker.

The Contingency Contract Some clinicians use a written stop-smoking contract signed by both the patient and the physician after setting a quit date. Some include the contract as a part of the medical record and ask the patient to sign the agreement to stop smoking. Whether writing a personalized note on a prescription blank or the clinician's letterhead, or using specially designed contracts as may be found in smoking cessation kits from a number of sources, something tangible for the patient to take home may enhance the effectiveness of the cessation attempt (Taylor, 1985). Such a contract also serves to communicate the important message that medical or dental practice goes beyond dispensing medicine and repairing damaged tissue.

Rewards Many physicians find rewards to be beneficial adjuncts for smoking cessation activities. We previously mentioned monetary rewards, such as putting the amount of money the patient would have spent on tobacco during 1 year into an escrow account to be used for a long-term goal—holiday gifts, a stereo, or a downpayment on a car. This can be broken down into smaller increments as well, with daily contribution to a nonsmoking fund. Other, nonmonetary rewards might mark the 1-day, -week, -month, or -year anniversary and include a new hairstyle, a facial, a trip to a favorite park, or the guarantee of a day off from child care (which involves family support). Creativity and engaging the patient in setting up a personalized reward system are important.

Followup After the quit date, followup is essential to reinforcing the message of smoking cessation to the patient. The physician or dentist should make the followup contact through a brief office visit or a personal phone call within a week or so of the quit date. If time constraints or schedules will not permit, the office staff may be just as useful in making these contacts. The perspective of Solberg and colleagues (1990) on the team approach to smoking cessation in the family physician's office is most instructive. At the followup visit, or if a future encounter reveals that the patient has relapsed by smoking one or more cigarettes, the physician or dentist must take care not to make the patient feel even more guilty about the relapse.

Many patients will assume that, because they have resumed smoking (even if it is at a much lower level), they have failed and cannot be helped. Rather, the relapse should be discussed in depth so that the patient can understand the circumstances under which smoking was resumed and create contingencies to address the situation that triggered the relapse. By building on what was learned during the smoking cessation effort, the patient should be encouraged to stop smoking again. Anticipatory guidance and warning the patient about tempting situations (being with smokers, attending parties, drinking alcohol—especially at bars) will assist the patient in dodging these bullets. A careful smoking history with a patient's smoking diary and recording the stimuli and situation associated with lighting up can be quite helpful to the clinician in this regard.

COMMUNITY AWARENESS AND ACTION

From auto races to rock concerts to athletic events, even community charity fundraising events, the promotion of tobacco products appears in the guise of corporate sponsorship. These events are intended to create social acceptance and complacency among users and non-users alike. The enormous economic power of the tobacco industry through sponsorship, taxes, and advertising revenues can make local prevention efforts very unpopular. Health professionals should be aware of, but not deterred by, those who either do not recognize the long-term health consequences that sponsorship of these events represents or who consider economic gain more important than health. Every physician and dentist is a potential smoking cessation specialist and should take advantage of opportunities to participate or take the lead in nontraditional activities in tobacco control.

Does everyone really know about the hazards of smoking? One need only consider the outcry by chain-smoking homeowners about radon vapors, by puffing parents over asbestos in the classroom ceilings, or by the news media over cyanide-tainted grapes, or the irony of tobacco-company-sponsored boat races to raise money for cerebral palsy before realizing that, although much is known, very little is perceived or believed. Surveys of relative risk in our society make it clear that the general public thinks tobacco smoking is much less dangerous than health professionals know it to be.

A letter to the newspaper editor or to the local sponsors of an event that uses tobacco products in association with sports or fitness can often prompt a turndown of tobacco company sponsorship. The letter can highlight the conflict between tobacco sponsorship and the health of the community's children and others attending the event.

Physicians and others concerned about health can make "house calls" to encourage good health; for example, protesting the Virginia Slims tennis tournament or comparable events by picketing while wearing white coat and stethoscope and holding placards (Figure 8). Other tactics include holding a health press conference at the event or volunteering for media talk shows (Richards et al., 1988). The credibility enjoyed by dentists and physicians in the community goes far beyond that of tobacco promoters. By using local media, the service club speaking circuit, volunteer agencies, and even solicitation among patients, corporations and bureaucrats can be mobilized and motivated to take up a call to ensure a smoke-free environment for all citizens. The prohealth community should not overlook bus benches, T-shirts, bumper stickers, notebook stickers for schoolchildren, and buttons as vehicles for antismoking messages (for example, the shirt in Figure 9).

Smoking cessation and tobacco control must become an integral part of clinical practice. The office should be an oasis of health-promoting ideas

Figure 8
Physicians picketing at the Virginia Slims tennis tournament in New Orleans

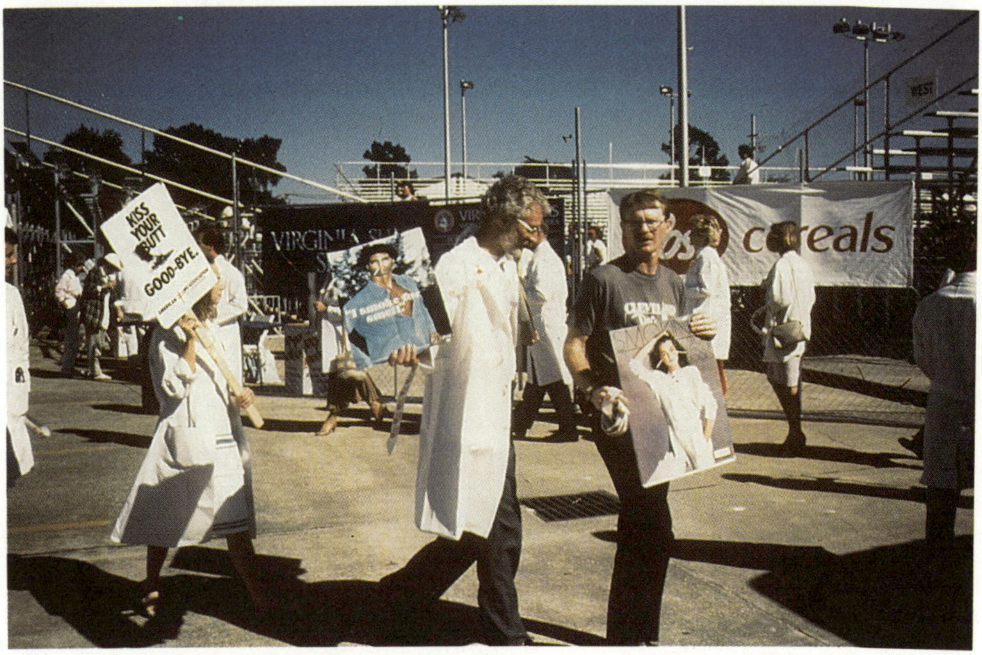

Source: Doctors Ought to Care; used with permission.

Figure 9
T-shirt bearing an antismoking message

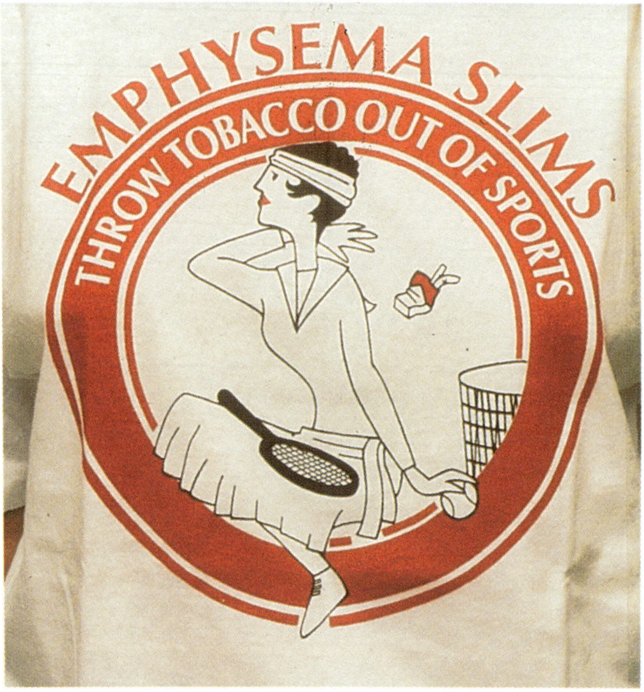

Source: Doctors Ought to Care; used with permission.

and messages for patients about the risks of smoking and the benefits of cessation. Beyond the traditional messages, however, the practitioner must accurately present the facts and statistics and change smokers' perceptions about the mystique of smoking. Practitioners must remember that smokers have been victimized by an industry that makes enormous profits from ill health, and they must create an alliance with patients against the tobacco industry. Health professionals bear a burden of responsibility about informing, educating, motivating, and working toward behavior change in their patients. To do less shortchanges patients and places practitioners in the unenviable situation of merely treating the resultant illness and comforting the families of those who have died prematurely.

Finally, we must not be afraid to go beyond the traditional activities that health professionals are expected to do and step outside the bounds of the individual doctor-patient relationship into the community. Participating with the local press, appearing on radio and television talk shows, going to civic clubs and churches, and organizing protests at tobacco-sponsored events all have their place in community and medical activism. The importance of these activities cannot be overstated, given the enormous burden of morbidity and mortality caused by smoking and the obvious benefits of cessation and the prevention of smoking initiation.

In many ways, the tobacco industry uses the community as a vector of the disease of nicotine addiction. Marketing pressures and social acceptance of smoking, exposure to environmental tobacco smoke, and the complacency of government, corporations, and even the medical community with respect to tobacco mandate action by the practitioner.

Individual clinicians can and do make a difference in community smoking control and individual smoking cessation. These two efforts are synergistic. The increased numbers of individuals who stop smoking add to the growing social unacceptability of smoking. Conversely, as community movements for smoking control gain momentum, individuals will become more motivated to seek advice on smoking cessation from physicians and dentists. To accomplish these joint tasks, we must first arm ourselves with the necessary skills, knowledge, and attitudes, then fully integrate smoking cessation counseling into everyday practice and work toward reducing the threat from the number one cause of morbidity and mortality.

Every physician and dentist can, should, and must become a smoking cessation expert. If we do not, who will?

REFERENCES

Anda, R.F., Remington, P.L., Sienko, D.G., Davis, R.M. Are physicians advising smokers to quit? The patient's perspective. *Journal of the American Medical Association* 257: 1916-1919, 1987.

Blum, A. The family physician and health promotion: Do-gooding or really doing well? *Canadian Family Physician* 28: 1613-1620, 1982.

Blum, A. Medicine vs. Madison Avenue: Fighting smoke with smoke. *Journal of the American Medical Association* 283: 739-740, 1980.

Blum, A. Would you buy bread lowest in carcinogens? *Advertising Age*, October 29, 1979, p. 86.

Brunton, S.A. Physicians as patient teachers. *Journal of Western Medicine* 141(6): 857-859, 1984.

Centers for Disease Control. Smoking-attributable mortality and years of potential life lost: United States, 1988. *Morbidity and Mortality Weekly Report* 49(4): 62-71, 1991.

Davis, R. Uniting physicians against smoking: The need for a coordinated national strategy. *Journal of the American Medical Association* 259: 2900-2901, 1988.

Fischer, P. Inappropriate magazines for the waiting room. *New York State Journal of Medicine* 85(7): 465-466, 1985.

Goldstein, B., Fischer, P.M., Richards, J.W., Goldstein, A., Shank, J.C. Smoking counseling practices of recently trained family physicians. *Journal of Family Practice* 24(2): 195-197, 1987.

Green, L.W., Eriksen, M.P., Schor, E.L. Preventive practices by physicians: Behavioral determinants and potential interventions. *American Journal of Preventive Medicine* 4(Suppl.): 101-107, 1988.

Harvey, L., Shubat, S. AMA Surveys of Physician and Public Opinion on Health Care Issues, 1987. Chicago: American Medical Association, 1987.

Horton, J. Education programs on smoking prevention and smoking cessation for students and housestaff in U.S. medical schools. *Cancer Detection and Prevention* 9: 417-420, 1986.

Houston, T.P. Priorities in health promotion. *Postgraduate Medicine* 76(5): 223-230, 1984.

Ockene, J.K. Smoking intervention: The expanding role of the physician. *American Journal of Public Health* 77: 782-783, 1987.

Owen, N., Davies, M.J. Smokers' preference for assistance with cessation. *Preventive Medicine* 19: 424-431, 1990.

Richards, J.W. Cancer screening in the office. *American Family Physician* 43: 1528, 1991.

Richards, J.W. A positive health strategy for the office waiting room. *New York State Journal of Medicine* 83(13): 1358-1360, 1983.

Richards, J.W. Words as therapy: Smoking cessation. *Journal of Family Medicine* 31(6): 687-692, 1992.

Richards, J.W., Blum, A., Houston, T., Fischer, P. DOC: A primer for social/health activism. In: *Smoking and Health 1987*. New York: Excerpta Medica, 1988, pp. 373-375.

Schwartz, J.L. *Review and Evaluation of Smoking Cessation Methods: The United States and Canada, 1987-1985*. U.S. Department of Health and Human Services, Public Health Service, National Institutes of Health, National Cancer Institute, Division of Cancer Prevention and Control. NIH Publication No. 87-2940, 1987.

Sexton, M., Fox, N.L., Hebel, J.R. Prenatal exposure to tobacco: I. Effects on physical growth to age three. *International Journal of Epidemiology* 19: 66-71, 1990a.

Sexton, M., Fox, N.L., Hebel, J.R. Prenatal exposure to tobacco: II. Effects on cognitive functioning at age three. *International Journal of Epidemiology* 19: 72-77, 1990b.

Solberg, L.I., Maxwell, P.L., Kottke, T.E., Gepner, G.J., Brekke, M.L. A systematic primary care office-based smoking cessation program. *Journal of Family Practice* 30: 647-654, 1990.

Taylor, R.B. Health promotion in clinical practice (seminar monograph). Portland, OR: Oregon Health Sciences University, 1985.

U.S. Department of Health and Human Services. *The Health Benefits of Smoking Cessation: A Report of the Surgeon General.* U.S. Department of Health and Human Services, Public Health Service, Centers for Disease Control, Center for Chronic Disease Prevention and Health Promotion, Office on Smoking and Health. DHHS Publication No. (CDC) 90-8416, 1990.

Wetzler, H.P., Cruess, D.F. Self-reported physical health practices and health care utilization: Findings from the National Health Interview Survey. *American Journal of Public Health* 75: 1329-1330, 1985.

APPENDIX A
Magazines Without Tobacco Advertising

FOR ADULTS

Accent on Living
Adirondack Life
Air & Space
Alaska Magazine
American Baby
American Health
American Heritage
American History Illustrated
American Square Dance
Americas
Animal Kingdom
Antique Automobile
Arizona Highways
Arthritis Today
Artist's Magazine
Audubon
Aviation Week & Space Technology
Backpacker
Bicycling
Business Week
Byte
Cars & Parts
Cat Fancy
Child
Christian Herald
Common Cause Magazine
Complete Woman
Consumer Reports
Cooking Light
Country Journal
Craftworks for the Home
Crafts
Cyclist
Dance Magazine
Diabetes Forecast
Dog Fancy
Down Beat
Down East Magazine
Elks Magazine
Exceptional Children
Exceptional Parent
Farm Journal
Final Frontier
Fishing Facts
Florida Sportsman
Flying
Flying Models
Freshwater & Marine Aquarium
The Futurist
Garbage
Garden
Golf Illustrated
Good Housekeeping
Good Old Days
Guideposts
Hadassah Magazine
Harvard Business Review
Harvard Lampoon
Harvard Medical School Health Letter
Health
Health News & Review
Hippocrates
Historic Preservation
Home Office Computing
Horn Book Magazine
Horse Illustrated
Horticulture
Income Opportunities
Instructor
International Travel News
Isaac Asimov's Science Fiction
Itinerary
Journal of Irreproducible Results
Kaleidoscope
The Lion
MacUser
MacWorld
MAD Magazine
Maine Fish & Wildlife
Maine Life Magazine
Mature Outlook
Mayo Clinic Health Letter
Men's Fitness
Men's Health
Midwest Living
Model Railroader
Modern Maturity
Montana Magazine
Mother Earth News
Mother Jones
Ms.
Muscle & Fitness
Nation
National Gardening
National Geographic
National Parks
National Wildlife
Natural History
The New Yorker
North American Review
Nutrition Action Healthletter
Oceans
Old House Journal
Organic Gardening
Parenting
Parents Magazine
PC Magazine
PC World
Personal Computing
Petersen's Hunting
Petersen's Photographic
Popular Communications
Popular Photography
Popular Woodworking
Prevention
Railfan and Railroad
Reader's Digest
Runner's World
Sail
Salt, Inc.
Satellite Orbit
Saturday Evening Post
Science
Science News
The Sciences
Scientific American
Sea Frontiers
Shape
Sierra
Single Parent
16 Magazine
Skin Diver Magazine
Smithsonian
Society
Southern Accents
Sports Afield
Stork
Sunset Magazine
Theatre Crafts
Threads
Travel Holiday
Travel & Leisure
Twins

Source: Medical news and perspectives: Magazines without tobacco advertising. *Journal of the American Medical Association* 226(22): 3099-3102, 1991.

FOR ADULTS (continued)

- Utah Holiday
- Vegetarian Times
- Venture Magazine
- Vermont Life
- Vibrant Life
- Video Review
- Walking Magazine
- The Washington Monthly
- Weight Watchers Magazine
- West Coast Review of Books
- Western Outdoors
- Westways
- Wildlife Conservation
- Women's Sports & Fitness
- Workbasket
- Workbench
- World Monitor
- Writer's Digest
- Yankee
- Zoogoer

FOR CHILDREN AND TEENS

- Big Bopper
- Black Beat
- Bop
- Boy's Life
- Cricket
- Highlights for Children
- Humpty Dumpty
- Jack and Jill
- Kid City
- Ladybug
- Ranger Rick's
- Right On!
- Sassy
- Sesame Street
- Seventeen
- Teen
- 3-2-1 Contact
- YM

Chapter 2

Recruitment and Training of Practicing Physicians, Dentists, And Their Office Staffs

CONTENTS

Introduction
Stuart J. Cohen 45

Effects of Training Family Physicians in a Comprehensive Smoking Cessation Intervention
Elizabeth A. Lindsay and Douglas M. Wilson 48
- Introduction 48
- Phase I Project (1984-1987) 53
- Phase II Project (1987-1989) 61
- References 67

Doctors Helping Smokers: Development of a Clinic-Based Smoking Intervention System
Thomas E. Kottke, Leif I. Solberg, Milo L. Brekke, Shirley A. Conn, Patricia Maxwell, and Mark J. Brekke 69
- Background: Doctors Helping Smokers 69
- A Meta-Analysis of Controlled Trials 71
- Nokomis Clinic Intervention Program 72
- Doctors Helping Smokers, Round III 75
- Lessons Learned 85
- Conclusions 89
- References 90

Prompting Smoking Cessation in Family Practice
William C. Wadland, John R. Hughes, and Roger H. Secker-Walker 92
- Introduction 92
- Recruitment in a Primary Care Trial 92
- Training on Brief Advice 94
- Summary of Pilot Trial Results 96
- Recommendations 97
- Future Pharmacological Therapy 98
- References 100

Smoking Cessation in Primary Care Practice: Summary of Results From the Quit for Life Project
Steven R. Cummings, Thomas J. Coates, Mort J. Stein, Neil D. Swan, and the Quit for Life Research Group 102
Introduction 102
Trials 103
Surveys 109
Other Analyses 110
Discussion 111
References 112

Physician and Dentist Interventions For Smoking Cessation
Stuart J. Cohen, George K. Stookey, and Sue A. Kelly 113
Background 113
Physician Interventions 113
Dentist Interventions 127
Differences Between Dental and Medical Programs 141
References 142

The Tobacco Reduction and Cancer Control (TRACC) Program: Team Approaches to Counseling in Medical and Dental Settings
Jack F. Hollis, Thomas M. Vogt, Victor Stevens, Anthony Biglan, Herbert Severson, and Edward Lichtenstein 143
Introduction 143
Nurse-Assisted Counseling 144
Intervention With Hospital Patients 151
ST Intervention for Dental Patients 156
Smoking Cessation Among Adolescents 162
Summary and Implications 165
References 167

Appendixes
A. Screening Form for Study on Assessing Patient's Health Risks 169
B. Study on Physician Advice for Smoking Cessation 170
C. Entry Questionnaire 171
D. Medical Screening Form 174
E. Generic Reminder Sheet 175
F. Reminder Sheet for Gum Group 176
G. Reminder Sheet for No-Gum Group 177
H. Physician Data: Initial Visit 178
I. Exit Questionnaire #1 (All Patients) 179
J. Exit Questionnaire #2 (No-Gum Group) 181
K. Exit Questionnaire #3 (Nicotine Gum Group) 182

L. One- to Two-Week Followup for Smoking Cessation Study 183
M. Six-Month Followup for Smoking Cessation Study 184
N. Followup Questionnaire on the Use of Nicotine Gum 185

Recruitment and Training of Practicing Physicians, Dentists, And Their Office Staffs

Editor: Stuart J. Cohen

INTRODUCTION This chapter contains a description of a series of research studies that involved the recruitment and training of practicing physicians, dentists, and their office staffs. The first section, by Drs. Lindsay and Wilson, describes the educational programs used to train community-based family physicians in Ontario, Canada, to help their patients stop smoking. Using the results of their experience with the first group of trainees, the investigators developed a more advanced and clinically effective 4-hour training program to assist a new cohort of community-based family physicians in helping their patients stop smoking. Of note in these investigations were the direct comparison of the performance and effectiveness of trained and untrained physicians, and an effort to assess the benefit of rescheduling patients for followup visits related to smoking.

In the second paper, Dr. Kottke and his colleagues describe the programs and results from a series of investigations in the Doctors Helping Smokers project, which involved more than 150 primary care physicians in Minnesota. The project emphasized the system for recruiting physicians and the establishment of a clinic environment system involving all office staff in the smoking cessation program. The clinical settings involved in the Doctors Helping Smokers project ranged from small private practices to large medical clinics. For the latter settings, the intensity of project support averaged 6 site visits, 24 telephone calls, and 6 mailings to help initiate the clinic smoking cessation program and sustain it for 18 months or longer.

In the chapter's third section, Drs. Wadland, Hughes, and Secker-Walker review the recruitment of smokers from a five-physician family practice in rural Vermont and from a six-physician academic general internal medicine practice. Their project attempted to assess the additional impact resulting from a prescription for nicotine gum on patients' efforts and success in quitting smoking and in their confidence in their physicians' advice. Of interest in the project was a 2- to 3-hour training program to help physicians in delivering smoking cessation advice and instruction in the proper use of nicotine gum.

The fourth paper, by Dr. Cummings and associates, describes the various studies and surveys involved in the Quit for Life project. The Quit for Life group conducted two randomized controlled trials to see if their program to train physicians in counseling patients about smoking cessation and to augment the training with involvement of their office staffs would result in greater smoking cessation among the patients of physicians in the training program than among the patients of physicians who did not participate. The cohorts of physicians consisted of 81 internists from the Kaiser Permanente Medical Group of Northern California and 44 private-practice internists and family practitioners. Three 1-hour training sessions were held; they included videotapes to demonstrate smoking cessation counseling, role-playing, and positive feedback. The correct use of nicotine gum and the benefit of followup visits were emphasized. Of note in the discussion are the problems of recruiting private-practice physicians to participate and of obtaining office staff support for implementing an office-based cessation program.

The fifth paper, by Drs. Cohen and Stookey and Ms. Kelly, describes parallel studies involving two cohorts of primary care physicians and two cohorts of private-practice dentists from Indiana. The first cohort of physicians involved residents in internal medicine and faculty general internists and their patients from the outpatient medicine clinic of a city/county teaching hospital. The second group of physicians were general internists and family physicians drawn from five sites of a large, freestanding HMO. Both cohorts of dentists were limited to private general dental practitioners and periodontists who primarily treated adult patients on a regular basis. The goal of the project was to develop, validate, and evaluate practical methods to help clinicians be more effective in helping their patients stop smoking. Of special interest was the impact of chart reminders and/or nicotine gum on the counseling provided by clinicians and on their patients' smoking cessation.

The final section describes the Tobacco Reduction and Cancer Control (TRACC) program developed by Dr. Hollis and his colleagues in Oregon and involving the clinical facilities of Kaiser Permanente. TRACC used a team approach to counseling smokers in a variety of situations and settings, including nurse-assisted smoking counseling for outpatient settings, smoking interventions for hospital patients, smokeless tobacco intervention for dental patients, and smoking cessation among adolescents. Some unique features of the TRACC program were the use of a videotape to teach smokers steps for quitting successfully and establishment of a centralized system to identify smokers and their quit dates so that supportive followup calls could be made by trained phone callers.

Collectively, the studies described here indicate that within the context of a 4-hour workshop, physicians and other health providers can be trained to be more effective in counseling their patients who smoke. Moreover, smoking cessation efforts in these projects appeared more likely to be successful when office systems were in place that involved the office staffs in the programs. Components of a successful office support system appear to include

- A way to readily identify patients who smoke and to highlight that information for the clinician;

- A method of triage so that the patients who are most ready to make an effort to stop smoking get more intensive counseling; and
- A followup procedure to support patients in their efforts to quit smoking.

Effects of Training Family Physicians in a Comprehensive Smoking Cessation Intervention[1]

Elizabeth A. Lindsay and Douglas M. Wilson

INTRODUCTION The McMaster/Waterloo[2] family practice studies were carried out between 1984 and 1989. The phase I study measured the impact on patient smoking cessation of a continuing education event with supporting educational materials and an office cueing system. Through the phase I studies, we learned that the physicians who were not provided training but were given a reminder system in their offices appeared to offer advice as effectively as trained physicians, because as many patients of untrained physicians expressed their intention to stop smoking: 82.2 percent of patients in the untrained group and 77.4 percent of patients in the trained group stated that they intended to quit after the physicians addressed the issue with them. It is noteworthy that the patients in this study did not have to make a commitment to stop smoking. Motivation to stop smoking was not part of the eligibility criteria.

Untrained physicians did not perform key elements of the intervention taught to trained physicians, such as setting stop-smoking dates, providing take-home material, and offering followup support; patients of untrained physicians reported being much less successful with smoking cessation at 2 months (6.6 percent) than those of trained physicians (16.5 percent). The 1-year cessation rates in the trained group were lower than the reported 2-month results but maintained statistical significance over the control condition. Following this successful outcome, the goal of the phase II study was to assess specific components of the experimental intervention tested in phase I. Because of the time and financial implications of offering long-term followup, we chose to compare the impact of short-term intervention (two visits) with a longer program offered by physicians.

In all of this work, the educational programs and resource materials enabled the physicians to intervene confidently in a systematic manner with their smoking patients. We found that physicians perceived the intervention to be helpful to them, that their compliance in delivering the specific elements of

---

[1] This research was supported by NIH grant no. CA-38334, by a Canadian National Research and Development Program Scholar Award to J.A. Best, and by Ontario Ministry of Health Research grant no. 01922.

[2] McMaster University, Hamilton, Ontario, and University of Waterloo, Waterloo, Ontario.

the intervention was at least 80 percent for each of the key elements, and that patients appreciated and responded well to their physicians' offer to help. Among the patients in the phase II study—who all had expressed an interest in stopping smoking—the 1-year, validated cessation rates averaged 13 to 14 percent. The long-term followup did not increase cessation significantly over the two-visit followup. However, we have strong evidence that many of the patients who were not intended to receive long-term followup actually did receive it through a natural sequence of followup appointments for other conditions.

This introduction is intended for program planners and educators who are responsible for providing education for physicians, residents, or the staffs who work with them. Recommendations for providing effective training in smoking cessation are presented here. The recommendations are grounded in the research described in this chapter and others in this monograph, but they also reflect our experience as workshop leaders in 20 states and 4 provinces in the United States and Canada.

Integration Into Practice

A review of recent physician intervention research projects leads us to conclude that making a measurable difference in the number of patients who have stopped smoking at the end of 1 year requires (1) an office system that will remind physicians to address the smoking issue and (2) the capacity to deliver an efficacious cessation intervention. A physician must be highly committed to the smoking issue to invest the time and energy required to set up a practice with a reminder system and to develop skills in effective counseling about smoking cessation. An educational planner must understand that the level of commitment to this issue, as well as knowledge and skills, will vary widely in a community of physicians; therefore, the objectives and format of educational sessions should vary as well.

Because there is a wide range of commitment and interest in smoking cessation among physicians and their office staffs, it is important that physicians know what they need to do to obtain different levels of impact. They may decide to limit their involvement in this issue to brief advice to stop smoking to all smoking patients, and others may decide to offer visits to patients that will focus on smoking cessation. Other physicians may choose to offer a long-term program that includes followup visits. For physicians to make choices about their level of involvement, they need to know the increases in cessation they can expect with increasing levels of intervention. We find that, among trained physicians, the level of involvement is an individual decision and depends on many factors. Educational planners can facilitate these decisions by what they include in their training sessions.

Clear Objectives

To help physicians be more effective, it will be important to set realistic objectives for specific educational programs. There will be a number of factors to consider as objectives are set; for example, time availability is a strong determinant of what can be accomplished. We find that several hours are needed to teach physicians how to set up their offices and how to deliver an efficacious intervention. In addition, to ensure that an office cueing system is set up, a personal visit to physicians' offices is often necessary. This comprehensive approach may be impractical in many continuing medical education situations. (See Chapter 5 for examples of how this can be accomplished.) Therefore, it is clear why it is important to teach physicians these skills while they are still in training.

Learning needs of the audience should be put together with time availability to determine what the objectives will be for a specific educational event. It will be important to consider the learners' level of motivation, their present skill level, and what is the most important material to be covered. For example, 30 minutes with a highly motivated physician might best be spent on helping the physician to be clear about what to do with a 10-minute office visit with a patient. In an hour with an audience that has gathered for a purpose unrelated to smoking cessation, the content might focus more on motivation for why smoking cessation is a good use of physician time. This type of audience will also need to hear a summary of an approach with practical tips that will demonstrate how to intervene effectively.

Features of The Program

The content of an educational presentation should cover the following elements: (1) motivational material, including scientific evidence, that will increase physicians' commitment to integrating effective smoking cessation interventions into their practice; (2) background material that will increase participants' understanding of smoking behavior, addiction, and behavior change; (3) the content and skills for delivering an effective intervention with patients; (4) knowledge and resources for creating a smoke-free office and an office system that cues and supports the intervention with patients; and (5) a description of the variety of roles that are possible for the physician as an influential figure in the community.

Areas of Emphasis

Physicians want to know what they should do with the brief time available to them. It is important to give specific structure to the patient visits and clearly defined content to cover. Our research to date has demonstrated that physicians are generally good at offering advice to stop smoking and indicating why patients should stop. Therefore, in our workshops we often move quickly through that aspect of an intervention and focus more on less familiar aspects of the intervention, such as the importance of setting a stop-smoking date, providing guidance for proper use of nicotine gum, advising patients on how to deal with withdrawal symptoms, and issues related to followup, such as weight gain and dealing with relapse.

How to deal with followup is confusing to some physicians. Our suggestion is to offer followup to any patient who is attempting to stop smoking. This can take the form of further visits or phone calls, the offer of which indicates continuing support that is perceived as important by patients. The research findings on the effect of this offer are mixed. We know that only some patients will attend followup visits and that those patients are more highly motivated than those who do not attend. We also know that followup sometimes is provided as part of future visits that are unrelated to smoking cessation. We believe that it is important for physicians and their health care teams to know how to deal with followup issues and to provide an opportunity for those patients who want this help to be able to obtain it easily.

Educational Methods We have found a combination of demonstration and practice with supportive print resources leads to high physician compliance with our approach to smoking intervention. It is this combination that requires more time than is available in a 1-hour presentation.

Physicians who have participated in this educational model rated the event highly in evaluations and often mentioned specifically the importance of having an opportunity to practice the intervention and use the support materials at the training session. Because the physicians have chosen to attend a workshop, they are probably not representative of the general population of physicians; however, their comments provide direction for the ideal model.

Flow of the Session For both 1-hour and longer sessions, it is important to involve participants and ask them to speak from their own experience. We have found it particularly helpful to ask physicians, very early in the session, what they have found to be obstacles to providing effective smoking cessation advice to their patients. We note these issues on a flipchart and assure participants that we will try to address all of the issues during the session.

There is an increasing use of technology at continuing medical education events that engages participants by asking key questions about the content to be covered in the session. Through the use of touchpads and computerized compilation of responses, answers are displayed on the screen within 30 seconds. This technique actively involves participants in the session and enables presenters to know the knowledge levels and practices of the audience.

The flow of the session should reflect the motivation and knowledge level of participants. Generally, we move from general background to the specific detail of what to do. The flow is also congruent with the sequence of the intervention. It is sensible to discuss how to address the smoking issue with patients, what to do with a followup visit, and then focus on specific difficult issues. Unfortunately, the introductory material sometimes takes longer than is intended and there is insufficient time for the important followup issues. This latter material is what physicians often need to know, and we suggest organizers take steps to ensure that time is carefully monitored.

A Range of Learning Opportunities Given the wide range of motivation to learn about smoking cessation, it is appropriate to offer different levels of learning opportunities to meet the needs and the practical considerations in most medical communities. (Chapter 5 demonstrates how this is being accomplished in the Community Intervention Trial for Smoking Cessation [COMMIT].)

The effort spent in marketing educational events will be an important determinant of attendance. We have learned, through a survey of physicians in 11 communities across the United States and Canada, that physicians believe they are addressing cessation with most smoking patients and that they feel adequately prepared to address the issue. If this is generally the case, it is probable that physicians will not see the need to attend a continuing medical education session on smoking cessation. We also know that they overreport the frequency of their interventions and that most do not include the ingredients we have found to be important for successful cessation. It will be important to help physicians assess accurately what they need to know about delivering an efficacious intervention and realize that they can make a significant impact by applying the intervention consistently.

The scheduling and the setting for CME events will be important determinants of who and how many will attend. In our research projects, when full attendance of participating physicians was critical, we offered several choices for attendance and chose the time for events after asking for "most convenient times" from potential participants. These choices should be determined by an analysis of your local customs and needs. It is always important to provide a comfortable learning environment and appropriate refreshments, and we have found that CME credits and financial incentives also can affect attendance.

Who Should Teach The leaders at educational sessions must have a depth of knowledge about smoking cessation so they can describe simply and clearly what physicians need to do in their brief time with patients. We have found that a team of a family physician and a behavioral scientist works very well, but the professional background of the leaders may be less important than their ability to deliver clear instructions, respond well to learner concerns, and help physicians see that smoking cessation is an effective use of their time.

Health Care Teams Smoking cessation interventions may be greatly enhanced by involvement of a receptionist, an office nurse, or other team member. In some cases, reimbursement considerations as well as interest and skills of a team member make this a feasible model.

It will rarely be enough to simply tell physicians how they can integrate their team in the smoking cessation initiatives. Other staff members need to attend training or receive training in their office environment. Any office system must be simple and nonintrusive to the regular work of the practice, and there must be a perceived payoff for putting the system in place. It may, therefore, be important to include a mechanism for keeping track of successful stop-smoking attempts to demonstrate the effect of their efforts.

PHASE I PROJECT (1984-1987)

McMaster/ Waterloo Project

The goals of the McMaster/Waterloo Family Practice Smoking Cessation Project were as follows: (1) to develop a smoking cessation intervention that could be delivered by community physicians within the context of regular office practice; (2) to design and deliver a continuing education session that increased the motivation, knowledge, and skills of the study physicians; (3) to create the print and audiovisual materials that would enable the effective delivery of the training session and the patient intervention; (4) to test the intervention package by means of a randomized controlled trial in which the physician was the unit of randomization; (5) to carry out both process and outcome evaluations to increase our understanding of physician compliance with the recommended changes in practices, the smoking cessation process, and the impact on patient behavior; and (6) to assess the role of the offer of further followup after two visits (phase II project).

Physician and Patient Recruitment

Eighty-three community family physicians and 1,942 smoking patients participated in this trial. We had invited 460 family physicians practicing within a 40-mile radius of McMaster University to participate. Their names were obtained from an Ontario Medical Association listing that includes the majority of family physicians in the area. One hundred two physicians responded positively, but 12 withdrew or, because of distance, were set aside for future studies, prior to randomization. The remaining 90 physicians, who represented 75 practices, were randomly allocated, by practice, to the three treatment groups; 7 physicians withdrew from the study after randomization. Comparison of characteristics of the physician dropouts and the study physicians (70 practices) revealed no significant differences that we feel would bias the composition of the experimental groups.

Patients entered the study when they visited their physician for a routine office appointment. We tried to recruit the most representative sample of smoking patients by asking all smokers to participate. Receptionists in all three groups recruited the study participants according to a standard protocol that started at the beginning of each family practice session by asking all patients if they were smokers. Receptionists asked each eligible smoker (not pregnant or breastfeeding, over age 16, and smoking at least one cigarette each day) to participate until a maximum of two smokers each day agreed to complete the questionnaire. The consent letter provided with the questionnaire asked patients to agree to be followed and emphasized that they were *not* agreeing to try to stop smoking.

The experimental variation in condition began when the patient went in to see the physician. In condition 1 (usual care), the physicians were not to know which of their patients had agreed to participate in the study. If it was part of their usual practice to address the smoking issue with patients, they did so. We gave no instructions to patients about whether they should mention their agreement to participate to their physician, and we had no way of assessing whether they did.

In condition 2 (cued only), the physicians were cued by a project document indicating the patient's agreement to participate. These physicians were instructed to advise the patient to quit smoking and offer nicotine gum as an aid to quitting. There were no further instructions given to these physicians.

In condition 3 (trained and cued), physicians had attended a training session to develop the knowledge and skills for delivering the intervention. A project flowsheet cued these physicians as to which patients were in the study and also helped them to remember the ingredients of the intervention. In addition, self-help materials were provided for distribution to patients.

Materials and Training Techniques

Training Program

The continuing medical education protocol was set up to enhance learning through attention to a comfortable setting and provision of time for the group to visit informally before the session began. Introduction material provided a context in which the intervention for smoking cessation could be seen as a worthwhile and appropriate activity for physicians. The protocol included (1) premailed background material that included several recent reprints from medical journals, (2) a 3- to 4-hour training session, and (3) materials that guided and reminded physicians of the maneuver taught in the training session.

Training Session

The purposes of the session were to increase (1) knowledge and understanding of the contents of the intervention, with particular emphasis on the rationale for and proper prescribing of nicotine gum; (2) skills for challenging smokers about quitting, negotiating a decision about quitting, and setting a quit date, as well as offering supportive followup visits; and (3) a positive attitude toward the importance of the physician's role in smoking cessation and toward implementing the intervention. The session began with an overview of the research project, including a brief discussion of the smoking cessation process, the literature on physician-delivered interventions, and a description of proper use of nicotine gum.

The experimental intervention included three types of visits. To teach the content and skills for these visits, the training session followed a loop-like format, in keeping with learning principles that support the need for information, demonstration, and practice. First, we described the protocol through slides and verbal instructions; then a physician-patient interaction was demonstrated on videotape, and participants experienced guided practice with surrogate patients. Through this sequence of description, demonstration, and practice, participants learned the procedures for *a challenge visit, a quit-date visit,* and *supportive followup visits.*

Intervention Taught

The full intervention, including six potential contacts, would be carried out over a 2-month period.

The first visit. When a patient agreed to participate, the receptionist attached project materials to the patient chart. The materials reminded the physician that the patient was a smoker and guided the discussion about smoking cessation. After the regularly scheduled office visit, the physician spent an additional 5 to 7 minutes with the patient, discussing the importance of stopping smoking and the advantages of quitting in terms of the individual's personal health and current symptoms related to smoking. The following were key parts of this discussion: (1) gathering a smoking history, such as the number of years of smoking and the quantity smoked each day, and (2) getting a sense of the patient's willingness to try quitting. It was also important to challenge the patient to make a clear decision about quitting and to set a date to stop smoking within the next month, when the patient would come back to see the physician.

During the initial visit, the physician informed the person about nicotine-bearing chewing gum as an aid to quitting and provided the patient with self-help materials. Before leaving the office, the patient set up an appointment for a quit-date visit and, if feasible, appointments for the four followup visits. The patient also received a document that resembled a contract, indicating his or her decision to try to stop smoking and dates of future appointments. Physicians did not receive reimbursement for this first visit, but the Ontario Health Insurance Plan reimbursed them for subsequent visits.

Quit-date visit. At the 10-minute quit-date visit, the physician reinforced and supported the patient's reasons for wanting to stop smoking, and the patient was to stop at that visit. For those patients who chose to use the gum, the physician explained its proper use while the patient tried a piece. Patients paid for the nicotine gum. In the training for this visit, we emphasized the importance of encouragement and building the patient's confidence. See Figure 1 for the patient chart that guided the content for this visit.

Supportive followup visits. The content of these four brief followup visits over the next 2 months varied, depending on the stage of the cessation process and the personal issues brought by the patient to each visit. Physicians assessed this stage by simply asking how the patient was doing with the smoking cessation program. A flowsheet for each patient provided guidelines for monitoring and supporting techniques. We encouraged physicians to listen carefully to the issues raised by the patient and to offer advice that was personal and supportive.

Print and audiovisual materials. For the purposes of training, we developed a slide presentation and demonstration videotapes. For the office maneuver, we developed a flowsheet for patient visits, a patient contract, and patient self-help "Tip Sheets." The patient materials were adapted from one-page summaries that were developed by the Stanford Cardiovascular Risk Reduction project for use with refrigerator magnets.

Results

Definition of Outcomes

The primary definition of successful cessation was self-reported sustained abstinence for 3 months prior to biochemically validated cessation after 1 year. However, we also included self-reported attempts to stop smoking and self-reported 2-month cessation.

Figure 1

Patient chart, quit-date visit and followup

PATIENT FLOW SHEET

Patient Name: ____________________	Major reasons for quitting	Health
Cigarette symptoms, e.g., cough		Other

	Quit Day	Post Quit Day	Post Quit Day	1 Month	2 Month
DATE:					
General well-being					
Average daily use of cigarettes over the past week					
Commitment to quitting (low, medium, high)					
Confidence to succeed (low, medium, high)					
Concerns about quitting					
Any strategies for getting ready?					
Average daily use of Nicorette over the past week					
Any side effects of Nicorette — Do you like the gum?					
Any withdrawal symptoms after stopping cigarettes?					
How often do you feel like smoking? How strong is this craving? (low, medium, high)					
Does the gum help you cope with this craving?					
Have you noticed any weight gain? Is this a problem? Need information?					
Do you spend a lot of time around other smokers?					
Are you feeling support from others at home or at work?					

Patient Response Patients' intentions to stop smoking with or without gum were recorded at the time of the initial visit. Of those who stated an intention to try to quit (approximately 80 percent), a significantly higher proportion of patients in the trained and cued group (71 percent) than in the cued-only group (61 percent) chose to stop smoking and to use nicotine gum. Gum use for greater than 2 weeks was less than 25 percent for both groups (Wilson et al., 1988). (See Tables 1 and 2.) Approximately 65 percent of patients in the trained and cued group returned for at least one followup visit. The 1-year cessation rate increased with the number of followup visits attended (Wilson et al., 1988).

On the 2-month questionnaire, 38.1 percent of the usual-care patients, 62.8 percent of the cued-only group, and 76.7 percent of the trained and cued group reported attempting to stop smoking for at least 24 hours. Successful cessation was reported by 3.8 percent in usual care, 6.6 percent of the cued-only group, and 16.5 percent of the trained and cued group (Table 3). Our primary definition of successful cessation was self-reported sustained abstinence for 3 months prior to biochemically validated cessation after 1 year. Validated 3-month sustained cessation rates at 1-year followup, adjusted for covariates, were 4.4 percent for usual care, 6.1 percent for the cued-only group, and 8.8 percent in the trained and cued group (Table 3).

The criterion for validation of smoking cessation was a saliva cotinine value of 0.057 μmol/L or lower, or a saliva thiocyanate level of 1,724 μmol/L or lower if the patient was still chewing nicotine gum. Approximately 92 percent of patients who reported they were not smoking were validated. Those not reached were classified as smokers. Of the patients who reported themselves as ex-smokers for at least 1 week and submitted to cotinine validation, 25 percent did not qualify as nonsmokers according to the validation criteria. Another 8 percent of those who reported themselves as nonsmokers would not submit to validation and thus were classified as smokers (Lindsay et al., 1989).

Physician Practices Counseling performance was measured by means of exit telephone interviews with a random 15 percent of patients and rated audiotapes of physician counseling with simulated patients. Physicians in the trained group were more likely than untrained physicians to use procedures they were trained to include, such as offering advice, inviting patients back for followup, setting stop-smoking dates, and providing take-home materials (Lindsay et al., 1989; Wilson et al., 1988).

Physicians who were cued to offer nicotine gum (both cued-only and trained and cued) offered nicotine gum at nearly the same frequency, whereas the usual-care physicians offered gum much less frequently (Wilson et al., 1988). Cueing and training each had highly significant effects on counseling performance, as demonstrated by the significant variations in performance between experimental conditions. Performance, as measured by exit interview scores, was associated with all short-term outcomes; however, in our first analysis of performance, the rated simulation performance scores were not.

Table 1
Patient's recall of office visit with physician[a]

	Percentage of Yes Responses				
	Usual Care (n=90)	Cued Only (n=94)	Trained and Cued (n=96)	Chi-Square[b]	p
Did Doctor Say Anything About Patient's Smoking?	31.1%	70.2%	85.4%	61.96	< 0.001
Suggested Quitting	24.4	64.0	84.4	59.72	< 0.001
Offered Help	12.2	61.7	84.5	106.93	< 0.001
Suggested Gum Method	8.9	58.5	62.5	38.15	< 0.001
Set Quit Date	2.2	11.7	54.2	80.84	< 0.001
Doctor Wants To See Again	4.4	22.3	83.3	137.22	< 0.001
Gave Reading Materials	2.0	17.0	80.2	144.07	< 0.001

[a] *Gathered through open-ended questions asked within 3 days.*
[b] *Chi-square based on differences among the three groups.*

Table 2
Stated intention to try to stop smoking in untrained (gum-only) and trained (gum-plus) groups and patient attendance at followup visits (gum-plus)

	Total n	Do Not Want To Quit n (%)	Try To Stop Without Gum n (%)	Try To Stop With Gum n (%)	Attended at Least One Followup Visit[a,b] n (%)	Attended Four or Five Followup Visits[b] n (%)	Unsure or No Data n (%)
Gum Only	726	108 (14.9)	171 (23.6)	425 (58.7)	ND	ND	21 (2.9)
Gum Plus	606	74 (12.1)	86 (14.2)	383 (63.2)	390 (64.3)	129 (21.3)	63 (10.4)

[a] *Includes those attending a quit-date visit.*
[b] *ND, no data available.*

Table 3
Smoking cessation attempts and proportion of ex-smokers in each of the treatment groups, as indicated in patient charts and 2-month questionnaire

	Total n	Physician Discussed Smoking With Patients[a]	Patient Intends To Quit[a]	Tried To Quit for 24 Hours[b]	Not Smoking at 2 Months (Self-Report)[b]	Adjusted Sustained 3-Month Cessation Rates at 1 Year (Validated)[b,c]
Usual Care	601	ND	ND	36.4%	3.8%	4.4%
Gum Only	726	98.0%	82.2%	60.7	6.6	6.1
Gum Plus	606	90.8	77.4	71.9	16.5	8.8

[a] *ND, no data available.*
[b] $p < 0.05$.
[c] *Analysis of covariance adjusted for differences at baseline.*

No performance indicator that we measured through exit interviews or simulated visits predicted long-term outcomes (J.A. Best and colleagues, unpublished data).

We were not satisfied with our first analysis of the audiotaped simulated visits, so a cooperating investigator conducted an innovative analytic procedure adapted from judging of technical and artistic merit in figure skating (Burgess, 1989). This analysis of 35 audiotapes of untrained and trained physicians to assess content and style of the delivery of a smoking intervention once again demonstrated a highly significant effect of physician training on the content of the intervention and on 2-month cessation rates. The analysis also revealed one measure of style, degree of empathy, and predicted enhanced 2-month cessation (Burgess, 1989).

Conclusions The research demonstrated that physicians will attend a half-day continuing education workshop to enhance their skills in smoking intervention. We found that the physicians integrated the maneuver into their practices but often needed the research staff to ensure that the project smoking cessation materials were used appropriately. When the materials were used with patient charts, physicians performed the intervention according to their training. Untrained physicians who were cued by project materials to address cessation with smoking patients performed several aspects of the intervention with the same frequency as trained physicians. Patients agreed to try to stop smoking as frequently in both groups, and similar numbers chose to use nicotine gum to try to stop smoking. Significantly fewer patients of physicians in the untrained groups reported trying to quit smoking for 24 hours. The trained group helped patients set a stop-smoking date, provided take-home materials, and offered followup support much more frequently than the untrained physicians. The trained, gum-plus group had much higher 2-month cessation rates than the other two groups, but the difference, although retaining statistical significance, was much smaller at the end of 1 year.

The influence of a physician intervention decreases with time. This is an expected finding, as the patient's daily social environment and other factors are likely to increase in relative influence as time passes after the physician intervention. We need to develop complementary interventions that will improve maintenance of the early effects of physician interventions.

Side Studies

Patients of Trained Physicians

We conducted a series of interviews over 1 year with patients whose physicians invited them to try to stop smoking (Willms et al., 1990 and 1991). The physicians in this study were trained in the same way as those in the main trial, but they were selected from a different community, distant from the main trial center. The interviews were designed to assess, from the patients' point of view, which were the most important components of the intervention. The interviews were transcribed and interpreted through application of a systematic approach for qualitative research methods (including ethnographic methods).

This research indicated that the most significant component of the physicians' intervention was the kind of support given. We describe the results of this study with the terms "interventionistic" and "personalistic." Although both aspects were important, patients emphasized the importance of the personalistic components. These activities include aspects of the physicians' work that are nurturing, egalitarian, and mutually communicative. It appears from this work that it is important for physicians to speak with biomedical authority, because our evidence suggests that patients expect a certain amount of that content and because there is need for emphasis on creating more organization- and clinic-based supports (Willms et al., 1991).

Nicotine Gum As an Adjunct

Another side study of the main trial assessed the intervention package tested in the main trial with and without the offer of nicotine gum (Gilbert et al., 1989). A separate sample of 12 community physicians selected previously for the main trial and set aside because of distance from the main center attended a 4-hour training session during which the maneuver was demonstrated and practiced. We taught physicians how to deliver the intervention both with and without the offer of nicotine gum. Receptionists were instructed to recruit the first two smokers visiting the practice each day. Patients (n=223) were randomized to receive the same intervention, but either including the offer of nicotine gum or without the offer of nicotine gum.

One-year smoking cessation was validated by cotinine saliva analysis. The validated 3-month sustained abstinence rates at 1 year were 8.1 and 9.8 percent in the gum and no-gum groups, respectively. The 95-percent confidence interval for this difference was -9.3 to 6.4 percent.

There was no evidence from this study that smoking cessation rates were enhanced by the offer of 2-mg nicotine-bearing gum, when added to a comprehensive intervention offered to all smokers in primary care. Insufficient power may be partially responsible for our findings; however, the trend in the findings does not support the additional usefulness of nicotine-bearing gum. It is also of interest that the other side study (described above)—which also tracked cessation rates for those offered and not offered gum—showed that cessation rates were higher but not statistically significant in the no-gum group.

PHASE II PROJECT (1987-1989)

Developing a More Effective Intervention

Structuring The Visits

Physicians in the phase I study found that the time they needed for talking to patients, when added to a regular visit, was quite disruptive to their practices. Therefore, we shortened the first visit to include only the following:

- An offer to patients to be part of the McMaster Family Smoking Cessation Program;
- Questions to patients about their interest in stopping smoking and the completion of a questionnaire;
- A clear statement of concern and support from the physician; and
- A request to come back and talk further about stopping.

Physicians offered patients an opportunity to come back for a separate visit to discuss their approach to cessation. At this second visit, a random selection of half of the patients were invited to come back for further followup.

Consideration of what is known about the cessation process can guide the selection of times that appear to be most appropriate to provide further physician support visits. These considerations led to the following recommendations for timing of the four followup visits:

- Close to the quit date (encouragement to get off to a good start, ensure proper use of gum, if appropriate);
- Seven to ten days after stopping (provide help with withdrawal symptoms);
- One month after stopping (patient may be able to give other lifestyle issues attention); and
- Two to three months after stopping (most relapses occur in first 3 months; the patient is learning to be a nonsmoker and is adapting to the nonsmoking culture).

The need for these visits and their timing are individually determined. Therefore, as with many aspects of the Family Practice Smoking Cessation Program, physicians offered opportunities for followup but let individual patient needs determine timing and content.

First return visit. If patients returned to discuss their smoking, physicians took a history of their smoking behavior, including information about previous attempts to stop smoking and what was helpful or not helpful in those attempts. Other key questions as well as a take-home questionnaire helped patients think about the reasons they smoked and why they wanted to stop. The ethnographic work in the first study suggested that patients appreciated a personal approach from their physicians that communicated a clear interest in individual concerns and advice that was relevant to their experience (Willms et al., 1991).

Assistance offered by the physician. The revised intervention recommended that physicians suggest several strategies for getting ready to stop smoking, including setting a stop-smoking date. The self-help materials available for each patient provided many tips on how to prepare, such as anticipating the discomfort of withdrawal symptoms. During the first week or two after cessation, an inability to handle withdrawal symptoms often undermines a smoker's good intentions. Guidelines recommended that physicians ask patients about previous experience with withdrawal and plan for how to deal with potential problems. This was in keeping with another finding from the ethnographic work, which indicated that patients expected and appreciated physicians focusing on the physiological aspects of the cessation process, especially regarding feeling better and becoming "healthier." The offer of nicotine gum with instructions for proper use was a part of this intervention, but because of the limitations of the evidence of its effectiveness in the previous study, physicians were advised to offer gum to smokers who seemed to be physically addicted to nicotine or who had previously made several unsuccessful attempts to stop smoking.

Office system for cueing and monitoring the intervention. A systematic approach to cueing and monitoring smokers was built into the Family Practice Smoking Cessation Program. The physician's office staff flagged all smokers' charts and appended flowsheets to guide the intervention in patient charts for the physician's attention.

Development of Training Session And Resources

Our previous study demonstrated that the training workshop provided to physicians led to changes in practice and ultimately led to higher smoking cessation rates among patients (Wilson et al., 1988). Review of continuing education intervention research indicates that physicians rarely change clinical practices through simple acquisition of knowledge (Fowler et al., 1989).

Through the first Family Practice Smoking Cessation Program, we learned that physicians without special training appeared to perform some of the elements of the intervention equally as well as the trained physicians (Lindsay et al., 1989). We found that physicians in both groups were almost equally successful at motivating patients to try to stop smoking and that they were equally persuasive about the use of nicotine gum. There were large differences in performance in the areas of setting stop-smoking dates, offering followup, and providing self-help materials to patients; and we also detected small differences in physician style in talking to patients (Burgess, 1989).

Less than half of the patients in the phase I study took advantage of the physicians' offer of followup visits. Little training time was spent on the followup visits, and physicians reported feeling least prepared for the followup element of the intervention. Because the focus of the present study was on the effect of followup and because of these weaknesses in the first study, a higher proportion (approximately 50 percent) of the content of the training was dedicated to content and process of the followup visits.

The training session followed the loop format used successfully in our prior work, which provided information, demonstration, and practice with feedback. By repeating this sequence for at least two types of visits, workshop participants had an opportunity to develop their skills in applying the intervention.

Teaching about style as well as content. Patients told us that physician style was important in their approach to smoking cessation. However, we were unable to quantify the characteristics of more successful approaches in the first study. The work of Ockene and colleagues (1990), in which a patient-centered intervention is taught to residents, emphasized the importance of asking questions and providing feedback to patients about their feelings. There is evidence in other areas of patient care that believing one is understood and receiving feedback about how the physician perceives the patient's feelings are related to both satisfaction and compliance by patients. The training included discussion of these style issues as well as a video demonstration of recommended interpersonal skills. These issues were reinforced through study materials provided for use during the patient visits.

Focus on key followup issues. The guidelines for the four followup visits were based on the cessation process and consideration of the amount of time physicians were likely to spend in these visits. Three key content issues and five style issues were the focus for followup visit training. Patients' interests and needs guided the content. The guidelines provided suggestions for how physicians could support patients in planning for and adapting to their new lifestyle as nonsmokers. The training session provided information on weight control, preventing and coping with relapse, and one method of relaxation to cope with stressful situations.

Study Design And Participants

This study tested the impact on smoking cessation of the offer and provision of several followup visits compared with attendance at one followup visit among patients who wanted to stop smoking.

Forty-one community family physicians agreed to participate in the study. They were recruited from the Hamilton, Ontario, area and were eligible if they agreed to attend the training session and provide administrative assistance through their office staff. Undoubtedly, these physicians were more interested than the average physician in providing smoking cessation assistance to their patients.

All of the physicians participated in a 4-hour training session designed to develop their ability to deliver two cessation interventions: one that included followup continuing for several months and one that did not. Six hundred forty-seven smoking patients participated and were randomly allocated to one of the two conditions.

Implementation Patients entered the study when they visited their physician for a regular office visit. The intention in this study was to attract people who were interested in stopping smoking. To qualify, patients had to smoke at least one cigarette every day (or most days), be 16 years of age or older, and not be pregnant or breastfeeding. Receptionists provided a copy of the consent form and the questionnaire to patients. Signs were posted in the offices to inform patients about the availability of the program.

Physicians spoke to consenting patients about their interest in stopping smoking. If patients expressed an interest in stopping, physicians invited them to return for a more in-depth discussion and development of a plan. When patients returned, receptionists provided physicians with the next in a sequence of numbered envelopes along with the patient chart. The materials for the two interventions were printed in different colors and were prepacked in envelopes that were placed in a random sequence determined by a computerized program and were numbered accordingly.

At the return visit, all patients were to receive the same intervention up to the point of the offer of further followup visits. In one group, the physicians completed their intervention at this visit. In the other group, the physicians offered to see patients four times over a 2- to 3-month period.

Process Measures And Baseline Characteristics Pretest questionnaires were completed to provide physician and patient characteristics. Interviews with patients, within 2 weeks of the quit-date visit and at 6 months after, provided information about patient perceptions about the visits with their physician and about their experience with attempting to stop smoking. The primary outcome in this study was sustained 1-year validated cessation rates, although we also provided 6-month self-reported data.

Results

Patient Reports of Physician Behavior

All physicians participating in the study attended the training session. Through exit interviews, patients reported what physicians included in the smoking cessation visit and their perceptions of its usefulness. At least 75 percent of the patients rated their physicians as very helpful, encouraging, and understanding. Patients who received the offer of followup rated their physicians as more helpful and encouraging than the ratings by patients who did not receive this offer (Gilbert et al., 1992). More than 90 percent of the time, physicians included advice about health risks, helped patients set a quit date, gave patients a stop-smoking contract, offered the use of nicotine gum, and provided self-help materials and reasons for the patient to stop smoking (Gilbert et al., 1992).

More than 80 percent of patients said their physicians discussed weight control, withdrawal symptoms, the role of planning and exercise, the importance of social support, and the role of spouses, as well as giving some attention to stress management. These first return visits averaged 16.5 minutes.

Patients' Perceptions

At the 6-month interview, we asked patients what aspects of the stop-smoking program had been the most helpful. At 6 months, physician advice and support were rated as the most helpful elements by patients in both groups; setting a quit date, having printed materials, and using nicotine gum were also rated highly. The usefulness of the contract and followup were rated lower.

Smoking Cessation

Although there were significant differences in self-reported cessation between the two experimental groups at 2 months and at 1 year, when the rates were validated at 1 year the differences lost statistical significance. We found considerable crossover had occurred between the two groups; that is, the group that was not to receive long-term followup often actually did receive it when they returned to their physician for other problems, and the long-term followup group often did not return for their followup visits. This blurring of the difference between the two groups makes interpretation of results difficult.

Elements of Successful Cessation

We also looked at the relationship between what elements of the intervention patients considered helpful or not helpful and whether they succeeded in stopping smoking. At the 6-month interview, patients rated the degree of helpfulness of various parts of the intervention. Physician advice and support were rated as the most helpful ingredients and followup visits as the least helpful. However, when we look at cessation rates at 6 months, we find that the patients who found the quit date, contract, and followup most helpful were also those with the highest cessation rates. This raises the question: Do patients who are highly motivated to stop smoking take advantage of all aspects of the program and therefore rate the components higher, or do the program components actually lead to higher cessation rates?

Approximately one-quarter of the patients at the 6-month interview rated nicotine gum as helpful. When asked at 1 year to describe their use of nicotine gum, slightly more than one-quarter of the patients (28 percent) reported using the gum for longer than 2 weeks. The cessation rate at 6 months for patients who rated the gum important was 27.3 percent.

Discussion

The purpose of this study was to determine the importance of long-term followup in relation to successful smoking cessation, to gather process data regarding the feasibility of incorporating this maneuver into regular office routines, and to determine the perceived relative importance of other ingredients of the intervention.

Cessation Rates The cessation rates in this study compare favorably with those in other studies. The 13- to 14-percent 1-year validated rate is similar to the rates for more motivated patients in our previous study and is in the same range as the results of other studies that have tested maneuvers of similar intensity. It is important for physicians to know that if they offer a smoking-specific visit to smoking patients, approximately 60 percent of those patients who have expressed an interest in stopping smoking will return, and the one visit will produce cessation rates in this range. It also appears that those patients who return for further visits are more successful in stopping smoking than those who do not return. Although we have not demonstrated the effectiveness of followup, the higher cessation rates will mean both physicians and patients may perceive this time as useful.

Structure of The Visits We found that physicians who attended the 4-hour training session set up their offices to accommodate the intervention, used the resource materials, and complied with the intervention. The brief introduction visit did not disrupt practice and the return visit focused on smoking, allowing physicians to take a smoking history, set quit dates, give instructions for gum use, and address other questions raised by patients. Although these visits were demonstrated in the training to be 8 to 10 minutes long, physicians estimated that they averaged 16.5 minutes. The visits were paid for by the provincial health insurance.

It appears that physicians offered patients long-term followup as indicated in the randomization process, but only 69 percent of those randomly offered followup attended more than one further visit. We discovered through chart audits that long-term followup happens naturally as patients return for future visits for other reasons (Gilbert et al., 1992). This natural followup within the no-followup group may explain why we found no differences in 1-year cessation rates. We should point out that the average duration of a scheduled followup visit was slightly more than 12 minutes. It is very unlikely that discussion about smoking on unscheduled followup was this long. However, we conclude that setting up smoking-specific followup visits after one smoking-focused visit may not be necessary for most people, as long as physicians are keeping good records and remember to check on progress at these other visits.

Personalized Advice And Support Project records and patient interviews indicate that physicians followed the recommended protocol and were perceived to be encouraging, understanding, and helpful. Patients reported that physician advice and support were the most important aspects of the intervention. This evidence validates the survey data that have indicated that patients do appreciate and value their physicians' interest in their smoking. Our data also indicate a high level of patient satisfaction with this particular maneuver; that is, patients gave high ratings of importance to their physicians' support in their cessation attempts.

Quit Date, Contracts, Gum — Our data demonstrate that most patients did set a stop-smoking date, but the effectiveness of the strategy was not tested in this study. In retrospect, only 140 indicated that the quit date was helpful, but 33 percent of those who found it helpful were successful at 6 months. As to the use of the contract and the nicotine gum, it appears that some individuals find each of these techniques helpful. This trial did not attempt to study those who selected these elements of the intervention.

Followup Visits — This study focused on the impact of physicians offering longer term followup, and we did search for differences between those who attended followup and those who did not. There is an overlap of the characteristics of those most likely to stop smoking and those who attended followup that confounds our ability to understand whether there are, in fact, differences. The primary overlapping characteristic is that those who are lighter smokers attended followup and also were more likely to be successful. This finding may be a little surprising, because one might expect the more addicted smoker to seek more medical assistance. Older, more educated patients with fewer friends who smoke tended to take advantage of followup visits. We might speculate that the more isolated smoker might seek ongoing support from his or her family physician.

Conclusion Physicians who attended training and used the program resources integrated the intervention into their practice fully when patients expressed an interest in participating. We do not know whether study physicians applied the intervention to patients not in the study or continued to use the resources after the study ended. Provision of a visit dedicated to smoking cessation produced substantial cessation rates, and the offer of subsequent smoking-specific followup visits did not increase those rates significantly.

REFERENCES

Burgess, S.C. Understanding physician-delivered smoking cessation counseling: An analysis of counseling style and content to predict outcome (Master of Science thesis). University of Waterloo, Ontario, Canada, 1989.

Fowler, G., Mant, D., Fuller, A., Jones, L. The "Help Your Patient Stop" initiative: Evaluation of smoking prevalence and dissemination of WHO/UICC guidelines in U.K. general practice. *Lancet* 1(8649): 1253-1255, 1989.

Gilbert, J.R., Wilson, D.M., Best, J.A., Taylor, D.W., Lindsay, E.A., Singer, J., Willms, D.G. Smoking cessation in primary care: A randomized controlled trial of nicotine-bearing chewing gum. *Journal of Family Practice* 28(1): 49-55, 1989.

Gilbert, J.R., Wilson, D., Singer, J., Lindsay, E.A., Willms, D.G., Best, J.A., Taylor, D.W. A family physician smoking cessation program: An evaluation of the role of followup visits. *American Journal of Preventive Medicine* 8(2): 91-95, 1992.

Lindsay, E.A., Wilson, D.A., Best, J.A., Willms, D.G., Singer, J., Gilbert, J.R., Taylor, D.W., Hannah, W.J., Vayda, E. A randomized trial of physician training for smoking cessation. *American Journal of Health Promotion* 3: 11-18, 1989.

Ockene, J.K., Ockene, I.S., Kabat-Zinn, J., Green, H.L., Frid, D. Teaching risk-factor counseling skills to medical students, house staff, and fellows. *American Journal of Preventive Medicine* 6(Suppl.): 35-42, 1990.

Willms, D.G., Best, J.A., Taylor, D.W., Gilbert, J.R., Wilson, D.M., Lindsay, E.A., Singer, J. A systematic approach for using qualitative methods in primary prevention research: A focus on smoking. *Medical Anthropology Quarterly* 4(4): 391-409, 1990.

Willms, D.G., Best, J.A., Wilson, D.M., Gilbert, J.R., Taylor, D.W., Lindsay, E.A., Singer, J., Johnson, N.A. Patients' perspectives of physician-delivered smoking cessation interventions. *American Journal of Preventive Medicine* 7(2): 95-100, 1991.

Wilson, D.M., Taylor, D.W., Gilbert, J.R., Best, J.A., Lindsay, E.A., Willms, D.G., Singer, J. A randomized trial of a family physician intervention for smoking cessation. *Journal of the American Medical Association* 260(11): 1570-1574, 1988.

Doctors Helping Smokers: Development of a Clinic-Based Smoking Intervention System[3]

Thomas E. Kottke, Leif I. Solberg, Milo L. Brekke, Shirley A. Conn, Patricia Maxwell, and Mark J. Brekke

BACKGROUND: DOCTORS HELPING SMOKERS

As with the other NCI-sponsored physician and dentist intervention trials, the goal of Doctors Helping Smokers was to determine how physicians might promote smoking cessation effectively among their patients. A decade before the Doctors Helping Smokers proposal was written, Russell and coworkers (1979) had already documented that a physician could make a small but significant impact on smoking cessation rates simply by advising patients to quit smoking and giving them a smoking cessation brochure. Additionally, the Multiple Risk Factor Intervention Trial had demonstrated impressive efficacy with its smoking intervention (Multiple Risk Factor Intervention Trial Research Group, 1982), and the Minnesota Heart Health Program had developed state-of-the-art self-help materials that could also be used in a one-to-one counseling session.

Because the first author had received a National Heart, Lung, and Blood Institute Preventive Cardiology Academic Award in 1981, we had already begun to work with primary care physicians at the time that we were preparing the Doctors Helping Smokers grant application. By analyzing the organizational context of angioplasty, the treatment of hypertension, advice to quit smoking, and advice to eat a low-fat diet, we identified nine factors that we believed must be considered in the implementation of any program (Kottke et al., 1987) (Table 4). This experience led us to formulate the problem of developing physician-based smoking interventions as a systems problem rather than a problem of selecting a single best solution from among a field of candidates (Kottke et al., 1990a).

We also recognized that any intervention must satisfy two conditions if it is to be effective—it must be efficacious (change patient outcomes when it is applied) and it must be acceptable to both the professional delivering the intervention and the patient who is the target of the intervention. We elected to focus Doctors Helping Smokers on the task of developing a solution to the problem that physicians tended not to use smoking interventions that were already available and of documented efficacy.

[3] Supported in part by National Institutes of Health grant no. CA-38361 and by Blue Plus Health Plan.

Table 4
Checklist for implementation of systematic smoking intervention protocols in medical practice

Knowledge of Relevance	Have we assured that the physician understands that his or her patients will benefit from a cue to stop smoking?
Skills	Have we given the physician the skills to advise the patient to stop smoking and help the patient develop problem-solving and maintenance skills?
Adequate Return	Have we designed a program that will either pay for itself or effectively serve as a practice-builder for the physician?
Organization	Have we designed an organization that will cue the physician to ask the patient to address smoking and to support the physician when he or she receives a request for help?
Perceived Effectiveness	Have we demonstrated to the physician that asking the patient to stop smoking increases the probability that the patient eventually will quit?
Perceived Patient Demand	Have we demonstrated to the physician that his or her patients want advice and help to stop smoking?
Perceived Legitimacy	Have we demonstrated to the physician that asking patients to stop smoking is a legitimate professional behavior?
Confidence	Have we given the physician the confidence to ask patients to stop smoking?
Commitment	Have we imparted to the physician the commitment to ask patients to quit smoking?

The proposal's original hypothesis was that physicians who attended a 6-hour training workshop and were supplied with the self-help booklet developed by the Minnesota Heart Health Program would so appreciate the negative health effects of smoking and be so convinced of the efficacy of their intervention that they would increase markedly the rates at which they gave advice to quit smoking. It was also hypothesized that this increase in physician activity would, in turn, lead to increases in patient smoking cessation rates.

As a test of recruitment strategies, physicians were recruited through one of three variations in a direct mail program. This recruitment program demonstrated that none of these direct mail interventions could recruit physicians at a rate that would have much impact on the patient or physician population. Regardless of the content of the particular mailing to a physician, only 10 percent of physicians responded, and 7 percent or fewer were willing and able to participate in the trial (Kottke et al., 1990c). Other investigators in this field have reported the same experience (Cummings et al., 1989a; McPhee et al., 1989; Wilson et al., 1988).

Rounds I and II of Doctors Helping Smokers asked the participating physicians to identify every smoker in their practices and ask them to quit smoking (Kottke et al., 1989). As part of the evaluation of our intervention, patients of those physicians were interviewed by telephone soon after their clinic visits and again a year later. Several findings emerged from this study:

- Even physicians who had promised to ask every smoker to quit smoking were unable to accomplish this task in more than 60 to 70 percent of cases.
- The proportion of patients who would agree to quit smoking when asked by a physician (approximately 30 percent) was far smaller than the proportion who would try to quit smoking during the subsequent year (approximately 50 percent).
- Quit attempts were frequently followed by rapid relapse. One-quarter of the patients who reported that they had quit smoking for at least 24 hours relapsed within 2 days, half relapsed within a week, and 65 percent relapsed within a month. If a patient was able to remain abstinent for 180 days, the probability of relapse within the next 180 days was low.
- Two factors had to be favorable if a smoker was going to quit smoking: the desire to quit smoking (in this case measured by the patient's response, on a 1 to 10 scale, to the question "How much do you want to quit smoking?") *and* the ability to deal with dependency on cigarettes (in this case measured by the length of time, after first rising, that the patient smoked his or her first cigarette). The desire to quit smoking was a necessary precursor of a quit attempt and was stimulated when the patient's spouse, significant others, or physician expressed a desire for the patient to quit smoking. However, even when the patient had a high desire to quit smoking, the probability of sustained abstinence was low if the patient smoked soon after first rising in the morning (Venters et al., 1990).
- The major source of disagreement between the physician and many patients was not whether patients should quit smoking but, rather, exactly how and when.
- Physicians disliked exhorting patients to quit smoking and would justify with multiple reasons why they did not perform that task. Conversely, physicians enjoyed assisting patients who wanted to follow their recommendations.
- Ongoing support from a physician reduced the probability that a patient who had stopped smoking would relapse.

A META-ANALYSIS OF CONTROLLED TRIALS

To better understand the source of apparent contradictions in the smoking cessation trial literature, Kottke organized a meta-analysis of 39 controlled trials that might possibly be delivered in a physician's office (Kottke et al., 1988). The same general pattern was observed for studies that reported their results after 6 months of followup and studies that reported their results after 12 months of followup. The fact that the intervention effects were uniformly stronger after 6 months of followup than after 12 months indicated that intervention effects decayed over time. No single intervention strategy was particularly more effective than all others. Success was associated with the following:

- Patient exposure to more than one intervention modality;
- Length of time that the subject was in contact with the program;
- Number of times that the subject was in contact with the program;
- Use of both physicians and nonphysicians; and
- Use of both group and face-to-face programs.

It was predicted from multivariate modeling that a program featuring two intervention modalities with six reinforcing sessions over a period of 1 year would produce a 43-percent success rate. This analysis demonstrated that the smoking cessation process has more characteristics of behavioral shaping (Skinner, 1959) than of health beliefs (Becker and Maiman, 1975).

NOKOMIS CLINIC INTERVENTION PROGRAM

During round I, we came to appreciate that physicians wanted to know precisely how to organize their practices to systematically provide smoking cessation advice; hypothetical situations did not convince most physicians that they should attempt an innovation in their own practices. We therefore used the storefront clinic directed by one of us to develop, test, and document whether our team-based smoking interventions produced success. This project demonstrated the following:

- Most smokers were willing to discuss smoking cessation, but only a few smokers could be recruited into formal programs.
- Just as a successful research program requires both testable hypotheses and a system to test them, the delivery of clinical smoking interventions required a system to deliver the intervention (Table 5).
- A clinical smoking intervention program could be described as containing five necessary components—identification of all smokers through a screening and labeling program, reminders to the physician, a brief message to quit smoking delivered by the physician, self-help materials, and followup (Table 6).
- The smoking intervention clinic environment program could be defined as consisting of seven necessary elements—policy establishment, coordination, an implementation plan, orientation and training, resources, audit, and maintenance (Table 7).
- When these conditions were implemented, almost 90 percent of smokers could be identified and almost the same proportion could be given a smoking cessation message at every encounter.

Table 5
Parallel components of supporting environments for testing the efficacy of interventions and delivering efficacious interventions as clinical programs

Research Environment	Clinical Environment
• Subject identification	• Identification of patients who smoke
• Standardized intervention	• Cessation message and application of patient-specific aids from a menu of efficacious interventions
• Data entry form	• Progress record
• Observation for effect of intervention	• Followup with patients
• Removal of environmental confounders	• Smoke-free clinic
• Official agreement to sponsor research	• Clinic endorsement
• Research personnel recruitment	• Necessary supporting staff
• Principal investigator	• Physician in charge
• Research assistants	• Clinical assistants/nurses
• Project coordinator	• Staff member in charge
• Manipulation protocol	• Physician role defined
• Manual of operations for research assistants	• Staff role defined
• Orientation and training	• Orientation and training
• Funding	• Cost-benefit adequacy
• Evaluation	• Evaluation
• Feedback	• Feedback
• Morale maintenance	• Spirit-building within team of providers

Table 6
Basic elements of patient-provider interaction for effective intervention

Screening and Labeling	• Routinely identifies at least all adult patients as to use or non-use of tobacco.
	• Labels charts for user or non-user status.
	• Re-screens users at each office visit for current usage.
Physician Reminders	• Reminds physicians at each visit of user status and current usage.
	• Reminds physicians of previous tobacco-related encounter attitudes and plans.
Physician Message	• Physician message during each visit that is brief, clear, supportive, and specific (negotiates specific plans, assistance, and followup).
Assistance	• Self-help guides, education, and counseling available to those who want or need them.
Followup	• Supportive communication (re-visit, phone call, or mail) near a promised quit date and after quitting.
	• Review of previous plans at all visits.

Table 7
Supporting elements needed to ensure application of the intervention

Policy Establishment	Clinic management clearly and specifically states the goal and timeframe of action. It names the individuals with authority to carry out the plan.
Coordination	Both a physician coordinator and a staff coordinator are identified to implement the policy. In large clinics, a committee or task force is desirable to support the coordinators.
Implementation Plan	A written plan is devised that identifies how each intervention element is to be performed, including the role definitions, job descriptions, financial aspects scheduling, and a timetable for startup.
Orientation and Training	Every physician and staff person affected by the plan is informed of it, given an opportunity to feel involved, and trained in the tasks that will be required of them.
Resources	All the materials needed are devised or obtained and distributed. Referral arrangements are identified (as needed).
Audit	Establishes a way to periodically assess both the end results and the process for both the overall clinic and for individual physicians and staff members.
Maintenance	Keeps the system going and improves its performance through a combination of feedback and audit information, spirit-building information and events, and repeat orientations and training as needed for both old and new clinic members.

- Not only was the program acceptable to smokers, but also they appreciated the assistance. Fewer than 5 percent of the smokers reported feeling that it was not appropriate for the clinic to ask its patients to stop smoking. Almost 80 percent reported that the program seemed to be about right, about 10 percent said it was too much, and 10 percent said it was too little. Three-quarters agreed that they were more satisfied with their overall care at the clinic because of the stop-smoking efforts there; one-quarter said that they would recommend the Nokomis Clinic to others because of those efforts.

Whereas the interventions used in round I and round II failed to produce sustained smoking cessation, the Nokomis Clinic project intervention system produced 1-year cessation rates of about 20 percent (Solberg et al., 1990). This project demonstrated that through development of a supportive environment and involvement of the entire clinic work unit in the smoking intervention effort, an effective and efficacious intervention effort could be incorporated into a busy family practice clinic, and it could be sustained there for more than 4 years.

When fully incorporated into an office practice, the smoking intervention system developed at the Nokomis Clinic would have the following features:

- Each adult patient would be categorized as a smoker or a nonsmoker and each medical record would be labeled accordingly.
- At every visit, each smoker would be asked about current tobacco use and be asked by the physician to quit smoking.
- The clinic would implement an intervention program that could respond to the particular needs of the individual smoker.
- A smoking cessation progress record would be kept for each smoker and used as a reminder to raise the topic as well as a simple way for physicians to review past actions and to arrange future assistance and followup.
- Self-help materials would be readily provided to interested smokers.
- The clinic would implement a process to assure that the progress of each smoker be followed and that quitters be reinforced for abstinence immediately after quit dates or as they visited the clinic for other reasons.

This smoking intervention system became the basis of the American Academy of Family Physicians Smoking Intervention Kit (AAFP Stop Smoking Program, 1987a and 1987b), and it provided much of the philosophical background for the National Cancer Institute publication, *How To Help Your Patients Stop Smoking* (Glynn and Manley, 1990). It also became the intervention program suggested to the clinics in the round III trial.

DOCTORS HELPING SMOKERS, ROUND III

For round III, Doctors Helping Smokers collaborated with Blue Cross/Blue Shield of Minnesota through its managed care plans, Blue Plus and HMO Midwest. Blue Cross/Blue Shield contracts with independent primary care practices in Minnesota through Blue Plus, and in Wisconsin through HMO Midwest, to provide health services to the individuals covered by these plans. In none of these medical practices do managed care patients make up more than 15 percent of all patients seen by the practice.

The target clinics of the round III intervention were all 11 Minnesota clinic organizations that provided service to enrollees living outside the Minneapolis-St. Paul metropolitan area but within a 2-hour drive of Minneapolis-St. Paul. At the beginning of the study, 126 primary care physicians were practicing in these clinics in 31 sites. Two sites closed during the period of the study.

The clinics in the control group were 10 clinic organizations in western Wisconsin that held contracts to provide services to individuals covered by the managed care contracts of Blue Cross/Blue Shield of Minnesota. These clinic organizations were somewhat smaller than the intervention group clinics; they averaged 7.7 primary care physicians per clinic and 1.5 sites per clinic.

The Patients When enrolling in Blue Plus or HMO Midwest, each enrollee is required to name a clinic that will be responsible for his or her primary care. (Because many individuals work in Minnesota while living in Wisconsin, it is not unusual for an individual covered by Blue Plus to name a Wisconsin clinic for primary care.) Blue Cross/Blue Shield has the names, addresses, and insurance claims of these enrollees and could survey them without the involvement of the physicians in either the intervention group or the control group clinics. This group of enrollees was used to evaluate the round III intervention.

In contrast to other programs that have tested smoking interventions in clinics (Cummings et al., 1989a; McPhee et al., 1989; Russell et al., 1979; Wilson et al., 1988), participating physicians consisted of an entire population, not volunteers from a population, and at no time did Doctors Helping Smokers provide salary support for any clinic employee, place a study employee in a clinic for the purpose of providing patient care, or have a Doctors Helping Smokers employee routinely monitor physician and staff activity.

Physician Recruitment The failure of rounds I and II to attract more than a small minority of physicians to give smoking cessation advice led us to develop a markedly different recruitment strategy for round III of Doctors Helping Smokers. While rounds I and II used direct mail contact with the individual physician, as described above, round III was based on developing a relationship with entire clinic groups over a period of time. Table 8 summarizes the differences between the recruitment strategies for the first two rounds and for round III of Doctors Helping Smokers. A letter was the initial contact for both, but the sponsoring organizations for round I did not have day-to-day interaction with the clinics as did the sponsors of round III. The initial response required of the physician in round I was the mailing of a postcard; aside from a reminder letter or two, Doctors Helping Smokers had no plausible explanation for attempting further contact with the physician if this card was not mailed. The letter in round III only advised the physician of the nature of an upcoming telephone call.

The second contact in both rounds I and II was a telephone call. However, the purpose of the telephone call in round I was to confirm that the physician was willing and able to participate in the randomized trial. In round III, the purpose of the telephone call was to ask the physician to name a date when the Doctors Helping Smokers team could visit the clinic to explain the study. The physician had to agree only to stay at the clinic over the lunch hour to meet with the Doctors Helping Smokers investigators.

The first face-to-face contact (third of all contacts) in round I occurred only if the physician attended the workshop. The first face-to-face contact (third of all contacts) with round III physicians was in their own clinics; they had to

Table 8
Summary of recruitment process for Doctors Helping Smokers

	Rounds I and II	Round III
Initial Contact	Mail	Mail
Organizational Relationship	No day-to-day contact about clinical matters	Day-to-day contact about clinical matters
Initial Response Required of Physician	Mail postcard	No response required
Second Contact	Telephone	Telephone
Second Response Required of Physician	Agree to come to workshop and participate in trial	Agree to stay at clinic to have lunch with Doctors Helping Smokers team
Third Contact	Face-to-face at nonclinic site if in workshop group; mail contact otherwise	Face-to-face in physician's own clinic
Third Response Required of Physician	Carry out trial in own office	Agree to ongoing negotiation of specific activities with Doctors Helping Smokers team

agree only to continue discussions with the Doctors Helping Smokers team about potential intervention strategies they might be willing to adopt for their clinical practices.

Using a philosophy similar to what later was called "the social learning model of consultation" (Brown and Schulte, 1987), which was based on Bandura's social learning theory (Bandura, 1977), we used the following recruitment process in round III: One of the Doctors Helping Smokers investigators contacted the medical director of each intervention group clinic with an introductory letter. The letter explained the study without asking for any commitment. We followed the letter with a telephone call to the medical director to arrange a site visit. The purpose of this visit was primarily informational but included four goals:

- To personally introduce the Doctors Helping Smokers investigators and the Doctors Helping Smokers agenda to the clinic physicians and administrators;
- To describe the commitment of Blue Plus to clinic-based smoking cessation interventions;
- To reach a consensus that smoking should be treated to the extent that it would not disrupt other clinic operations; and

- To ensure that the effort would be a true collaborative effort,
  - The physicians in each clinic would agree to consider implementing the Doctors Helping Smokers program, but individual physicians or the entire group would be free to start or stop at any time without a requirement to justify the action to Doctors Helping Smokers.
  - The clinic personnel would be seen as contributing depth of knowledge about the personnel, organization, and patient preferences at that particular clinic: Doctors Helping Smokers would be seen as contributing breadth of knowledge and special expertise about smoking intervention techniques and activities based on experience at multiple sites.
  - Doctors Helping Smokers would provide a recommended approach and provide intervention and training materials, training programs, audits, feedback, and consultation at the desire of the clinic.
  - Doctors Helping Smokers would advocate only interventions of documented feasibility.

To avoid having the physicians hold back for fear of being trapped into undesired or nonproductive commitments, the Doctors Helping Smokers team explicitly told each clinic that they did not need to even start the project unless they wished to and that they would be free to stop at any time.

Complimentary workshops, in which physicians, nurses, administrators, and other clinic personnel received instruction and exchanged experiences with each other, were provided three times a year at Blue Plus headquarters. The workshops were usually organized into three components. First, a national expert (e.g., Ronald Davis, M.D.; Stuart Cohen, Ed.D.; Thomas Glynn, Ph.D.) was brought in to discuss smoking intervention from a national perspective; this gave the attendee a sense of interacting in an important, high-level, national process. Second, the Doctors Helping Smokers investigators would discuss their new procedures and findings; this allowed the investigators to transfer information to attendees and give them a sense that they were essential participants in the local program. Finally, the individual attendees would present their own activities; this created a sense of commitment and competence in the attendees and allowed them to learn from each other's experiences.

Newsletters were mailed bimonthly to all key personnel at the clinics, and the two nurse-educators employed by Doctors Helping Smokers telephoned or visited each clinic site at regular intervals to provide help with problem-solving, to assess program progress, and to provide feedback and reinforcement. The newsletters provided information about the project to those who were not currently involved and provided information and a sense of belonging to office personnel who had become active in Doctors Helping Smokers. The site visits were essential for recruitment of the clinic personnel and to reinforce their commitment to the project. The site visits served particularly to signify to the clinic personnel that they were important to the project as individuals and that the project staff valued their contribution highly.

The Patient Intervention Program

The clinics could adopt any patient intervention program that they wished. However, we strongly advocated the above-described program developed at Nokomis Clinic. Rather than trying to recruit smokers into formal cessation programs, the patient intervention program designed for Doctors Helping Smokers was based on consistent and repeated advice to the smoker to quit smoking. The entire clinic was involved, and the clinic's task was defined as working with patients who wanted help rather than trying to convince resistant patients to quit smoking.

The Clinic Environment Program

The goal of the clinic environment program was to provide the physicians and medical staff with an environment that made it easier to give the advice than not to give it. It was also the intent of the program to reinforce clinic staff members when they gave smoking cessation advice. In designing the system, the investigators looked to the organization of surgical operating rooms, coronary care units, hypertension treatment programs, and other successful interdisciplinary medical systems as models to be emulated.

In the specific case of a clinical smoking intervention program, we postulated that a supportive environment would have to include 14 elements (Solberg et al., 1990):

- A smoke-free clinic;
- Formal clinic endorsement of the program;
- Staff support;
- Physician support;
- A physician coordinator;
- A staff coordinator;
- Definition of the physician's role and responsibility;
- Definition of staff roles and responsibilities;
- An orientation program;
- Cost-benefit adequacy;
- Program evaluation;
- A system to feed results back to the physicians and staff;
- A spirit-building program; and
- A program to market and advertise the program.

The purpose of a *smoke-free clinic* was to avoid giving the patient conflicting messages about the importance of being a nonsmoker. A clinic was considered smoke-free if patients, physicians, and employees were prohibited from smoking in all clinic buildings and on clinic grounds.

We believed that *clinic endorsement* of the program was essential if the clinic was to be committed to the program. Clinic endorsement was considered present if the clinic management had developed systems and procedures to incorporate smoking interventions into the daily clinic routine and had announced the formation of a smoking intervention program.

Staff support was considered present if staff members encouraged each other to perform the program well; if there was no negativity or sabotage by staff members; if nurses, medical records personnel, and receptionists were all involved and supportive of the program; and if personnel wore symbols (pins and T-shirts) associated with the program.

Physician support was considered present if the physicians were positive about the program and encouraged each other to participate in the program; if no physicians were negative about the program or sabotaged the program; if physicians exhibited leadership to their employees; and if physicians wore symbols of the program.

Many observers of innovation and product development have observed that new products languish if they don't have a "product champion," and all successful medical programs—for example, operating rooms, coronary care units, and emergency rooms—have both a physician coordinator and a staff coordinator. The *physician coordinator* was expected to be the "product champion" for the smoking intervention program. The physician coordinator was expected to meet with the staff on a regular basis, discuss the program at the physicians' meetings, and take supportive action when required. The *staff coordinator* was expected to champion the product among the employees and to bring the employees' problems to the attention of the physician coordinator.

The *physician role* was to give a brief smoking cessation message, to ask the patient if he or she were willing to set a quit date, to give the patient self-help materials, to reinforce those who had quit smoking, and to document the encounter on the smoker progress record. The *staff role* included identifying smokers, documenting the patient's history of tobacco use, and carrying out the activities identified by the Nokomis Clinic project.

The physicians and staff could not be expected to participate in the program if they did not understand what was expected of them. Therefore, the purpose of the *orientation program* was to train the physicians and staff who worked in the clinic at the beginning of the project and train new physicians and staff as they were hired by the clinic. The orientation program was also expected to follow up with physicians and staff as required by special circumstances.

Programs that do not have *adequate cost-benefit ratios* can be expected to disappear in times that the clinic is in a crisis. Therefore, it was a goal to have the smoking program benefit the clinic financially and benefit the staff emotionally. Benefits had to exceed costs in terms of fiscal return, production of health to the patient, and emotional reward to the staff. Cost-benefit adequacy also was considered to require a method to recover the program costs, definition of service charges, billing and receipt of payments, and administrator satisfaction that the program was not an undue financial burden on the clinic.

Preventive medicine programs like the smoking intervention program tend to give only negative feedback. Smokers who are resistant to the smoking cessation message create a stronger impression than those who quit smoking because they were given advice to quit. Therefore a formal *program evaluation, feedback system*, and *spirit-building program* were considered necessary to demonstrate that the program was being carried out and that it was successful. Program evaluation required the development of a plan to evaluate whether the patients were being identified as smokers or nonsmokers, whether the charts were being labeled, whether patients were being given a smoking cessation message, whether patient progress was being documented, whether patients were quitting smoking, and whether patients were getting positive reinforcement for quitting. It was expected that both individual and group performance of these tasks was to be evaluated.

The *feedback* component of the program was expected to present program results to the clinic management, physicians, and staff groups at regular intervals. It was also expected that feedback be provided to individual physicians and staff.

The goal of the *spirit-building* component of the intervention was to reinforce the positive aspects of the intervention for the clinic as a group and for individuals in the clinic. The spirit-building component was also expected to create incentives for participating in the program.

Physicians respond to patient demand for services, so it would be ideal if patients would ask for smoking cessation assistance. If the program is to be sought by the patients, it must be advertised and marketed to the patient community. The *marketing and advertising* component of the program was expected to generate demand for the program among the patient population and community. Also, it was expected to prime the smoker so that he or she expected to be asked about smoking when coming to the clinic for other reasons.

Round III Results

Clinic Recruitment

All medical directors in the 11 intervention clinics agreed to an initial meeting with a Doctors Helping Smokers/Blue Plus physician and the nurse-educator. The presence of the nurse-educator at this meeting reinforced our intentions to use a team approach, and it introduced her as the individual who would be making the site visits. At some of the initial meetings, only the medical director represented the clinic. At some of the clinics, a few additional physicians joined the medical director, and at others, nearly the entire medical staff was present. Although only 6 of the 126 primary care physicians (5 percent) attended the first workshop and only 13 physicians (10 percent of the total) attended any workshop, all 11 clinic groups were represented by at least some clinic personnel at the first training workshop. The members of the Doctors Helping Smokers intervention team made 177 site visits, 759 telephone calls, and 175 mailings to the intervention clinics between May 1, 1987, and October 31, 1988. This was an average of 5.7 site visits, 24.0 telephone calls, and 5.6 mailings per practice site.

Approximately 6 months after the initial contact with the clinics participating in round III, an audit of the Doctors Helping Smokers patient encounter records demonstrated that 68 percent of the primary care physicians were completing the Doctors Helping Smokers records for at least some of their patients. On the survey that was mailed at the same time that the medical records were audited, more than 90 percent reported that they had heard of a systematic program in their clinic to identify and help patients who smoked (Kottke et al., 1990c) (Table 9). None expressed a belief that their clinic should not be involved with such a program, and 69 percent reported using the program with their patients who smoked. One-third of the physicians reported that the program had helped them deal with the problem of smoking among their patients. Fewer than 10 percent of the physicians reported that they had been very much involved with developing the program.

Eighteen months after initial contact, physicians in 25 of the 31 sites were participating in the implementation of a smoking intervention system similar to, or exactly the same as, the Doctors Helping Smokers program. All 11 clinic systems were represented by at least one active site. Although 2 sites had closed, physicians in 24 of the remaining 29 sites were participating in the implementation of a smoking intervention system similar to, or exactly the same as, the Doctors Helping Smokers program. Five sites never started any component of the Doctors Helping Smokers program.

One of the investigators conducted site visits during February, March, and April 1989 to assess the level of implementation at each of the other 24 sites. Although the rates of implementation varied for the different components of the patient intervention program, between 40 and 50 percent of the 29 clinic sites showed very little evidence of implementing the program (Kottke et al., 1992). About one-quarter of the 29 sites systematically identified smokers and noted the smoking intervention encounter at every visit. Fewer than 20 percent of the 29 sites kept complete smoker progress records, but almost half of the sites had implemented a cessation intervention plan and a patient followup plan. Three-quarters of the 29 sites made self-help materials available for their patients.

Table 9
Self-reported participation in round III[a]

Physician has heard of Doctors Helping Smokers.		
Yes = 79 percent	No = 5 percent	Uncertain = 2 percent
Physician believes clinic should be involved with Doctors Helping Smokers.		
Very much = 53 percent	Quite a bit = 21 percent	Somewhat = 10 percent
Not at all = 0 percent	Not answered = 2 percent	
Physician uses the program with patients who smoke.		
Now and in past = 59 percent	Past only = 2 percent	Never = 25 percent
The extent to which physician identifies patients who smoke and offers them help to stop smoking:		
All patients = 26 percent	Most patients = 46 percent	
Some patients = 13 percent	No patients = 1 percent	
Program has helped physician to deal with patients who smoke.		
Yes = 30 percent	Uncertain = 28 percent	No = 5 percent
No experience = 24 percent		
Physician reports being involved in development of program.		
Very much = 8 percent	Quite a bit = 8 percent	Somewhat = 36 percent
Not at all = 34 percent		

[a] *105 of the 122 primary care physicians returned the survey. The response to each variable plus the 14-percent nonresponse rate totals 100 percent.*

Clinic Environment Program

Between one-quarter and one-third of the 29 clinic sites showed little or no evidence of adopting the clinic environment program. About 15 percent of the 29 sites adopted all aspects of the clinic environment program. Adoption of individual components varied from a high of 80 percent for a smoke-free clinic to a low of 14 percent for formal endorsement of the program, evaluation of the program, adoption of a spirit-building program, and development of a marketing program.

The reasons for not adopting the clinic environment program differ for each site, and the investigators have not yet been able to develop a mathematical model that explains the reasons for adoption or nonadoption by each of the sites. We believe that four major factors contributed to the problem of nonadoption: (1) the instability of the regional medical environment at the time of the study, (2) the investigators' inability to visit the clinics more frequently to provide them with help and reinforcement, (3) the investigators' inability to reimburse clinics for even the modest extra effort required by each of the physicians, and (4) the generally held attitude that giving smoking cessation advice is optional in clinical practice.

Patient Experience

Although only 10 percent of physicians ever attended a workshop, the inclusion of office staff as part of the intervention team and the use of site visits created avenues of communication with the clinics that could be used to foster adoption of the Doctors Helping Smokers intervention. Therefore, round III changed the experience of patients who attended the intervention group clinics during the intervention period (Kottke et al., 1992). For those who had visited their clinic in the 6 months prior to the preintervention survey, the proportion reporting that tobacco use had been brought up by the physician or clinic staff was equally low (about 22 percent) for both cohorts (Table 10). The two cohorts did, however, report significantly different experiences during the intervention. The mean proportion of patients who reported on the postintervention survey that someone asked them if they smoked was about 14 percentage points higher for the intervention clinics than for the control clinics ($p < 0.05$). The mean proportion of patients who reported on the *preintervention survey* that *no one* had asked if they smoked at their last clinic visit, and subsequently reported on the *postintervention survey* that *someone* had asked if they smoked when they last visited the clinic, was also higher for intervention group clinics in comparison to control group clinics ($p < 0.05$).

The mean proportion who reported on the postintervention survey that they had been asked if they smoked when they last visited the clinic, and who reported on the preintervention survey that no one had asked if they smoked, was about 8 percentage points higher for the intervention cohort than for the control cohort ($p < 0.05$). The mean proportion of patients who reported on the postintervention survey that their doctor had advised them to stop smoking was about 14 percentage points higher for intervention group clinics than for control group clinics ($p < 0.05$).

The difference in the mean proportion reporting that the smoking cessation advice was helpful when given was about 50 percent higher for the intervention group cohort than for the control group cohort, and the rate at which specific help was offered was nearly twice as high for respondents in the intervention group cohort than for respondents in the control group cohort. Because of the small sample sizes, these differences only approached statistical significance ($p < 0.10$).

In comparison to patients of control group clinics, patients of intervention group clinics who were not smoking at their last visit were more than twice as likely to report that *someone* had commended or complimented them at their last visit for not smoking and were almost three times as likely to report that *their doctor* had commended or complimented them at their last visit for not smoking (both $p < 0.05$). About twice as many of the members of the intervention cohort reported that they felt helped by the clinic or doctor in some way to remain an ex-smoker. Because of the small sample sizes, the difference in this rate for the two cohorts was not statistically significant.

Table 10

Activities of the control and intervention clinics, as reported by regular smokers[a]

	Control[b]	Intervention[b]	
(Number of Clinics Analyzed)	(8)	(10)	
Prior to the Intervention			
Tobacco use was brought up by a physician or staff at any visit in the 6 months prior to intervention.	22.9%±11.2	21.9%±9.6	0.84
At the Last Clinic Visit During the Intervention Period			
Someone asked whether the patient used tobacco.	26.0±12.2	39.8±12.3	< 0.05
Patient was asked if he/she used tobacco when he/she hadn't been asked before the intervention.	20.4±6.9	28.7±8.5	< 0.05
The doctor advised the patient to quit smoking if he/she was still smoking at the last clinic visit.	26.4±14.6	40.5±12.1	< 0.05
The patient considered advice helpful if given.	16.4±9.0	23.9±8.0	< 0.10
The patient was offered specific help if he/she expressed interest in quitting.	13.4±11.1	22.8±11.5	< 0.10
If the Patient Was Not Smoking at Last Clinic Visit			
Someone commended or complimented the patient for not smoking.	11.3±11.8	28.2±19.9	< 0.05
The doctor commended or complimented the patient for not smoking.	9.5±11.4	25.9±19.8	< 0.05
The patient felt helped in some way to remain an ex-smoker.	6.6±9.8	13.0±16.9	0.33

[a] *Regular smokers were those who smoked one or more cigarettes every day for the 7 days prior to the preintervention survey.*

[b] *Column entries are percentages of patients responding affirmatively.*

LESSONS LEARNED Through an iterative cycle of hypothesis formulation, program development, hypothesis testing, and hypothesis reformulation as suggested by Argyris et al. (1985), Doctors Helping Smokers was able to develop a clinic-based intervention that increased the rate at which smoking patients received advice to quit when they sought care from a group of nonvolunteer medical clinics. We feel that the following observations are the most important lessons to be learned from this study.

Requirements for Recruitment

Positive, Ongoing Relationship

The success of recruitment in round III is predicted by the literature on the relationship between social contacts and successful recruitment. Green (1970) found that perceived expectations of the subject's friends is an important modifier of behavior, and Rogers (1983) noted that innovations are most likely to diffuse when individuals are alike in personal and social characteristics. Gerlach and Hine (1970) found in their studies of Black Power and Pentecostal organizations that recruitment predictably takes place through preexisting, significant social relationships of positive affect; mass media are rarely the source of recruitment. In their studies, the type of relationship (brother, spouse, parent, fellow church member, neighbor, patron, peer) was a less important predictor of recruitment than either the *frequency of interaction* between recruiter and potential member or the *affect of the relationship* (positive or negative) with the potential convert. Recruitment was always achieved by those with whom the relationship had been very positive; negative relationships, even between kin supposedly important to each other, did not result in recruitment.

Face-to-Face Interaction

Factsheets, letters, brochures, articles, and other mass media only provide information (Gerlach and Hine, 1970). Rogers (1983) has found that without regard to the type of innovation, only 5 to 10 percent of individuals will respond to information in the absence of peer group support. The responders represent members of two groups: information seekers, who wish to find out more about the activities being promoted, and individuals who are already active and are seeking reinforcement. The implication is that mailed materials can provide support for the already active or information for those not active, but any differences among mailed materials will result only in minor differences in recruitment rates.

Repeated Contacts

The Doctors Helping Smokers experience is consistent with Rogers' observation that adoption of innovation requires ongoing contact between the change agents and the adopter. Rogers (1983) noted that the requirement of more than 20 contacts per year between an early adopter and a change agent is not atypical if an innovation is to be diffused. Without a similar level of investment, apparently one cannot expect adoption even if recruitment is initially successful. The 177 site visits, 759 telephone calls, and 175 mailings from Doctors Helping Smokers to the clinic sites between May 1, 1987, and October 31, 1988, were inadequate to produce full adoption.

Entire Work Unit

Although similar proportions of physicians attended workshops in all three rounds, round III resulted in recruitment of 10 times as many physicians because the recruitment effort was directed toward the entire clinic and took place in the clinic. Doctors Helping Smokers is not the only trial where it was observed that recruiting whole work units was far more successful than recruiting individual physicians (Cummings et al., 1989a).

An effective program involves recruiting the entire unit, because peers and employees who are not part of a new program will be working against it if they do not understand how it contributes to the mission of the clinic. The surgeon

Charles H. Mayo, the sociologist Eliot Freidson, and others have all appreciated the impact that the organizational base of the medicine work unit has on the ability to complete a desired task (Freidson, 1970; Mayo, 1988; McDonald et al., 1984).

Behavior Shaping

A model that assumes that patient behavior is primarily motivated by attempts to avoid disease makes patient behavior appear irrational. The vast majority of smokers acknowledge that smoking is a health hazard, that quitting smoking would benefit their health, and that they would like to quit smoking. Even so, they claim that they are unable to stop smoking for extended periods of time.

The data from the meta-analysis (Kottke et al., 1988) and from Doctors Helping Smokers (Kottke et al., 1989, 1990c, and 1992) demonstrate that smoking and smoking cessation behavior is rational if it is viewed as a process of behavior shaping (Skinner, 1959) or social learning (Bandura, 1977). Patients give priority to achieving goals that are more immediate than the maintenance of physical health into the far future. The smoker may feel that smoking increases the probability of attaining these short-term goals. It is up to the smoking intervention program to help the patient learn ways to achieve short-term goals without smoking and to come to believe that smoking interferes with the attainment of short-term goals.

Desire and Ability To Quit

Our experience with transdermal nicotine patches is consistent with the observation that a way of countering the factors of habit and addiction and a way of maintaining a high desire to quit smoking must be present if a smoker is to remain abstinent. Almost 80 percent of patients on the active patch, compared with 40 percent on the placebo, quit smoking while on the patch, but the long-term success of the two groups was identical (Hurt et al., 1990). The nicotine patch offered the smokers a way to deal with the addiction but could not maintain their desire to abstain from smoking. The desire to quit smoking, independent of habituation or addiction, is a product of the social environment and must be continuously reinforced by the social environment and support system.

Physician and Staff Behavior

If viewed from a "rational" perspective, failure to adopt a smoking intervention of documented efficacy is an enigma: Addressing matters that affect a patient's health is a physician's responsibility. Physicians believe that smoking is among the most harmful of the behaviors that their patients can practice (Orleans et al., 1985; Wechsler et al., 1983), and more than half of American smokers try to quit each year. Why, then, is it so remarkably difficult to get physicians to give smoking cessation interventions to their patients (Cummings et al., 1989a; Kottke et al., 1990c; McPhee et al., 1989; Wilson et al., 1988)? Why do patients continue to report that their physicians still do not routinely give them advice to stop (Anda et al., 1987)? And, why do physicians not adopt smoking cessation interventions that have been documented to be both efficacious and cost-effective (Cohen et al., 1989;

Cummings et al., 1989b; Kottke et al., 1989; Ockene et al., 1991; Strecher et al., 1991)? From the perspective of the health belief model (Becker and Maiman, 1975), physician behavior is as irrational as patient behavior.

However, physicians are not typically irrational and, viewed from another perspective, their behavior is not mysterious. American medicine is driven primarily by patient expression of demand for service, not unexpressed patient need for service (Kottke et al., 1990b). Viewed in this context, physicians can truly want their patients to quit smoking but fail to act because they expect their patients to follow the convention used for almost all medical encounters: They expect their patients to broach the subject of smoking cessation as a signal that they want and will accept help with the problem.

Although physicians enjoy special status in society (Freidson, 1986), it appears that their behavior is determined by the same factors that determine patient behavior. The physician never has adequate time to complete all possible tasks, and some rewards can be increased only at the cost of other rewards. Time spent talking with patients about smoking means time not spent seeing patients who are presenting undiagnosed symptoms and signs. The physician's diagnosing conditions tends to increase patient satisfaction; trying to convince patients to stop smoking tends to upset and anger patients. Behavior shaping predicts that, given a choice, physicians would tend to choose the behavior that is emotionally reinforcing, making diagnoses, over the behavior that is emotionally punishing, advising people to quit smoking. The observation that physician performance at the task of asking patients if they smoke and advising them to quit tends to decay over time (Ewart et al., 1983) corroborates this explanation.

Mutual Acceptability Of the Encounter

Patient-physician interaction takes the form, almost exclusively, of a patient seeking out a physician and asking for help through the making of a "chief complaint." The physician responds by telling the patient if and how he or she is willing to provide help. It is the exceptional situation in which the physician acts against the will of the patient. These situations are limited to incarceration when the patient is mentally incompetent, notification of contacts when the patient poses an infective threat to the community, and pediatric immunization. In the first, the physician must obtain a court order to act. In the second, the private physician almost always lets the public health officials take over responsibility for care. On the basis of this observation, we can expect that physicians will always try to avoid conflict with the patient and take action only if it is in response to a patient request or is likely to be accepted by the patient.

In the case of advice to quit smoking, if the physician is expected to take action, that action must be defined as *advice* to the patient to quit smoking. There is little reason to believe that physicians will ever adopt the practice of routinely attempting to *convince* their patients to quit smoking. Even if the physician is not considered obligated to convince the patient to stop smoking, it is appropriate to obligate the physician to carry out six smoking intervention tasks (Kottke et al., 1990b): (1) understand why people smoke and how they quit; (2) identify patients who smoke; (3) advise those patients to quit; (4) enable them to stop smoking by prescribing services or by imparting them with the knowledge, skills, and confidence to stop; (5) help those patients to maintain abstinence by providing positive reinforcement both in the examining room and in the community; and (6) establish, support, and maintain a system to facilitate tasks 2 through 5.

CONCLUSIONS On the basis of the empirical evidence gathered in Doctors Helping Smokers, we have markedly reformulated the way in which we see the smoker, the physician, and the environment in which they interact:

- The smoker, rather than being an individual lacking in knowledge about the harmful effects of smoking who would quit if he or she were aware of these facts, almost always knows about the harmful effects, usually would like to quit, has a 40-percent probability of trying to quit in a given year, but is unlikely to remain abstinent after any single attempt.
- The physician, rather than being an autonomous individual who would try to convince the smoker to quit if he or she were aware of the harmful effects of smoking, is an individual who is highly aware of the harmful effects of smoking but operates under a number of misconceptions about how to help smokers quit, lacks the resources to identify the smokers who want to quit and provide them with help, and experiences intense competition for his or her time and attention.
- The environment, designed to help the physician meet the demands of the patient for acute care, currently offers little support to the physician who would like to help patients stop smoking.

We therefore designed an interdisciplinary clinic-based program that (1) identified all smokers but focused on providing help to the smokers who wanted to quit smoking, were trying to quit smoking, or who had recently quit smoking; (2) conceived of the physician as an individual who is highly dependent on office staff for support and, therefore, involved the entire office staff in the effort to identify smokers, advise them to quit, and provide them with the help they might want or need in the smoking cessation effort; and (3) provided a clinic environment that cued the staff to act and reinforced them when they did act. Through the Doctors Helping Smokers program, we have demonstrated, in a group of nonvolunteer clinics, that at least some clinics can be recruited to adopt the program described above and that this adoption, even at incomplete levels, results in significant increases in the rates at which smokers are identified, advised to quit, and reinforced in their quit attempts.

ACKNOWLEDGMENTS The authors wish to thank the Minnesota Academy of Family Physicians and the health care professionals who participated in this study.

REFERENCES

AAFP Stop Smoking Program. *Patient Stop Smoking Guide.* Kansas City, MO: American Academy of Family Physicians, 1987a.

AAFP Stop Smoking Program. *Physician and Office Staff Manual.* Kansas City, MO: American Academy of Family Physicians, 1987b.

Anda, R.F., Remington, P.L., Sienko, D.G., Davis, R.M. Are physicians advising smokers to quit? The patient's perspective. *Journal of the American Medical Association* 257: 1916-1919, 1987.

Argyris, C., Putnam, R., Smith, D.M. *Action Science.* San Francisco: Jossey-Bass, 1985.

Bandura, A. Theories must demonstrate predictive power. In: *Social Learning Theory,* S. Finnemore (Editor). Englewood Cliffs, NJ: Prentice-Hall, 1977, p. 5.

Becker, M.H., Maiman, L.A. Sociobehavioral determinants of compliance with health and medical care recommendations. *Medical Care* 13: 10-24, 1975.

Brown, D., Schulte, A.C. A social learning model of consultation. *Professional Psychiatric Research and Practice* 18: 283-287, 1987.

Cohen, S.J., Stookey, G.K., Katz, B.P., Drook, C.A., Smith, D.M. Encouraging primary care physicians to help smokers quit: A randomized controlled trial. *Annals of Internal Medicine* 110(8): 648-652, 1989.

Cummings, S.R., Richard, R.J., Duncan, C.L., Hansen, B., Vander Martin, R., Gerbert, B., Coates, T.J. Training physicians about smoking cessation: A controlled trial in private practice. *Journal of General Internal Medicine* 4(6): 482-489, 1989a.

Cummings, S.R., Rubin, S.M., Oster, G. The cost-effectiveness of counseling smokers to quit. *Journal of the American Medical Association* 26(1): 75-79, 1989b.

Ewart, C.K., Li, V.C., Coates, T.J. Increasing physicians' antismoking influence by applying an inexpensive feedback technique. *Journal of Medical Education* 58(6): 468-473, 1983, p. 88.

Freidson, E. *Profession of Medicine: A Study of the Sociology of Applied Knowledge.* New York: Dodd, Mead, 1970, p. xi.

Freidson, E. *Professional Powers.* Chicago: University of Chicago Press, 1986, p. 137.

Gerlach, L.P., Hine, V.H. *People, Power, Change: Movements of Social Transformation.* Indianapolis: Bobbs-Merrill, 1970, pp. 79-97.

Glynn, T.J., Manley, M.W. *How To Help Your Patients Stop Smoking: A National Cancer Institute Manual for Physicians.* U.S. Department of Health and Human Services, Public Health Service, National Institutes of Health, National Cancer Institute. NIH Publication No. 90-3064, 1990.

Green, L.W. *Status, Identity, and Preventive Health Behavior.* Pacific Health Education Reports. Berkeley: University of California School of Public Health, 1970, p. 32.

Hurt, R.D., Lauger, G.G., Offord, K.P., Kottke, T.E., Dale, L.C. Nicotine-replacement therapy with use of a transdermal nicotine patch: A randomized double-blind placebo-controlled trial. *Mayo Clinic Proceedings* 65: 1529-1537, 1990.

Kottke, T.E., Battista, R.N., DeFriese, G.H., Brekke, M.L. Attributes of successful smoking cessation interventions in medical practice: A meta-analysis of 39 controlled trials. *Journal of the American Medical Association* 259: 2882-2889, 1988.

Kottke, T.E., Blackburn, H., Brekke, M.L., Solberg, L.I. The systematic practice of preventive cardiology. *American Journal of Cardiology* 59: 690-694, 1987.

Kottke, T.E., Brekke, M.L., Solberg, L.I., Hughes, J.R. A randomized trial to increase smoking intervention by physicians: Doctors Helping Smokers, round I. *Journal of the American Medical Association* 261: 2101-2106, 1989.

Kottke, T.E., Solberg, L.I., Brekke, M.L. Beyond efficacy testing: Introducing preventive cardiology into primary care. *American Journal of Preventive Medicine* 6(Suppl. 1): 77-83, 1990a.

Kottke, T.E., Solberg, L.I., Brekke, M.L. Initiation and maintenance of patient behavioral change: What is the role of the physician? *Journal of General Internal Medicine* 5(Suppl.): S62-S67, 1990b.

Kottke, T.E., Solberg, L.I., Brekke, M.L., Conn, S., Maxwell, P., Brekke, M.J. A controlled trial to routinize smoking cessation advice by 11 clinics: Doctors Helping Smokers, round III. *Journal of Family Practice* 34: 701-708, 1992.

Kottke, T.E., Solberg, L.I., Conn, S., Maxwell, P., Thomasberg, M., Brekke, M.L., Brekke, M.J. A comparison of two methods to recruit physicians to deliver smoking cessation interventions. *Archives of Internal Medicine* 150: 1477-1481, 1990c.

Mayo, C.H. As quoted in *Mayo Alumnus.* Rochester, MN: Mayo Foundation, Summer 1988.

McDonald, C.J., Hui, S.L., Smith, D.M., Tierney, W.M., Cohen, S.J., Weinberger, M., McCabe, G.P. Reminders to physicians from an introspective computer medical record: A two-year randomized trial. *Annals of Internal Medicine* 100: 130-138, 1984.

McPhee, S.J., Bird, J.A., Jenkins, C.N.H., Fordham, D. Promoting cancer screening: A randomized, controlled trial of three interventions. *Archives of Internal Medicine* 149: 1866-1872, 1989.

Multiple Risk Factor Intervention Trial Research Group. Multiple Risk Factor Intervention Trial: Risk factor changes and mortality results. *Journal of the American Medical Association* 248: 1465-1477, 1982.

Ockene, J.K., Kristeller, J., Goldberg, R., Amick, T.L., Pekow, P.S., Hosmer, D., Quirk, M., Kalan, K. Increasing the efficacy of physician-delivered smoking intervention: A randomized clinical trial. *Journal of General Internal Medicine* 6: 1-8, 1991.

Orleans, C.T., George, L.K., Houpt, J.L., Brodie, K.H. Health promotion in primary care: A survey of U.S. family practitioners. *Preventive Medicine* 14: 636-647, 1985.

Rogers, E.M. *Diffusion of Innovations* (3rd edition). New York: Free Press, 1983, pp. 253, 275-277.

Russell, M.A.H., Wilson, C., Taylor, C., Baker, C.D. The effect of general practitioners' advice against smoking. *British Medical Journal* 2: 231-235, 1979.

Skinner, B.F. *Cumulative Record.* Cambridge, MA: Harvard University Press, 1959, p. 21.

Solberg, L.I., Maxwell, P.L., Kottke, T.E., Gepner, G.J., Brekke, M.L. A systematic primary care office-based smoking cessation program. *Journal of Family Practice* 30: 647-654, 1990.

Strecher, V.J., O'Malley, M.S., Villagra, V.G., Campbell, E.E., Gonzalez, J.J., Irons, T.G., Kenney, R.D., Turner, R.C., Rogers, C.S., Lyles, M.F., White, S.T., Sanchez, C.J., Stritter, F.T., Fletcher, S.W. Can residents be trained to counsel patients about quitting smoking? Results from a randomized trial. *Journal of General Internal Medicine* 6: 9-17, 1991.

Venters, M.H., Kottke, T.E., Solberg, L.I., Brekke, M.L., Rooney, B. Dependency, social factors and the smoking cessation process: The Doctors Helping Smokers Study. *American Journal of Preventive Medicine* 6: 185-193, 1990.

Wechsler, H., Levine, S., Idelson, R.K., Rohman, M., Taylor, J.O. The physician's role in health promotion: A survey of primary care practitioners. *New England Journal of Medicine* 308: 97-100, 1983.

Wilson, D.M., Taylor, D.W., Gilbert, J.R., Best, J.A., Lindsay, E.A., Willms, D.G., Singer, J. A randomized trial of a family physician intervention for smoking cessation. *Journal of the American Medical Association* 260(11): 1570-1574, 1988.

Prompting Smoking Cessation In Family Practice

William C. Wadland, John R. Hughes, and Roger H. Secker-Walker

INTRODUCTION The primary aims of this project were to determine the effect of a prescription for nicotine gum when added to brief physician advice and followup on (1) smoking cessation, (2) quit attempts, (3) intentions to quit, (4) self-efficacy about the ability to quit, and (5) confidence in physician advice. The study design was a randomized clinical trial where adult smokers receiving routine health care from their family physician were assigned to either the group receiving physician advice against smoking and followup (advice alone) or the group receiving physician advice against smoking and followup plus a prescription for nicotine gum (advice plus gum). Subjects were expected to fill the prescription at their own expense. Verification of smoking cessation was done at 6 months by self-report, observer report, and carbon monoxide (CO) monitoring. The intentions to quit, self-efficacy, and confidence in physician advice were measured by brief questions given before and after the physician visit. The secondary aims were to describe and compare the rates of recruitment between two intervention sites. As a pilot project, the study generated information useful for further clinical trials on smoking cessation in primary care medicine. Because of the varied success of nicotine replacement therapy in general medical practice, there is a need to assess alternative pharmacological measures for smoking cessation in the same setting.

RECRUITMENT IN A PRIMARY CARE TRIAL Physicians in two primary care practices in Chittenden County, Vermont, agreed to participate in this pilot project on smoking cessation. The first practice (site 1) was a private family practice with 5 physicians (aged 35 to 62) and about 15,000 patients, including children. The clinic is located in a semirural town near Burlington. At this site, the study was conducted during 34 working days from February through April 1987.

The second practice (site 2) was an academic general internal medicine practice with 6 physicians (aged 32 to 58) and about 16,000 patients, not including children. The practice was located in the University Health Center in Burlington. Site 2 had a history of research efforts related to smoking cessation and adult comprehensive care (Bronson and Omeara, 1986). The study described here was carried out during 53 working days from July through October 1987.

All adult patients entering the practices for routine, nonemergency care, including new and return appointments, received a screening questionnaire to identify health risks (see Appendix A at the end of this chapter). The screening form asked all potential subjects about their age, gender, and general health risks, including smoking. Because both smokers and nonsmokers completed the screening form, it allowed for gathering of information on both groups without embarrassing smokers by being the only group completing forms. The screening of potential subjects was done either by the practice receptionists at the first site or by trained study coordinators at the first and second sites. All study forms were color-coded to make filing easy for the coordinators.

At the private-practice site, 576 adult patients were screened, of whom 128 (22 percent) were smokers (Figure 2). Among the 128 adult smokers screened, 54 percent consented to enter the study (see consent form, Appendix B). Among those who consented, 11 smokers (9 percent) failed to meet the inclusion criteria, as determined by an entry questionnaire and a medical screening form (Appendixes C and D). The forms were color-coded for easy reference. A total of 58 smokers (45 percent of those eligible) enrolled in the clinical trial.

Initially at site 1, the receptionists screened 287 patients over 21 days, or 13.7 patients per day; whereas the study coordinators screened 267 patients over 13 days, or 20.5 patients per day. The receptionists received only a brief orientation to the project. They were instructed to hand out forms to interested smokers and refer them to the coordinators for more instruction. The rate of enrollment was 1.7 patients per day.

At site 2, the screening form was offered to 2,050 adult patients, of whom 358 (17.5 percent) refused to read it, and 1,692 (82.5 percent) completed it. Of those completing the form, 274 (16.2 percent) were smokers. Site 2 had already done a study on smoking cessation (Bronson and Omeara, 1986) that may have affected the overall prevalence of smokers in the practice. Among the smokers screened, 19 percent consented to enter the study. A total of 38 smokers (14 percent of those eligible) enrolled in the trial. The rate of enrollment was 0.7 subjects per day.

It was hypothesized that the impersonal nature of handing out a consent form discouraged enrollment. To test this hypothesis at site 2, 104 interested patients were randomly assigned to have the study coordinators either actively read the informed consent form to them or to have subjects read the consent form on their own. The actively informed group had 51 patients, of whom 27 consented (53 percent). The self-informed group had 53 patients, of whom 25 consented (47 percent). The difference between the two methods of gaining consent was not found to be significant.

The conclusions of tracking recruitment in this clinical trial on smoking cessation in two general medical practices were as follows: (1) the rate of enrollment was 3.3 times as great in the private practice as in the academic practice (45 vs. 14 percent); (2) trained coordinators were better recruiters than practice receptionists; and (3) having the study personnel actively involved in obtaining informed consent did not improve recruitment. This study has been described in more detail by Wadland and colleagues (1990).

Figure 2
Comparative depiction of recruitment to a smoking cessation trial at two sites

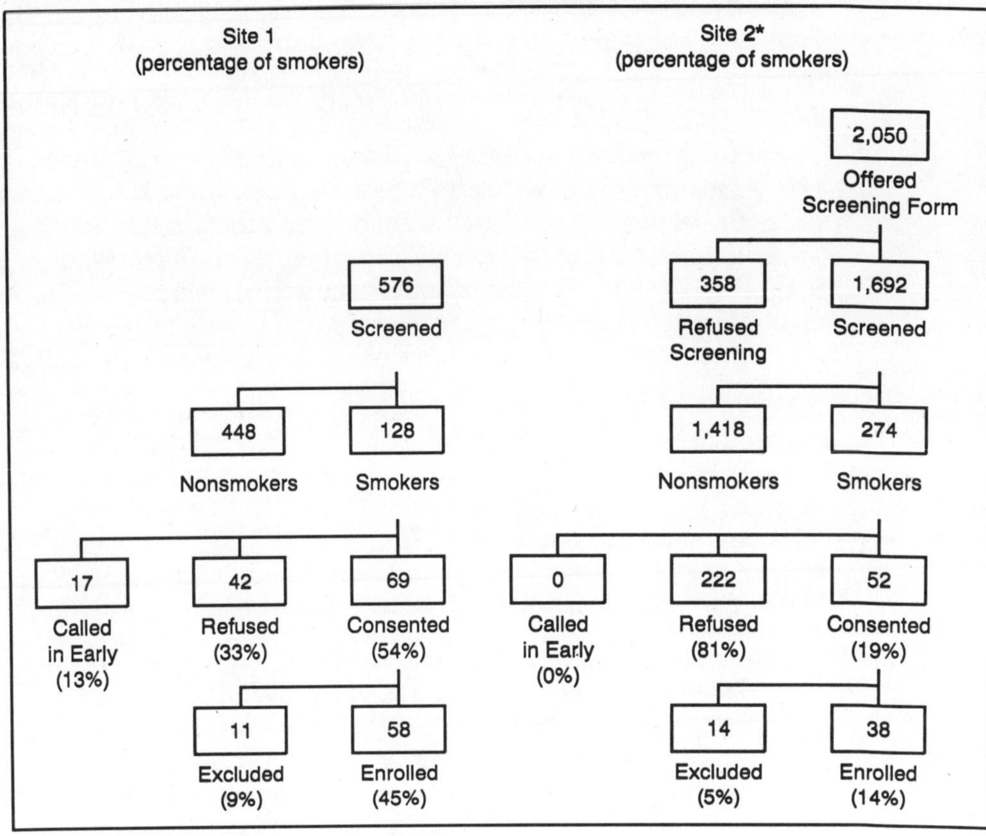

** Refusal to general screening was monitored only at site 2.*
Source: Wadland et al., 1990; used with permission of the authors.

TRAINING ON BRIEF ADVICE As part of the current trial, participating physicians attended a 2- to 3-hour workshop training them to (1) elicit a health problem that is a reason for smoking cessation; (2) state the reversibility of the problem; (3) provide a previously tested cessation booklet, "Quit and Win"; (4) give a prescription for nicotine gum and instructions on its proper use; (5) ask for a commitment to quit smoking; (6) ask for a quit date; (7) make an appointment for followup at 1 to 2 weeks after the quit date; and (8) congratulate the patient for trying to quit. The physicians received continuing medical education credit and refreshments for attending the session, which was held in their offices after patient care hours. Prior to the session, they had received a packet of information explaining the study rationale, review articles on nicotine replacement therapy, expected time commitment of the physician and practice personnel, and payment for participation—

$10 per subject receiving physician advice against smoking. The physicians were invited to comment on the study protocol and to make suggestions for applying it in their practices.

Common scenarios were role-played. For example, a patient wants to quit because of frequent coughing and easily sets a quit date. Another patient has no real reason to quit and is not sure of committing to an exact date to quit. A third patient wants to quit but is not sure of the date. A fourth patient really likes smoking and believes it is a personal right. Physicians watched the project directors play out such scenarios, and then they role-played themselves. Finally, the physicians viewed a slide-tape show on nicotine gum and its proper use. There was ample time for questions and answers.

During the course of the study, the office coordinators provided qualified subjects with an envelope containing different instructions to the physicians, based on the randomization schedule. After the physicians dealt with the primary reason for each visit, they reviewed the degree of smoking dependency, provided by the entry questionnaire (Appendix C). The entry form included information on the type of cigarettes smoked, average number of cigarettes per day, and Fagerstrom tolerance questions for assessing the degree of dependency. All subjects received generic advice suggesting reasons to quit and stating the reversibility of symptoms. A generic reminder sheet was used to prompt physicians (see Appendix E).

The physicians then opened a randomization envelope that stated whether the patient was to receive a prescription for nicotine (gum group) or further advice only (no-gum group). Reminder sheets for the gum group (Appendix F) and no-gum group (Appendix G) were provided, depending on the assignment. Subjects in both groups were asked for a commitment to quit and a quit date, and they were offered followup by appointment or phone. To equalize the duration of contacts, patients in the no-gum group, instead of receiving instructions on the gum, were asked about their biggest fear related to quitting and received further coping tips and advice about weight control with smoking cessation. Both groups received about 5 to 10 minutes of physician advice. To verify that they provided advice, the physicians completed a form documenting each patient's quit date (Appendix H). All patients completed an exit questionnaire (Appendix I) verifying the content of the physician advice. All patients answered postadvice questions on intentions to quit, self-efficacy, and confidence in the physician advice. The no-gum group completed a separate exit form to verify the physician advice content (Appendix J). The gum group completed a similar form, verifying that a prescription and instructions for nicotine gum were provided (Appendix K). All subjects were offered a followup visit in 1 to 2 weeks after quitting.

At 1 to 2 weeks after the physician visit, all subjects received by mail a questionnaire (Appendix L) that served as a reminder to subjects and as a log of quit attempts and cessation. At 6 months, subjects received a questionnaire

(Appendix M) asking similar questions to document quit attempts and cessation. All subjects who did not complete the forms were called by telephone. Family observers were asked to verify cessation in those who stated that they had quit. A followup questionnaire on gum use (Appendix N) asked about filling and using the prescription. All subjects stating they had quit at 6 months were invited to receive $25 for verifying cessation with a CO breath test.

SUMMARY OF PILOT TRIAL RESULTS

After recruitment and screening, 94 subjects entered the clinical trial. There were no significant differences between sites with respect to sociodemographic variables, rates of quitting, or quit attempts. Observer verification was always in agreement with subject reporting.

At the 6-month followup, there was information on 43 subjects in relation to smoking cessation. The results are in Table 11. The numbers were small, and there was clearly no significant difference.

The quit attempts were reported by subjects answering the questions in Table 12 at 2 weeks and at 6 months. There was no significant difference between the groups in quit attempts. This may be the result of small numbers, as the mean number of quit attempts was greater in the gum group.

There were no differences in change from before to after the interventions between the gum and no-gum groups with respect to their intentions to quit, self-efficacy about the ability to quit, and confidence in the physician's advice.

Table 11
Cessation at 6-month followup

	Quit	Not Quit
Gum Group	2	20
No-Gum Group	4	17

Table 12
Quit attempts

	Did Patient Make Quit Attempt?		How Many Quit Attempts?	
	Yes	No	Mean	S.D.
Gum Group	21	11	3.35	6.37
No-Gum Group	19	15	1.78	0.94

The gum and no-gum groups were combined in the analysis of preintervention and postintervention changes in intentions to quit and self-efficacy. Concerning prechange and postchange on the intention-to-quit question ("Do you intend to quit?"), 22 subjects reported no change, 3 subjects reported decreased intention to quit, and 40 reported greater intention to quit (Wilcoxon signed-rank test, $p < 0.001$). Concerning prechange and postchange in the self-efficacy question ("Will you succeed if you try?"), 33 subjects reported no change, 4 subjects reported lower self-efficacy, and 24 subjects reported higher self-efficacy (Wilcoxon signed-rank test, $p < 0.001$). These results are encouraging in suggesting that even brief physician advice on smoking cessation will enhance intentions to quit and self-efficacy.

The initial sample size and power calculation to complete the project called for 219 subjects per treatment arm to show a 10-percent difference (10 percent in the no-gum group and 20 percent in the gum group) in quit rate with a power of 80 percent and an α of 5 percent. It was estimated that at least 600 subjects were required for the entire study to allow for refusal and loss to followup. With the recruitment data from this pilot project, a more accurate prediction of the total cost and scope of the project can be made. Using only private practices with 4 to 5 physicians and a population base of 12,000 to 15,000 patients, and assuming 1.5 true subjects enrolled per day, it would take 10 similar practices 40 days, or about 2 months, to accrue 600 subjects.

RECOMMENDATIONS The experience of this project provides an opportunity to share suggestions for other investigators based on what did not work, what worked, and what could be done differently.

The following approaches did not work:

- Using untrained receptionists for recruitment of subjects; and
- Reading the informed consent to subjects (made no difference in recruitment).

The following approaches did work:

- Having trained research coordinators at the practice site and using a generic screening form enhanced recruitment of subjects.
- Color-coding physician and research assistant prompts was helpful.
- Training sessions of physicians at the practice site enhanced study interest.
- Giving feedback to individual physicians seemed to enhance their motivation to continue the study.

The following approaches are suggested for future studies:

- Include the practice personnel in the practice orientation and training sessions about the project.
- Choose sites that have not had prior smoking cessation studies that may have decreased the interest and prevalence of potential subjects.
- Include more sites and longer study periods to enhance sample size.

FUTURE PHARMACOLOGICAL THERAPY

The success of nicotine gum replacement in general medical practice has been marginal at best. Several prior studies (see Table 13) have reported improved quit rates (from 1 to 7 percent better) with the use of nicotine gum versus placebo (Hughes et al., 1989; Fagerstrom, 1988). Studies have been criticized for sample sizes inadequate to detect differences of less than 10 percent. However, a 10-percent difference may be necessary for physicians to sustain an interest in the use of nicotine replacement therapy. Clearly, the effect of nicotine chewing gum is far greater in combination with group therapy in heavily dependent smokers (Tonneson et al., 1988). Many general physicians who tried nicotine replacement therapy with brief advice against smoking are now seeing a number of return smokers who failed nicotine gum therapy. Failed smokers and their physicians are expressing frustration and looking for options. Referring patients to costly behavioral treatment programs is an option, but fewer than 7 percent of those referred actually attend (Hughes et al., 1989). Because more than 70 percent of all smokers see their physician every 2 years, the rationale for a simple, effective pharmacological aid to physician's advice against smoking remains attractive (Pederson, 1984). There is less patient effort and cost and better availability than with psychological treatment.

Physicians should be discouraged from using some pharmacological measures. Silver salts combined with tobacco smoke cause unpleasant metallic tastes and appear ineffective. Sedatives to relieve anxiety have not been effective. Pentobarbital and alcohol do not decrease smoking, and they increase it in abusers of those substances. Diazepam abates the first 24 hours of withdrawal and craving only. Meprobamate shows quit rates similar to no-drug and inferior to placebo treatment. Antidepressants show some promise, but the side-effects profile may be prohibitive. Stimulants such as amphetamines increase smoking. Beta-blockers show no decrease in craving and no long-term quit rates. Narcotic agonists such as naloxone have showed increased smoking and mixed results. Over-the-counter medications such as lobeline have questionable efficacy, in light of poor study designs (Jarvik and Henningfield, 1988).

Though it is not an approved indication for the drug, physicians are using transdermal clonidine in treatment failures with nicotine replacement. Transdermal clonidine is available for the treatment of hypertension and is well tolerated with minimal side effects. There is no need to taper off of

Table 13
Long-term abstinence in randomized trials of nicotine gum with brief advice

	Setting	n	Percentage Abstinent[a] 6 months Nicotine	6 months Control	1 year Nicotine	1 year Control
Nicotine Gum vs. No Gum						
British Thoracic Society (1983)	Pulmonary clinic	777	-	-	10%	9%
Campbell et al. (1987)	General practice	573	-	-	3	1
Fagerstrom (1984)	General practice	145	-	-	25[b,c]	9[e]
Gilbert et al. (1989)	General practice	223	-	-	6	7
Harackiewicz et al. (1988)	University health center	151	-	-	13	15
Page et al. (1986)	General practice	289	12[c,d]	8	-	-
Russell et al. (1983)	General practice	1,354	-	-	9[c]	4[e]
Shaughnessey et al. (1987)	General practice	99	-	-	10	20
Sutton and Hallett (1987)	Worksite	270	-	-	9	2[e]
Sutton and Hallett (1988)	Worksite	161	-	-	9	2
Wilson et al. (1988)	General practice	1,933	-	-	9	4
Nicotine Gum vs. Placebo						
British Thoracic Society (1983)	Pulmonary clinic	802	-	-	10	11
Campbell et al. (1987)	General practice	836	-	-	3	2
Fortmann et al. (1988)	Public health clinic	600	30[b]	22[e]	22[b]	18
Hughes et al. (1989)	General practice	315	29	19	10	7
Jamrozik et al. (1984)	General practice	200	10[b]	8	-	-

[a] *Percentage continuously abstinent and biochemically verified except as noted.*
[b] *Point prevalence rather than continuous abstinence.*
[c] *Biochemically verified in only a subset of claimed abstainers.*
[d] *No biochemical verification.*
[e] *$p < 0.05$ by chi-square test.*

transdermal clonidine as there is with oral clonidine, where abrupt withdrawal can provoke hypertensive rebound. Clonidine, an α_2-antagonist, blocks firing in the locus ceruleus, which is the major controller of sympathetic activity in the brain. It has been used to counter symptoms of withdrawal from alcohol and morphine. Most studies on the use of clonidine in smoking cessation have been limited to oral use, short-term followup, and withdrawal effects (Davison et al., 1988; Franks et al., 1989; Glassman et al., 1984 and 1988; Ornish et al., 1988; Sees and Clark, 1988). There is a growing need for long-term efficacy and safety trials in involving transdermal clonidine as an aid to smoking cessation in general medical practice. Some creative study designs may consider combinations of pharmacological therapy such as transdermal clonidine with nicotine gum.

Transdermal nicotine replacement may be an attractive alternative for smoking cessation in general medical practice. The transdermal approach improves compliance dramatically and produces more stable blood levels of nicotine than does nicotine chewing gum. Initial reports (McNabb et al., 1982) of short-term success with extensive behavioral therapy are encouraging (Buchkremer et al., 1989; Rose et al., 1985). A preliminary study in general medical practice by Abelin and cowokers (1989) demonstrated 3-month abstinence rates of 36 percent for the nicotine group versus 23 percent for the placebo. There is a definite need to test the long-term efficacy and safety of transdermal nicotine replacement therapy in general medical practice. Mixed study designs using nicotine gum and transdermal nicotine in selective smokers may prove most effective.

Other possible nicotine replacement therapies include nicotine aerosols, inhalers, and nasal sprays; however, social acceptability and potential abuse limit their efficacy. With the advent of transdermal nicotine, future studies on smoking cessation in general medical practice are necessary and the prospect seems promising.

REFERENCES

Abelin, T., Buehler, A., Müller, P., Vesanen, K., Imhof, P.R. Controlled trial of transdermal nicotine patch in tobacco withdrawal (comment). *Lancet* 1(8628): 7-10, 1989.

British Thoracic Society. Comparison of four methods of smoking withdrawal in patients with smoking-related diseases: Report by a subcommittee of the Research Committee of the British Thoracic Society. *British Medical Journal* 286: 595-597, 1983.

Bronson, D., Omeara, K. The impact of shared medical records on smoking awareness and behavior in ambulatory care. *Journal of General Internal Medicine* 1: 34-37, 1986.

Buchkremer, G., Bents, H., Horstmann, M., Opitz, K., Tölle, R. Combination of behavioral smoking cessation with transdermal nicotine substitution. *Addictive Behaviors* 14: 229-238, 1989.

Campbell, I.A., Lyons, E., Prescott, R.J. Stopping smoking: Do nicotine chewing gum and postal encouragement add to doctors' advice? *Practitioner* 231: 114-117, 1987.

Davison, R., Kaplan, K., Fintel, D., Parker, D., Anderson, L., Haring, O. The effect of clonidine on the cessation of cigarette smoking. *Clinical Pharmacology and Therapy* 44: 265-267, 1988.

Fagerstrom, K.O. Effect of nicotine chewing gum and followup appointments in physician-based smoking cessation. *Preventive Medicine* 13: 517-527, 1984.

Fagerstrom, K.O. Efficacy of nicotine chewing gum: A review. In: *Nicotine Replacement: A Critical Evaluation* (Progress in Clinical Biological Research Series, volume 261), O.F. Pomerleau and C.S. Pomerleau (Editors). New York: Alan R. Liss, 1988, pp. 109-128.

Fortmann, S.P., Killen, J.D., Telch, M.J., Newman, B. Minimal contact treatment for smoking cessation. *Journal of the American Medical Association* 260: 1575-1580, 1988.

Franks, P., Harp, J., Bell, B. Randomized, controlled trial of clonidine for smoking cessation in a primary care setting. *Journal of the American Medical Association* 262: 3011-3013, 1989.

Gilbert, J.R., Wilson, D.M., Best, J.A., Taylor, D.W., Lindsay, E.A., Singer, J., Willms, D.G. Smoking cessation in primary care: A randomized controlled trial of nicotine-bearing chewing gum. *Journal of Family Practice* 28(1): 49-55, 1989.

Glassman, A.H., Jackson, W.K., Walsh, B.T., Roose, S.P., Rosenfeld, B. Cigarette craving, smoking withdrawal, and clonidine. *Science* 226: 864-866, 1984.

Glassman, A.H., Stetner, F., Walsh, T., Raizman, P., Fleiss, J., Cooper, T., Covey, L. Heavy smokers, smoking cessation, and clonidine. *Journal of the American Medical Association* 259: 2863-2866, 1988.

Harackiewicz, J.M., Blair, L.W., Sansone, C., Epstein, J.A., Stuchell, R.N. Nicotine gum and self-help manuals in smoking cessation: An evaluation in a medical context. *Addictive Behaviors* 13: 319-330, 1988.

Hughes, J.R., Gust, S., Keenan, R., Fenwick, J., Healey, M. Nicotine vs. placebo gum in general medical practice. *Journal of the American Medical Association* 261: 1300-1305, 1989.

Jamrozik, K., Fowler, G., Vessey, M., Wald, N. Placebo contrôlled trial of nicotine chewing gum in general practice. *British Medical Journal* 289: 794-797, 1984.

Jarvik, M., Henningfield, J.E. Pharmacological treatment of tobacco dependence. *Pharmacology, Biochemistry and Behavior* 30: 279-294, 1988.

McNabb, M.E., Ebert, R.V., McCusker, K. Plasma nicotine levels produced by chewing nicotine gum. *Journal of the American Medical Association* 248(7): 865-868, 1982.

Ornish, S., Zisook, S., McAdams, L. Effects of transdermal clonidine treatment on withdrawal symptoms associated with smoking cessation. *Archives of Internal Medicine* 148: 2027-2031, 1988.

Page, A.R., Walters, D.J., Schlegel, R.P., Best, J.A. Smoking cessation in family practice: The effects of advice and nicotine chewing gum prescription. *Addictive Behaviors* 11: 443-446, 1986.

Pederson, L.L. Role of physicians in smoking cessation. In: *The Health Consequences of Smoking: Chronic Obstructive Lung Disease. A Report of the Surgeon General.* U.S. Department of Health and Human Services, Public Health Service, Office on Smoking and Health. DHHS Publication No. (PHS) 84-50205, 1984.

Rose, J.E., Herskovic, J.E., Trilling, Y., Jarvik, M. Transdermal nicotine reduces cigarette craving and nicotine preference. *Clinical Pharmacology and Therapy* 38: 450-456, 1985.

Russell, M.A., Merriman, R., Stapleton, J., Taylor, W. Effect of nicotine chewing gum as an adjunct to general practitioner's advice against smoking. *British Medical Journal* 287(6407): 1782-1785, 1983.

Sees, K., Clark, H.W. Use of clonidine in nicotine withdrawal. *Journal of Psychoactive Drugs* 20: 263-268, 1988.

Shaughnessy, A.F., Davis, R.E., Reeder, C.E. Nicotine chewing gum: Effectiveness and the influence of patient education in a family practice. *Journal of Family Practice* 25: 266-269, 1987.

Sutton, S., Hallett, R. Randomized trials of brief individual treatment for smoking using nicotine gum in a workplace setting. *American Journal of Public Health* 77: 1210-1211, 1987.

Sutton, S., Hallett, R. Smoking intervention in the workplace using videotapes and nicotine chewing gum. *Preventive Medicine* 17: 48-59, 1988.

Tonnesen, P., Fryd, V., Hansen, J., Gunnersen, A.B., Forchammer, H., Stockner, M. Effect of nicotine chewing gum in combination with group counseling on the cessation of smoking. *New England Journal of Medicine* 318: 15-18, 1988.

Wadland, W.C., Hughes, J.R., Secker-Walker, R.H. Recruitment in a primary care trial on smoking cessation. *Family Medicine* 22: 201-204, 1990.

Wilson, D.M., Taylor, D.W., Gilbert, J.R., Best, J.A., Lindsay, E.A., Willms, D.G., Singer, J. A randomized trial of a family physician intervention for smoking cessation. *Journal of the American Medical Association* 260(11): 1570-1574, 1988.

Smoking Cessation in Primary Care Practice: Summary of Results From the Quit for Life Project

Steven R. Cummings, Thomas J. Coates, Mort J. Stein, Neil D. Swan, and the Quit for Life Research Group

INTRODUCTION Most American physicians believe that cigarette smoking is an important threat to health and that efforts to encourage smoking patients to quit the habit should have a high priority in the practice of medicine. Physicians are generally aware that cigarette smoking is the single most important avoidable cause of premature death and disability in the United States (US DHEW, 1979). Because some 70 percent of smokers visit a physician each year, patients could be influenced to quit smoking by the physician's counseling or other smoking cessation strategies (Ockene, 1987). Most physicians, however, report that they feel poorly prepared to counsel smoking patients to stop, and only a few say they believe their smoking cessation efforts to be very successful (Cummings et al., 1989d; Ockene et al., 1988; Wechsler et al., 1983).

The literature suggests that physicians can effectively help their patients to quit smoking by routinely asking whether patients smoke, counseling and otherwise motivating patients to quit, helping smokers to commit themselves by establishing a date on which they will stop smoking, getting the patients' further commitment by persuading them to return for a followup office visit, and providing self-help materials and support from the physician's office staff (Orleans, 1985; US DHHS, 1986). Physicians rarely use any of these strategies (Cummings et al., 1989d), however, and the value of training physicians to use these approaches had not previously been tested in a rigorous randomized trial.

We tested the value of these approaches in two groups: (1) internists in a large hospital-based health maintenance organization and (2) internists and family practitioners in private practice. We also conducted surveys of physicians and dentists to describe their current attitudes and practices about smoking cessation, analyzed the cost-effectiveness of counseling about smoking cessation, and, as an underpinning for our research, estimated the best cutoff points for biochemical tests of smoking cessation used in intervention trials. This review summarizes the 10 papers that resulted from the Quit for Life project and offers further observations on the processes used in the studies.

TRIALS

Trial Objectives

The main goal of the trials was to test the value of a combination of commonly advocated strategies for brief physician counseling, using rigorous methods with adequate power to reveal even small effects. addition, we aimed for generalizable results: We sought to create a program that could be adopted by anyone and to test its value in samples of internists in different practice settings.

We developed a standardized continuing education program (Quit for Life) to teach physicians how to counsel smoking patients to quit. The counseling protocol was designed to be concise, to have an impact, and to fit into doctors' busy schedules. We set out to test the hypothesis that physicians who received controlled and standardized training in effective counseling about smoking cessation—in combination with intensified office support and followup counseling—would show higher rates of smoking cessation among their patients than do physicians who do not receive such counseling training combined with heightened staff involvement and patient followup.

Quit for Life Training

We created a standard training program in smoking cessation based on commonly advocated principles of brief counseling. To test the value of the program, we conducted parallel trials, one involving private-practice physicians (internists and family practitioners) and one involving HMO internists. From four medical centers of the HMO, the Kaiser Permanente Medical Group of Northern California, 81 internists were recruited; 40 were randomly assigned to the training program and 41 served in the control group, receiving no counseling training (Cummings et al., 1989a). In the second trial, we recruited private-practice internists and family practitioners, 44 in all; 24 were randomly assigned to the experimental (training) group and 20 to the control group (Cummings et al., 1989b). All physicians in the two experimental groups attended three 1-hour training seminars led by an internist or a psychologist. The seminars demonstrated the five steps that have been advocated as part of brief physician counseling about smoking cessation (Cummings et al., 1989a and b). In the first seminar, the instructor presented a systematic approach to counseling smoking patients to quit. Physicians viewed a videotape illustrating effective counseling approaches and then rehearsed their own counseling techniques through role-playing.

The first Quit for Life seminar focused on five steps in the counseling process:

- Ask all patients whether they smoke.
- Ask all who do whether they are interested in stopping.

For those who say they are interested in quitting, continue with the next three steps:

- Reinforce smokers' motivations to quit. Ask questions about their own reasons for wanting to quit and demonstrate the personal benefits of cessation, rather than making general statements about the consequences of smoking.
- Help those interested in quitting to commit to a specific quit date. Dramatize the quit date as a tangible goal by presenting the patient with a signed physician's prescription form with the patient's name and the quit date written on it.
- Offer a self-help booklet to all smokers, even those who say they are not interested in quitting.

The physicians were urged to practice the five-step counseling approach at once, before the second training seminar.

During training, the physicians practiced these steps in role-plays. The sessions ended with positive feedback from the participants and the instructor for use of the suggested steps during the role-play session.

At the second seminar, 1 or 2 weeks later, the participants discussed their experiences in counseling patients. They related and discussed obstacles faced by patients trying to quit—fear of failure; apprehension about gaining weight; the reactions of spouses, friends, and coworkers who continue to smoke; and the discomfort of withdrawal symptoms. The instructor suggested specific ways to overcome each obstacle discussed. Nicotine gum was recommended as an adjunct to counseling for smokers showing clinical evidence of addiction, and instructions for how to use nicotine gum were reviewed. The instructor also discussed the importance of scheduling followup office visits with the counseled smokers and ways that physicians might respond to problems encountered in followup visits.

The experimental group also attended a third session (a booster) 4 to 12 weeks later, discussing their experiences in counseling smokers. The instructor congratulated those who had tried the suggested approaches and described the medical significance and cost-effectiveness of persistence in counseling smokers to quit, emphasizing the importance of followup office visits.

Recruitment for Two Trials

For the HMO trial, we enrolled nearly 50 percent of the eligible Kaiser Permanente HMO internists with relatively little effort (Cummings et al., 1989a). We first obtained the support of the HMO chiefs of medicine and patient education, enlisted an investigator from each of the Kaiser Permanente groups of internists to help contact colleagues about the study, sent a letter describing the trial to HMO internists, and then made a single presentation to the regular physician staff meeting at each participating hospital. The fact that all HMO physicians practice in one building, where the Quit for Life training was conducted during the time usually devoted to CME, made participation very easy for the Kaiser Permanente physicians.

Recruitment of private-practice physicians for the trial was much more difficult (Cummings et al., 1989b). We enrolled only about 5 percent of eligible private physicians, despite our using more intensive enlistment efforts than those employed with HMO internists. We first enlisted the support of the local medical associations, obtained letters of support from the chief of staff of each major hospital in the region, sent those endorsements in a letter (addressed by hand to prevent its being treated as junk mail) to all primary care physicians in the target region, enclosed a stamped and preaddressed response card and a phone number to call for those interested, conducted a followup mailing, and made presentations to many of the hospitals' staff meetings. In retrospect, we believe it would be more productive to target a smaller, randomly selected group of physicians with personal contacts, perhaps "dear colleague" phone calls from a physician-investigator.

We tried two approaches to recruiting patients for the study. First, we asked the physicians' staff members to help recruit; they were instructed to ask all patients whether they smoke and to invite them to participate in the studies. Patients who agreed were enrolled and then filled out a baseline information questionnaire. Despite intensive efforts to enlist the cooperation of office staffs (see below), recruitment proceeded slowly and unevenly from office to office. We found that it was better to hire research assistants to identify smokers in each office, and most participants were enlisted by research staff. Patients were enrolled until we had accrued from 15 to 30 smokers per physician in 6 weeks.

Data Collection All physicians completed a baseline questionnaire about their training, type of practice, smoking history, and opinions about and practices for counseling smokers. Selected questions were administered a second time to physicians in the experimental group after their training.

Prior to seeing their physicians, participating smokers answered questions about the extent of their commitment to quitting and their level of confidence in their ability to do so. As soon as possible after each patient's visit to the physician, a member of the research staff, who was not aware of the patient's assignment to the experimental (physician training) group or the control group, interviewed each smoker by telephone. The interviewer asked whether smoking had been discussed during the visit, how many minutes had been spent in the discussion, what steps the physician had recommended, what the smoker had agreed to do, and whether the patient had received a self-help booklet or a followup appointment about smoking cessation.

One year after the first telephone interview, smokers were interviewed again by telephone to determine their current smoking habits and how many times they had tried to quit smoking (a single attempt was defined as abstinence for at least 24 hours). Those who said they had not smoked a cigarette during the past 7 days were defined as self-reported nonsmokers; they were offered $25 to have a breath test and give a saliva sample. Investigators analyzed results of patients' self-reported and biochemically validated abstinence from smoking. All those lost to followup or who refused biochemical testing were counted as smokers.

Conducting the Trials

From the 125 participating physicians, we enrolled 3,004 smokers in the two trials of private-practice physicians and those in an HMO. We interviewed more than 90 percent of the smoking patients after they first received office counseling from their physicians and then interviewed more than 80 percent of those patients again 1 year later. Of those who claimed to have quit smoking, 80 percent completed biochemical tests to confirm that claim, and 10 percent were reclassified as smokers after the testing (Cummings et al., 1989b). Detailed results of these trials have been published (Cummings et al., 1989a and 1989b).

These separate trials had three characteristics in common. First, the smoking cessation counseling and other interventions were designed to be convenient, specific, and standardized. The training was presented in short sessions to fit into physicians' CME schedules. The office materials employed were simple, inexpensive, and easy to use in a physician's office without special training.

Second, the intervention combined many of the elements of other NCI-supported trials—a reminder system and training about counseling involving videotape demonstrations, rehearsals and role-playing, and building upon feedback from the smokers, from other physicians in training, and from the instructor's exercises in reinforcing positive elements of the continuing intervention process.

Third, the trials adhered to rigorous principles of randomized studies. For example, randomization was blinded, all data about cessation outcomes were collected by research assistants who were blinded to the assignment of patients to treatment or control groups, and all data were analyzed by initial assignment (in compliance with the "intention-to-treat" principle).

Office Staff Involvement

We had difficulty in enlisting and maintaining consistent office staff support of physician counseling and other cessation efforts. One member of the research staff spent at least 1 hour in the office of every experimental group physician in the trials. Recruitment in private offices was slow and uneven, with varying levels of cooperation. We also became concerned about biased sampling because at least one physician instructed his staff to enlist only smokers he had counseled who seemed likely to quit smoking.

We had further difficulty enlisting cooperation from the Kaiser Permanente office staff, because staff members frequently rotate from office to office and station to station within the HMO. Staff members who had been trained for the trial were frequently replaced by temporary or "float" personnel. Many HMO staff members expressed the feeling that they were overworked and said they did not regard participation in the trial as "part of [their] job description."

The problem of office staff cooperation was compounded at the HMO by the fact that staff members' loyalties do not focus on a specific physician because they are not employed or supervised by the physicians; they are instead employees of the HMO nursing service and hospital administration. Trying to overcome the lack of cooperation, the research staff offered incentive payments to private and HMO staff members for enrolling smokers and gave periodic gifts of appreciation; but those inducements seemed to make little difference. At the HMO, there was poor compliance by staff in identifying smoking patients, and the prescribed use of stickers to remind physicians of their counseling obligation was ignored consistently by the staff at two-thirds of the nursing stations.

In retrospect, the investigators concluded it would be better to work through the hierarchy of the HMO nursing service from the beginning of the trial and to invite all staff members to participate in the training seminars and in the design of the office staff intervention support system.

To test the hypothesis that a different approach to staff involvement might have a degree of success with staff intervention, we conducted a small controlled trial with Kaiser Permanente after completion of the main trial. This trial included intensive staff involvement in planning and carrying out the intervention as well as designation of followup visits specifically for counseling about smoking. We found that such an approach enhanced the identification of smokers and the use of recommended counseling techniques (Duncan et al., 1991).

Results

In the trial involving physicians in private practice, we found, on the basis of 1-year followup interviews with patients, that physicians in the experimental group who received the special smoking cessation training were more likely to discuss smoking with patients who smoked than were the physicians in the control group (64 vs. 44 percent), spent more time counseling smokers about quitting (7.5 vs. 5.2 minutes), helped more smokers set dates to quit smoking (29 vs. 5 percent of smokers), gave out more self-help booklets (37 vs. 9 percent), and were more likely to make a followup appointment about smoking (19 vs. 11 percent of those counseled) (Cummings et al., 1989b). In the trial involving internists in HMOs, 1-year followup interviews with patients showed that physicians in the experimental group who received the special smoking cessation were more likely to discuss smoking with their patients than were the control group physicians (50 vs. 45 percent), spent more time counseling smokers (5.4 vs. 4.2 minutes), were more likely to write a prescription establishing a quit date (16 vs. 1 percent), and were more likely to schedule follow-up appointments to discuss smoking (15 vs. 4 percent) (Cummings et al., 1989a).

In two categories studied, however, there was no significant difference in smoking cessation efforts between the physicians who received training and those who did not. Physicians in the experimental group wrote prescriptions for nicotine gum for 10.2 percent of their patients, the control group for

10.4 percent; and 25.6 percent of experimental group physicians suggested a treatment program for their patients, while 25.4 percent of the control group did the same.

Thus, we found that a 3-hour continuing education program about how to counsel smokers, combined with supportive materials for use in the physicians' offices, substantially changed the way physicians counseled patients about smoking. In both trials, with physicians in private practice and those in HMOs, those who received the Quit for Life training counseled patients more often and longer. Physicians in private practice who received the training helped six times as many patients set dates to stop smoking and gave self-help materials to four times as many patients as did physicians in the control group. Among HMO physicians, those who received training helped six times as many patients set quit dates and gave self-help material to three times as many patients as did physicians who did not receive the training.

In both trials, counseling resulted in slightly higher rates of long-term (9-month) abstinence from smoking, but only among patients who specifically expressed a desire to quit. Among counseled patients most interested in quitting, there was a small (2.0 percent) increase in long-term cessation in the private-practice physicians' trial; there was a similar small (1.6 percent) increase in long-term cessation among those most interested in quitting in the HMO trial.

In the overall patient population, however, the trials showed that improved counseling, as reflected in changes in physician behavior, had very little impact on patients' smoking habits. Rates of long-term smoking cessation, confirmed by biochemical tests of patients who report they have quit, were only 1.1 percentage points higher in the HMO experimental group than in the control group (2.6 vs. 1.5 percent), and only 0.7 percentage points higher in the private-practice experimental group (3.2 vs. 2.5 percent). Neither result was statistically significant.

We found that more intensive staff involvement, combined with diligence in scheduling followup counseling appointments ("training-plus") increased the level of physician counseling beyond that seen with the Quit for Life training alone. Those physicians receiving "training-plus" staff support counseled more patients, set more quit dates, and scheduled more followup appointments to deal with smoking cessation than did those who received the training without the coordinated staff support. This pilot study of the effect of staff cooperation and support of physician counseling efforts was too small to determine whether these changes resulted in higher rates of smoking cessation.

The investigators found that convincing patients to set quit dates appears to be an effective technique for encouraging patients to make smoking cessation attempts; patients in the HMO trial who agreed to set quit dates were about four times more likely to attempt to quit for at least 24 hours, even after results were adjusted to account for evaluations of *desire* to quit, *confidence* in the ability to quit, and *number of cigarettes* smoked per day.

SURVEYS

In addition to the controlled trials, investigators conducted surveys of random samples of internists, dentists, and nurse practitioners to assess and describe their office-practice use of smoking cessation counseling and other interventions. The response rate for the survey of internists was 92 percent—higher than that of any similar previous survey of physicians' smoking cessation practices. We believe the high response rate resulted from the strategy of targeting a random sample of physicians, one small enough for the survey staff to pursue responses aggressively, with hand-addressed letters, multiple telephone calls, and even personal visits (if necessary) from a doctor on the survey team.

The authors found that the internists, dentists, and nurse practitioners surveyed believe that smoking is extremely dangerous to health and that counseling about smoking cessation is important and just as worthwhile as other, more widely practiced preventive procedures, such as mammography. On the other hand, a substantial proportion of physicians *never* use counseling strategies that might help patients to quit smoking. Dentists were even less likely to use counseling strategies such as setting quit dates, providing self-help booklets, or scheduling followup counseling.

In the dentists' survey, only 17 percent of San Francisco Bay area dentists said they frequently discussed smoking cessation with their patients who smoke, in contrast to 58 percent of a similar group of Bay area internists, who said they frequently counsel smokers (Gerbert et al., 1989). Dentists attributed their lack of counseling to inadequate insurance coverage, insufficient time, lack of training, and apprehension that patients might become irritated and leave their dental practices.

Nurse practitioners, however, are more likely than physicians to adopt smoking cessation counseling techniques introduced through CME, investigators found (Zahnd et al., 1990). A study and patient surveys determined that nurse practitioners are more likely than physicians to counsel smokers to quit. Internal medicine nurse practitioners and internists at four HMO centers received training in the Quit for Life program, and their patients were then surveyed about their counseling practices. It was found that nurse practitioners discussed smoking with patients more often than did physicians (64 vs. 50 percent), asked patients more frequently whether they were interested in quitting (49 vs. 40 percent), distributed more smoking cessation literature (37 vs. 25 percent), and made more followup appointments about smoking (36 vs. 19 percent). These results support the view that nurse practitioners, because of greater emphasis on counseling during their professional training, more readily incorporate counseling about cessation into their medical care of smokers than do physicians.

We found in another survey that physicians only infrequently prescribe nicotine gum to their smoking patients, and that a large minority of physicians (20 to 35 percent) are unfamiliar with important features of how the gum should be used as an adjunct to smoking cessation counseling (Cummings et al., 1989c). Thus, there is evidence of a need for physician education about how to use nicotine gum more effectively. The advent of transdermal delivery systems for nicotine may, however, circumvent this gap in physicians' knowledge.

Although more than 90 percent of internists (in HMOs and in private practice) questioned in another survey believe that smoking is extremely dangerous to health, fewer than half believed they were effective at motivating patients to quit smoking, and most felt that counseling about smoking was extremely frustrating because of the minimal success rate relative to the time invested with patients (Cummings et al., 1989d).

A majority of private-practice internists believed that physicians are not adequately reimbursed for counseling about smoking, a sentiment shared by only 28 percent of the HMO internists surveyed. Only a minority of internists in both groups thought that insurance coverage would actually increase the amount of time that they spend counseling smokers. Most internists indicated that insufficient time was an important barrier to helping smokers quit. This may partly explain why, when they do discuss smoking with patients, most internists and other physicians spend fewer than 3 to 5 minutes on counseling. Few internists ever schedule visits with patients primarily to address smoking cessation, perhaps because such visits are not reimbursed by third-party payers. Consistent with previous surveys, we found that HMO internists were much more likely to refer patients to smoking cessation programs. This is probably because such programs are often provided on-site at HMO centers and are at least partially covered by the health plans, which typically provide more preventive care benefits than do traditional health insurance plans.

OTHER ANALYSES In preparation for the trials, we demonstrated that test cutoff points for biochemical validation of smoking cessation used in previous studies were too high (Cummings and Richard, 1988). We devised a method for calculating the optimum cutoff point for these tests to take into account the prevalence of deception among those who claim to have stopped smoking. On the basis of this method, we recommended revised cutoff points for future studies of smoking cessation.

We also analyzed the cost-effectiveness of counseling about smoking cessation, as reflected in longer life expectancy among smokers who succeed in quitting (Cummings et al., 1988). We found that, in terms of cost per years of life saved, counseling about smoking cessation was more cost-effective than treatment of moderate hypertension or hypercholesterolemia. If brief counseling motivated only 1 percent of smokers to quit, the cost per year of life saved was $2,020 for one middle-aged man among the successful 1 percent. We estimated that scheduling a single followup counseling session would also be quite cost-effective when total population costs of therapy are divided and expressed as costs of counseling the successful 1 percent—$5,051 per year of life saved. By way of comparison, we estimated the cost-effectiveness of treating moderate hypertension at $11,300 per year of life saved.

In additional analyses of data from the Quit for Life trials, we described racial differences in smoking behavior among patients who smoke (Vander Martin et al., 1990). Whites were heavier smokers and more likely to feel addicted to cigarettes. Blacks believed that they were more likely to quit smoking and felt less addicted than whites. Hispanics were lighter smokers, and both Hispanics and Asians rated family pressures as an important reason for wanting to quit smoking.

From our patient questionnaires at baseline and at 1-year followup, we also found that patients' concern about their health was the single most important motivating reason to quit; about three-quarters of those who quit cited a health-related reason. Most commonly, they said that disturbing symptoms and diseases related to their smoking led them to quit. However, most smokers gave more than one reason, often citing social pressures, dislike of the negative aesthetic image, and the feeling of being the victim of addiction.

We also analyzed factors influencing whether patients participating in the two main trials received prescriptions for nicotine gum as a physical adjunct to counseling (S.R. Cummings, unpublished data). Of all the patient factors analyzed, a patient's belief that he or she is addicted to cigarettes appeared to be the most important influence upon physicians to prescribe the gum. In addition, black smokers were less likely to receive a prescription for the gum than were members of other racial groups. Physicians were much more likely to prescribe gum if they were confident of their ability to instruct patients to use it effectively.

DISCUSSION While many physicians say, when questioned, that they are making an effort to counsel smoking patients, a substantial proportion of physicians never use commonly advocated counseling strategies with their smoking patients. Using rigorous randomized trial methodology, we tested the hypothesis that training physicians to use strategies such as quit dates would substantially improve their success in helping smokers quit and remain abstinent. However, the Quit for Life trials confirmed earlier findings about other types of CME: Such programs can substantially change physicians' clinical practices but those changes do not necessarily result in comparable improvements in patient outcomes (Haynes et al., 1984).

Nevertheless, even very small effects from counseling smokers make the effort worthwhile. Primary care providers and those who reimburse medical providers should note that even marginally effective smoking cessation programs are among the most cost-effective interventions in medicine.

REFERENCES

Cummings, S.R., Coates, T.J., Richard, R.J., Hansen, B., Zahnd, E.G., Vander Martin, R., Duncan, C., Gerbert, B., Martin, A., Stein, M.J. Training physicians in counseling about smoking cessation: A randomized trial of the "Quit for Life" program. *Annals of Internal Medicine* 110(8): 640-647, 1989a.

Cummings, S.R., Hansen, B., Richard, R.J., Stein, M.J., Coates, T.J. Internists and nicotine gum. *Journal of the American Medical Association* 260(11): 1565-1569, 1988.

Cummings, S.R., Richard, R.J. Optimum cutoff points for biochemical validation of smoking status. *American Journal of Public Health* 78(5): 574-575, 1988.

Cummings, S.R., Richard, R.J., Duncan, C.L., Hansen, B., Vander Martin, R., Gerbert, B., Coates, T.J. Training physicians about smoking cessation: A controlled trial in private practice. *Journal of General Internal Medicine* 4(6): 482-489, 1989b.

Cummings, S.R., Rubin, S.M., Oster, G. The cost-effectiveness of counseling smokers to quit. *Journal of the American Medical Association* 261(1): 75-79, 1989c.

Cummings, S.R., Stein, M.J., Hansen, B., Richard, R.J., Gerbert, B., Coates, T.J. Smoking counseling and preventive medicine: A survey of internists in private practices and a health maintenance organization. *Archives of Internal Medicine* 149(2): 345-349, 1989d.

Duncan, C., Stein, M.J., Cummings, S.R. Staff involvement and special followup time increase physicians' counseling about smoking cessation: A controlled trial. *American Journal of Public Health* 81(7): 899-901, 1991.

Gerbert, B., Coates, T., Zahnd, E., Richard, R.J., Cummings, S.R. Dentists as smoking cessation counselors. *Journal of the American Dental Association* 118(1): 29-32, 1989.

Haynes, R.B., Davis, D.A., McKibbon, A., Tugwell, P. A critical appraisal of the efficacy of continuing medical education. *Journal of the American Medical Association* 251(1): 61-64, 1984.

Ockene, J.K. Smoking intervention: The expanding role of the physician. *American Journal of Public Health* 77: 782-783, 1987.

Ockene, J.K., Aney, J., Goldberg, R.J., Klar, J.M., Williams, J.W. A survey of Massachusetts physicians' smoking intervention practices. *American Journal of Preventive Medicine* 4: 14-20, 1988.

Orleans, C.T. Understanding and promoting smoking cessation: Overview and guidelines for physician intervention. *Annual Review of Medicine* 36: 51-61, 1985.

U.S. Department of Health and Human Services. *Clinical Opportunities for Smoking Intervention: A Guide for the Busy Physician.* U.S. Department of Health and Human Services; Public Health Service; National Institutes of Health; National Heart, Lung, and Blood Institute. PHS Publication No. (NIH) 86-2178, 1986.

U.S. Department of Health, Education, and Welfare. *Smoking and Health: A Report of the Surgeon General.* U.S. Department of Health, Education, and Welfare; Public Health Service; Office of the Assistant Secretary for Health; Office on Smoking and Health. DHEW Publication No. (PHS) 79-50066, 1979.

Vander Martin, R., Cummings, S.R., Coates, T.J. Ethnicity and smoking: Differences in white, black, Hispanic, and Asian patients who smoke. *American Journal of Preventive Medicine* 6(4): 194-199, 1990.

Wechsler, H., Levine, S., Idelson, R.K., Rohman, M., Taylor, J.O. The physician's role in health promotion: A survey of primary care practitioners. *New England Journal of Medicine* 308: 97-100, 1983.

Zahnd, E.G., Coates, T.J., Richard, R.J., Cummings, S.R. Counseling medical patients about cigarette smoking: A comparison of the impact of training on nurse practitioners and physicians. *Nurse Practitioner* 15(3): 10-18, 1990.

Physician and Dentist Interventions For Smoking Cessation[4]

Stuart J. Cohen, George K. Stookey, and Sue A. Kelly

BACKGROUND As a result of funding from the National Cancer Institute, parallel studies involving primary care physicians and private-practice dentists were initiated in August 1984. The goal of the projects was to develop, validate, and evaluate practical methods to help physicians and dentists encourage their patients to stop smoking cigarettes and remain nonsmokers. The studies were designed in two stages. The first stage involved efficacy studies to determine which office-based interventions had the greatest impact. For the second stage, effectiveness studies were conducted to determine whether office staff would adopt and incorporate into routine care the interventions that had been successful elsewhere and whether the results from the interventions supported by the office staff would be comparable to the results obtained in practices receiving the support of the research project staff. This paper describes the stage I and II studies involving physicians and the parallel studies with dentists in private practice.

PHYSICIAN INTERVENTIONS

Purpose of Project: Stages I and II

The goal of the stage I project was to develop, validate, and evaluate practical methods to help physicians encourage their patients to stop smoking cigarettes and remain nonsmokers. To determine the most effective intervention method, participating physicians and their patients who smoked cigarettes were randomly assigned to one of the following conditions: (1) control (usual care), (2) nicotine polacrilex available to patients at no charge, (3) a reminder system for following a practical protocol to help patients stop smoking, or (4) both nicotine polacrilex and the reminder system.

The purpose of the stage II trials was to determine the extent to which the "best" smoking cessation intervention identified in stage I was adaptable and generalizable to medical office settings. When stage II began, the stage I trials still had 1 year of data collection remaining; therefore, the "best" intervention method for stage II was determined according to data developed during the first 20 months of stage I. Preliminary analysis of these data determined that for the physicians, all three interventions were equally effective and each was better than the control (Cohen et al., 1989b). However, for the dentists, the nicotine polacrilex intervention either alone or with the reminders was the "best" method (Cohen et al., 1989a). To keep the physician and dentist stage II studies parallel, the method selected as "best" was the nicotine

4 Supported by National Institutes of Health grant no. R01-CA38337.

polacrilex (group 2 from stage I). In stage II, new cohorts of participating physicians and their panel of patients who smoked were randomly assigned to one of three intervention conditions: (1) control (usual care), (2) nicotine polacrilex program supported by project staff (as in stage I), or (3) nicotine polacrilex program supported by office staff.

Stage I Components

Target Audience And Clinical Setting

The stage I cohort involved 97 residents in internal medicine and 15 faculty general internists who staffed the outpatient general medicine clinic of a city/county teaching hospital. The outpatient clinic was structured so that physicians could provide continuity of care to their patients. A computerized scheduling system increased the likelihood that the same physician-patient dyad would remain together throughout the duration of a physician's residency in the program. The clinic was divided into four different areas or teams, each with its own nurses, clerks, and panel of physicians. To foster the research mission of the clinics and to minimize selection bias, all new patients were randomly assigned to available patient slots across teams, as were new physicians. For the stage I study, the intervention conditions (four groups) were randomly assigned such that each team was assigned to one condition only.

The ambulatory clinics served a predominantly indigent patient population. Patients were eligible for participation in the study if they were between the ages of 18 and 64, reported smoking one or more cigarettes daily, and had an alveolar breath carbon monoxide determination of more than 8 parts per million. Patients were excluded if any of the contraindications for the use of nicotine polacrilex pertained. The sociodemographic characteristics of the 1,420 patients who agreed to participate (the refusal rate was less than 5 percent) were as follows: the mean age was 46.2 (SD 11.6); the mean number of office visits per year was 2.2 (SD 2); 39 percent were white, and 61 percent black; 63 percent were female; the median education level was 10th grade; and the median annual income was $2,500.

Recruitment Procedures

The stage I physicians were all affiliated with the Department of Medicine at Indiana University School of Medicine. The project had the expressed support of the chairman of that department, as well as the section chief of the Division of General Internal Medicine. Consequently, there was considerable pressure to participate in the study, and no one refused. When senior residents left at the end of their program, their panel of patients was retained in the appropriate study condition and assigned to the incoming replacement physician. The replacement physician was oriented into the appropriate study condition and became the physician of record. Rarely did patients change physicians. In the event that a patient was transferred to a physician in a different study condition, the patient was removed from the study but was retained in the data analysis up until the time of removal (e.g., included in 6-month data on smoking status but not in 12-month analysis if the transfer occurred before the 12-month interval).

Specially trained research assistants conducted patient recruitment after an extensive training program in how to approach and interview patients. The research assistants memorized a script that explained to patients the purpose of the study and the fact that people who agreed to participate were agreeing only to have their smoking status assessed; participation did not require an attempt to quit smoking. Each research assistant role-played interviewing and recruiting the other research assistants, who in turn role-played patients who were illiterate, uncooperative, or too ill to be interviewed. Each research assistant spent at least 2 weeks working with his or her assigned clinic teams to learn the entire office system before contacting any patients for recruitment into the study. All patients were screened for eligibility for the study, and they signed an informed consent form that indicated that their smoking habit would be monitored at each regularly scheduled clinic visit regardless of their decision to quit or to continue smoking. Patients were notified that they would be asked to provide a breath sample for carbon monoxide analysis at each regularly scheduled clinic appointment and to answer questions immediately after seeing their physician.

Nature of Training Program

The training program for physicians consisted of two parts: a 1-hour lecture during medical grand rounds and then a special in-clinic followup session to orient each team to its specific study condition. The intent of the first part of the training program was to provide a common educational background on smoking and its management. Because each of the four intervention methods involved different procedures, the physicians received the condition-appropriate orientation at the start of their clinic sessions. The orientation lasted from 10 to 25 minutes, depending on the nature of the intervention. Prior to the grand rounds, all physicians completed a two-page attitude and practice questionnaire about their personal smoking histories, their current smoking management practices for patients, and their current interests and beliefs in effectively helping patients to stop smoking. The 1-hour general lecture presented evidence of the health consequences of smoking, the benefits of quitting, the addictive nature of nicotine, and the effect of nicotine polacrilex on smoking cessation. Also discussed was the available evidence that physicians' advice can be effective in helping counsel patients. Physicians were encouraged to use a four-step counseling protocol developed at the National Heart, Lung, and Blood Institute for counseling smokers: (1) Ask your patients about smoking; (2) deliver a firm quit-smoking message; (3) mutually agree on a quit date; and (4) check your patient's progress at each regularly scheduled visit. Physicians were also given a copy of a National Cancer Institute pamphlet, "Quit for Good," and were informed that copies would be provided to their offices for use with their patients who smoke.

The small group presentations centered on providing specifics for each intervention technique. Physicians in the control group were given a booklet containing the four-step protocol and were encouraged to counsel their patients who smoke. Neither the physicians nor their staffs were informed as to which of their patients had agreed to participate in the project. Physicians in the other three study conditions (nicotine polacrilex, reminders, both nicotine polacrilex and reminders) received the same instructions as the control group plus additional instruction based on their assigned experimental condition.

For the nicotine polacrilex group, physicians were instructed on the use of fluorescent red stickers to flag the charts of patients who were eligible to receive the nicotine replacement product. Physicians were told that research assistants would place the stickers and remove them after the patient had received the product. The uses, indications, contraindications, and side effects of nicotine polacrilex were discussed in detail. Research assistants dispensed the product at no cost when it was requested by a physician for an eligible patient (i.e., one with an appropriate sticker on the chart and a medication request initialed by the physician). The education of the patient as to the use of the nicotine substitute remained the responsibility of the physician or his or her designee. Physicians were also encouraged to record on the patient's chart when the product had been dispensed.

In the reminder condition, physicians were instructed on the use of two fluorescent chart stickers to help remind them to follow the four-step protocol. A green sticker was used to remind them to ask the patient about smoking, and an orange sticker reminded them to ask the patient to set a quit date. Physicians were informed that a feedback report issued to them bimonthly would provide the names of smoking patients they identified as well as the quit dates they established with their patients.

Physicians in the combined condition (nicotine polacrilex plus reminder) received instruction on the use of all three stickers.

Results

Table 14 shows how physicians behaved under each of the interventions (Cohen et al., 1989b). The impact of the interventions on the smokers is shown in Tables 15 and 16.

Because cigarette smokers often quit smoking and later have relapses, the prevalence of smoking was estimated for two subsequent periods. The prevalence of smoking at 6 months was defined as the smoking status determined at any visit that occurred at least 3 months after the initial appointment but not more than 9 months after it. The second estimate was at 1 year, defined as at least 9 months and 1 day after the initial visit and up to 15 months after the initial visit. If there was more than one visit during a time interval, the smoking status was determined by the status of the last visit during that interval. For patients who had a regularly scheduled appointment during the critical period, their smoking status was confirmed through carbon monoxide assessment, the procedures for which are described elsewhere (Stookey et al., 1987). Patients who did not visit a physician during the 6- or 12-month period were assumed to be smokers. Thus, the results are

Table 14
Reported physician counseling about cigarette smoking

	Percentage of Patients Reporting Actions		
	Asked About Smoking	Advised To Quit	Asked About Setting a Quit Date
Physician Group			
Advice	41%	27%	2%
Gum	84	61	10
Reminder	75	66	33
Both	95	84	58

Table 15
Confirmed success rates at the 6-month visit for each physician intervention[a]

	Percentage, Returnees Only (n=895)	Percentage, All Enrollees (n=1,420)
Physician Group		
Control	1.3%	0.9%
Reminder	7.0	4.2
Gum	7.7	5.0
Both	6.3	3.8

[a] *A generalized linear model was applied separately to returnees only and to all enrollees. The significant p values were 0.005 for the reminder by gum interaction for both analyses.*

Table 16
Confirmed success rates at the 12-month visit for each physician intervention[a]

	Percentage, Returnees Only (n=764)	Percentage, All Enrollees (n=1,420)
Physician Group		
Control	2.7%	1.5%
Reminder	15.0	7.9
Gum	8.8	4.7
Both	9.6	5.2

[a] *A generalized linear model was applied separately to returnees only and to all enrollees. The reminder by gum interaction was significant for returnees only (p=0.002) and for all enrollees (p=0.004).*

reported both for returnees, for whom biochemical validation was possible, and for all enrollees, based on the assumption that a patient was a smoker unless there was biochemical evidence to the contrary.

The range of patients per physician who quit at the 6-month interval was zero to three and at the 12-month interval was zero to four. Thus, smoking cessation by patients was widely distributed across physicians and not clustered into the practices of a few "effective counselors." A generalized linear model was used to analyze the results of the quit-smoking rates. The 6-month results are shown in Table 15. There was a significant negative interaction between nicotine gum use and reminders, both for returnees and for all medical patients. The combination of nicotine gum and reminders did not produce a higher rate of patients who quit smoking than the rate for either condition alone. Pairwise comparisons among the groups (adjusted for multiple tests with the Bonferroni inequality) showed a significant difference ($p < 0.05$) between each of the three intervention groups and the control group for analyses based on patients who had a scheduled return visit and for all patients.

The results at 1 year, shown in Table 16, also produced a significant negative interaction between nicotine gum and reminders. Pairwise comparisons among the groups showed that the three intervention groups were not significantly different from each other; however, each of them was significantly different from the controls for analyses based on returnees and on all patients. (For greater detail, see Cohen et al., 1987 and 1989b, and Stookey et al., 1987.)

Special Resources Or Procedures

For a program of this size, involving 112 physicians, lasting 3 years, and involving more than 1,400 patients, special resources were necessary to achieve sufficient cooperation from the general medicine clinics. Most critical was the use of research assistants who were permanently based in the clinics. Although there were four clinic teams and four research assistants, the responsibilities of the research assistants were divided so that they worked with one team 2 days a week and with another team 3 days a week. This was done so that there was always a backup person familiar with the operational procedures of each team. This rotation also helped dissipate any effect that a particular research assistant might have on patient recruitment or implementation of the study conditions.

For stage I, given the emphasis on training only the physician rather than the office staff, research assistants concentrated their efforts on integrating the program into the regular office routines. This was accomplished in two ways. First, each research assistant spent 2 weeks as an apprentice with his or her designated team, learning all of the office routines and helping with minor chores. For example, the research assistant would occasionally volunteer to assist the check-in clerk or the nurses with clerical duties such as filing charts or helping patients complete registration forms. This work not only relieved the office staff of these tedious tasks but also provided the research assistant with an opportunity to blend the program functions into the regular office routine. While research assistants were helping to file charts, they were able to find the best occasion to place stickers on the charts of newly recruited patients.

The working relationship that developed among the office staff helped facilitate program implementation. As part of their job responsibilities and throughout the study, when research assistants had free time available, they were expected to help the clinic staff in performing chores that would not interfere with their primary responsibilities. This system of volunteerism helped reduce occasions during which the clinic staff members were overburdened and the research assistants were idle. Conversely, when too many study patients were in the clinic for the research assistant to manage at one time, the office staff would often keep the patients occupied until the research assistant could see them. This system of reciprocity helped to build a supportive relationship between the project and the clinic staff.

Barriers or Problems Overcome

There were few problems to address in the stage I study. In all cases, the research staff learned to adjust to the demands of the clinic setting. For example, the research assistant usually tried to enroll patients before they were seen by the physician. However, whenever an examining room became available, a patient was taken to that room even if the research assistant was in the middle of explaining the study. Some of these procedures were established initially by the clinic directors, but other procedures evolved as more efficient ways of operating became evident.

The training of new office personnel presented some problems. Each year as interns replaced senior residents, about one-third of the physicians were new to the clinic. The training of all new physicians was done by blocking out time in the patient schedule for orientation instructions that lasted from 15 to 30 minutes, depending on the intervention condition. The physicians, in turn, were expected to educate their new staff members on the components of the program, but they often relied on the research assistant to educate new members. Not only were new staff members not trained for their responsibilities in the program, but also many were not informed of the program on accepting the position. Changes in personnel usually slowed the progress of implementing the smoking cessation program. The orientation of new physicians was given by one of the senior research staff members. Followup instruction usually was provided by a research assistant.

One effort to minimize confusion about the nature of the study was the use of a one-half page yellow sheet presenting the goal of the project, the eligibility and exclusion criteria for patients, and a telephone number to call if there were questions. This information was posted on the bulletin board above each physician's desk in the staffing rooms. Despite a careful effort to explain that the research assistants were not smoking counselors, some physicians attempted to refer their patients to the research assistants for help in quitting. Such requests usually resulted in a re-explanation of the program for the physicians.

Stage II Components

Target Audience And Clinical Setting

The second cohort of physicians consisted of 39 general internists and family physicians who saw adult medicine patients at 5 sites of a freestanding HMO serving central Indiana. At the start of the stage II study, more than 80,000 patients were active enrollees in the 9 sites of the HMO. Each of the five largest HMO sites participating in the project contained two adult medicine clinics. Each adult medicine clinic had its own check-in clerk, nurses, physician assistants, and physicians. Patients were scheduled to see a primary health care provider only within their designated clinic. The interventions were assigned such that at each site two different interventions were conducted, one at each clinic. All combinations of two of the three study conditions were determined and then randomly assigned to each of the five sites of the HMO. This procedure helped offset the fact that there could be differences in the sociodemographic characteristics of the patients, depending on the location of the site they visited for care. For the most part, those patients enrolled in the HMO were from working class or professional class backgrounds.

Recruitment Procedures

Stage II was initiated 1 year before the completion of the 3-year stage I study. The HMO's medical director and director of adult medicine were enthusiastic supporters of the project. Through their efforts, all physicians in adult medicine were notified about the project during a routine monthly staff meeting and asked to share any concerns or reservations about participation in the study. The only concern that physicians voiced was the extent to which their workload would be affected. They were assured that the study was designed to help them clearly identify which of their patients were smokers and that they would then determine the extent to which counseling was appropriate as part of those patients' visits. All physicians were also informed that they were expected to attend a site-specific special orientation meeting. At each of the five sites, the nurse manager was recruited to serve as the project liaison during a special meeting held with the principal investigator of the project and the chief of adult medicine at the HMO. The function of the liaison was to help arrange the logistics of integrating the project into the routines of that site. No additional compensation was offered for that effort.

Unlike the orientation in stage I, stage II orientation emphasized the level of team commitment required of the office staff. Project orientation luncheons were held at each site and included physicians, nurses, other health care providers, receptionists, medical records clerks, and other pertinent support staff. The chief of adult medicine stressed the importance of the project in terms of the benefits to patients at the HMO. He also noted that what staff members were being asked to do should be considered the standard for good care. No one overtly refused to participate in the study.

Nature of Training Program

The educational seminar used a format similar to the stage I training session. Physicians completed an attitude and practice questionnaire at the beginning of the meeting. A general orientation seminar on smoking and its management was followed by the breakup of the group into two smaller groups to discuss the details of the particular intervention.

The first half of the program lasted about 30 minutes and included the same information as the stage I general seminar but emphasized the team approach. The team approach required the involvement of most staff members, in particular the check-in clerk and the nurse manager. In addition, physicians were encouraged to tailor the smoking cessation program to maximize the resources, skills, and interests of the team. At all sites, the site nurse manager was asked to serve as a program coordinator and to be responsible for maintaining the program and providing communication between the office staff and research personnel.

During the general seminar, the emphasis was on specific techniques for physicians to use when counseling their patients who smoke. A videotape, developed at the University of California at San Francisco, was used to show physicians talking with patients about smoking. Shown is an interaction to assess a patient's interest in quitting, establishing a quit date, and receiving educational materials and encouragement. Also shown is an interaction between a physician and a patient who had made a quit attempt and then relapsed before the office visit. One segment depicts a conversation with a patient who is interested in discussing exercise but not smoking. The videotape illustrates a positive, nonthreatening approach to smoking counseling. For example, rather than lecturing patients and emphasizing the health consequences of smoking, the physician role models engage in asking questions such as, "Have you thought about quitting?" and "Are you ready to make another quit-smoking attempt?" The vignettes illustrate how to tailor the counseling for patients who have varying degrees of interest in stopping smoking. Physicians were encouraged to use these skills with their patients who smoke.

At the conclusion of the general seminar, attendees were given a copy of the "Quit for Good" pamphlet. They were informed that copies would be provided at no charge for their patients who smoke.

During the second half of the instructional program, specific techniques pertaining to each intervention condition were outlined and discussed. Persons in the control group were given the same booklet as was given the stage I group, and they were encouraged to follow the step-care protocol for counseling their patients who smoke. Those in the other two interventions received the same instruction as the control group plus additional instruction based on their assigned condition.

Those individuals in the free nicotine polacrilex group supported by research staff were instructed in basically the same manner as their counterparts in stage I. They were informed that red fluorescent stickers would be placed by research assistants on the charts of patients who were eligible to receive the nicotine replacement product. Physicians were made aware that the stickers would be permanently removed once the product had been prescribed. The uses, indications, contraindications, and side effects of nicotine polacrilex were discussed in detail. This small group instruction took about 20 minutes.

Physicians assigned to the nicotine polacrilex prescription method supported by office staff were instructed on the use, indications, contraindications, side effects, and recordkeeping procedures for nicotine polacrilex in a manner identical to the free-product group described above. However, because the purpose of this trial was to determine the feasibility of having a physician and his or her office staff carry out the step-care protocol of a cessation program with only minimal support from the research team, this group of participants was taught how to perform the procedures needed to support the program on their own. Instead of offices being provided with free nicotine polacrilex to dispense to patients, this group was instructed on how to prescribe the product and instruct patients in its use. Staff members were provided with a one-page handout about use of nicotine polacrilex, which reviewed basic information such as "quit smoking before starting to use the product." Office staff members (usually check-in clerks) were instructed to insert a copy of the handout in the chart of all eligible patients and to review the items with them when nicotine polacrilex was prescribed. Check-in clerks were instructed in the method for placing stickers on the charts of eligible patients. They were informed that the research assistant permanently assigned to their site would provide a list of patients recruited that week who were eligible for a prescription and who should have a sticker placed on their chart. Research assistants periodically checked charts to determine if stickers had been placed. As with the second group, physicians or their designees were encouraged to review the product usage instructions with the patient and to record in the chart when the product had been prescribed. Those physicians and staff members unable to attend the regular orientation meeting were given a personalized presentation before their involvement in the project. This was required for approximately 15 percent of the staff, and 15 to 20 minutes were scheduled before the morning or the afternoon clinic for this small group orientation.

Results

To determine the extent to which the office staff performed the tasks requested of them, the research staff examined the office charts of the patients enrolled in the study. In comparison with the 100 percent of charts that were flagged in the research-support condition, only 43 percent of the charts were flagged in the office-staff condition, and only 31 percent of appropriate charts had nicotine polacrilex instruction sheets attached to them. These results were much lower than anticipated and could be attributed in part to the numerous changes in management and high staff turnover of the HMO during the course of the project.

Not surprisingly, the behavior of the physicians in counseling smokers was affected by the intervention condition. Office exit interviews of patients showed that 44 percent of control group patients, 41 percent of office-staff patients, and 61 percent of research-support patients reported that their physician had talked to them that day about smoking. Also, the percentages of patients who were given or prescribed the nicotine substitute were 15 percent, 22 percent, and 39 percent, respectively, for the control, office-staff, and research-support conditions. Neither the 6- nor 12-month smoking cessation results produced statistically significant differences among the three groups.

Special Resources Or Procedures

In stage II, the emphasis was on working with the entire office staff in a team approach. Developing a rapport with the entire office was a major priority. Research assistants worked at making staff members feel that they were an integral part of the success of the program. In addition, for each HMO site, the nurse manager who already had supervisory responsibility for most of the office staff was designated as the office program coordinator. Communication on specific program details was relayed through the program coordinator. In return, any problems or concerns regarding the in-office mechanisms of the program were communicated to the research staff through the program coordinator. The use of this new position was vital for clarifying the lines of communication and avoiding the misunderstandings that sometimes occurred during stage I. For example, some of the stage I physicians did not want the research assistants to start interviewing patients about study participation until patients had finished their visit with the physicians. Other physicians did not care, so long as their patient flow was not interrupted. A program coordinator would have been helpful in establishing appropriate procedures to reduce potential conflict between the research assistants and clinic staff.

As in stage I, the research assistants were solely responsible for recruiting patients who smoked into the study and obtaining signed informed consent forms. Research assistants were responsible also for conducting all patient exit interviews after patients had been seen by their health care provider and for biochemically verifying the smoking status of those who claimed that they were no longer smoking cigarettes or using other tobacco products.

Barriers or Problems Overcome

Stage II presented some new barriers that had not existed in stage I. Before the study was initiated, the HMO had been locally owned and operated for 13 years. During the 3-year course of the study, the HMO changed management three times. These changes, and the uncertainties they produced, created problems such as low staff morale and subsequent high staff turnover. In this context, the requirements of the study, such as flagging charts of smokers, frequently became viewed as an additional burden and source of frustration.

These changes placed additional demands on the diplomacy of the research assistants. In some cases, research assistants took office staff members to lunch. Also, in an effort to engender rapport and support, research assistants contributed to all office social events, such as pitch-in lunches. Despite these efforts, the requirements for maintaining an office-based smoking cessation program, such as flagging charts and having an instructional system in effect, were never made part of the job descriptions and responsibilities of the new staff. Had such changes occurred, some of the problems caused by high staff turnover might have been prevented.

What Worked And Why

Much of the success of stage I can be attributed to the support of the directors of the general medicine clinic. They made sure that all new physicians were aware of the project and its importance to the Department of Medicine, making the task of orientation much easier for the research staff.

The fact that much of the logistical support (e.g., putting stickers on charts and attaching nicotine polacrilex instruction sheets to the charts of eligible patients) was performed entirely by the research assistants probably expedited their receptivity by the clinic staff. Another essential ingredient for success was the ability of the research assistants to work without disrupting the routines of the clinic. In time, they became viewed as part of the staff in their teams. When the project concluded, there were requests for them to stay and work as regular staff members on their respective teams.

For stage II, the initial attempt to create a team spirit and orientation appeared to be successful. Having one staff member in each practice serve as the program coordinator expedited communication with the office. Unfortunately, the subsequent frequent changes in management made the continuation of this approach difficult, if not impossible. The coordinators' efforts were shifted toward dealing with morale problems and training new clinic staff members in their routine functions. Thus, little time was left to help resolve problems pertaining to the study. Obviously, medical practices that are in flux are poor candidates for taking on additional projects. However, determining in advance which practices will remain stable is easier said than done. The general principle is that the best predictor of future behavior is past behavior. Thus, for subsequent projects, an examination of staff turnover rates could be helpful in determining which practices to select and which to avoid.

What Did Not Work and Why

Obviously the concentration of the training on the physician in stage I, compared with training the office team in stage II, affected the rate of integration of the program into routine care. Physicians were simply too busy with patient care to concentrate their efforts on all the details of providing orientation to their staffs. The investigators' short-sighted approach to training was, in part, compensated by the continuing presence of the research assistant who often became the primary source for educating the office staff. Thus, for the second study, the investigators opted to provide orientation and training for the entire office staff and not just the physicians.

In stage II, the goal was to foster a team approach. Unfortunately, the unforeseen changes in management of the HMO in large part undermined that effort. The high staff turnover meant that much time was required by the research staff to ensure that new personnel received an orientation to the project. In hindsight, one additional step should be considered: namely, insist that the changes in responsibility required for the smoking cessation program become part of the written job description of all pertinent employees. Had that been done, the study might have fostered the continuity of effort and commitment to tasks required by the project coordinator, the check-in clerks, the nurses, and the physicians.

Another consequence of the changes in management was that the medical director and the director of adult medicine became absorbed with the logistics of changing administrative systems such as billing and reporting responsibilities and were diverted from providing the project with the additional support it needed. At one point, a new medical director was hired, and his first project-related action was to suspend the ongoing project and prevent the research assistants from gathering any information on the patients. About 2 weeks' work was lost. Reinstatement occurred only after one of the senior research staff and the director of adult medicine convinced the new director that patients participating had signed consent forms and that the project had been approved by the Institutional Review Committees of both Indiana University and the HMO.

What Would Be Done Differently Now

Two areas should be emphasized in implementing office-based smoking cessation programs. The first is the fostering of a team approach and a team spirit to implement the program. The second is the creation of conditions so that the program not only is integrated into routine care but also is sustained after the project support system is no longer present. Were the program to be implemented again, the investigators not only would continue to emphasize the team approach but also would concentrate more on having each of the roles involved in the office-based system for smoking cessation become clearly defined and part of the written job roles and responsibilities for appropriate office staff. Furthermore, one of the roles that needed to be assigned was that of instructor for new office staff members about their program responsibilities. Ideally, this instructional role would be the responsibility of the program coordinator.

One task that could have been performed better was the instruction of patients in the use of a nicotine substitute. To increase the likelihood of patients' adherence to the proper use of a nicotine substitute, free, individually packaged samples (from the manufacturer) could be provided to each office for trial use. This would allow the physician or other health professional to field questions concerning the correct usage of the product before the prescription is purchased.

Another task that could have been improved was the use of chart reminders. In both stages I and II, stickers were provided to flag the charts of patients who were smokers. When a chart did not have a sticker, it was not apparent whether the patient was a nonsmoker or had never been asked about smoking. Ideally, receptionists could be trained to use stickers that identify patients as smokers or nonsmokers. This system immediately distinguishes smokers from nonsmokers and identifies those patients whose smoking status has not yet been determined. This type of reminder system requires commitment on the part of the receptionist and office team, but it is an appropriate measure in determining long-term commitment by the practice to a smoking cessation program.

Because of the investigators' interest in having a sample size sufficient to test the hypotheses under investigation, they enrolled all practices interested in participating. Had this not been a research study, the investigators might have produced better results by establishing a certain number of prerequisites before allowing a practice to participate. Just as the time and effort to counsel smokers will produce maximal results with those most ready to change their behavior, so too the time and effort needed to train practices may be best spent with those most receptive to making changes. In making such a determination, it may be best to avoid offices that have a high level of staff turnover and to assess in advance the extent to which physicians and their office staffs have both the time and interest to establish a smoking cessation program as part of routine care. A preassessment questionnaire might identify those ready for change and those disinclined to change. For example, the physicians might be asked, "Are you willing to use office staff time to put smoking identifiers on all patient charts?" A question to front office staff might be, "Are you willing to put smoking identifiers on all patient charts?"

In working with physicians in future cessation programs, the nature of the training sessions could be modified to produce a more individualized training session. The office could be given a list of very specific job duties to be distributed to all staff members with the understanding that a commitment to each person's responsibilities is necessary to make the program work under a team approach. Specific emphasis would be placed on a team member's accepting the role of "trainer" when new office personnel are hired. This list would go one step beyond telling the office to make it a team commitment by demonstrating how the roles can be distributed. Also, group training in the office could be more effective than a large group session held away from the clinic environment. The general background seminar could still be accomplished through a large group program, but individual intervention techniques might be better demonstrated in smaller site visits to further personalize the program. Although these changes would increase considerably the time demands on the research team, the final payoff of increased team commitment would make the initial investment of time worthwhile.

DENTIST INTERVENTIONS

Purpose of Project: Stages I and II

The goal of the stage I project was to develop, validate, and evaluate practical methods to help dentists encourage their patients to stop smoking cigarettes and remain nonsmokers. To determine the most effective intervention method, participating dentists and their panel of patients who smoked cigarettes were randomly assigned to one of the following conditions: (1) control (usual care), (2) nicotine polacrilex available for patients at no charge, (3) a reminder system for following a practical protocol to help patients stop smoking, or (4) both nicotine polacrilex and the reminder system.

The purpose of the stage II trials was to determine the extent to which the "best" smoking cessation intervention method identified in stage I was adaptable and generalizable to private dental practice settings. When stage II began, the stage I trials still had 1 year of data collection remaining. Thus, the "best" intervention method for stage II was determined on the basis of data developed during the first 20 months of stage I. Preliminary analysis of these data for dentists determined that the nicotine polacrilex intervention alone or with the reminders was the "best" method, and it was, therefore, applied in stage II (Cohen et al., 1989b). In stage II, new cohorts of dentists in private practice and their panel of patients were randomly assigned to one of three intervention techniques: (1) control (usual care), (2) free nicotine polacrilex program supported by the project staff (as in stage I), or (3) prescription nicotine polacrilex program supported by the office staff.

Target Audience: Stages I and II

For both phases of the study, participation was limited to private dental practitioners who primarily treated adult patients on a regular basis. Thus, the participating dentists were general practitioners and periodontists. Excluded were dentists specializing in oral surgery, pedodontics, orthodontics, and removable prosthodontics.

Clinical Setting: Stages I and II

All participating dental offices were in Indianapolis and adjacent suburban areas. Practice size ranged from offices with single practitioners to clinic or group practices. The number of established patients, the number of staff members employed, and the use of a hygienist varied from office to office, as did the use of a recall system and a means for identifying smokers.

To minimize practice size as a potential bias source, offices were stratified on the basis of the number of eligible and interested practitioners at each site. They were then assigned to an intervention condition according to random permutations of four for stage I and random permutations of three for stage II.

Patients were eligible for participation in the study if they were between the ages of 18 and 64, reported smoking one or more cigarettes daily, and had an alveolar breath carbon monoxide determination of more than 8 parts per million. Patients were excluded if any of the contraindications for the use of nicotine polacrilex pertained.

The sociodemographic characteristics of the 1,027 stage I patients who agreed to participate (less than a 10-percent refusal rate) were as follows: the mean age was 37.1 (SD 10.4); the mean number of office visits per year was 1.2 (SD 1.2); 95 percent were white, and 4 percent black; 57 percent were female; the median education level was 1 year of college completed; and the median income was $40,000 annually.

Stage I Components

Recruitment Procedures

Procedures to recruit the dentists for participation in stage I began in August 1984. With names drawn from the American Dental Association's Directory of Practicing Dentists in Indianapolis, more than 350 letters of introduction, briefly explaining the proposed program, were sent to eligible area dentists. Two weeks later, a followup telephone call was made to each eligible dentist; 297 offices were reached by telephone and 92 expressed an initial interest in participating. Next, either the project coordinator or project dentist met with each practicing dentist to further discuss and describe their potential for participation. During this meeting, a brief overview of the project was given, and the role of the dentist in the program was emphasized; 54 dentists agreed to participate and signed up to attend the educational seminar.

The dentists were motivated to participate in the program for a number of reasons. One important factor was the encouragement of the chairman of the Department of Preventive Dentistry, a long-term advocate for a more active role by dentists in smoking cessation. In general, those dentists who had a sincere interest in working with the researchers and in developing a successful cessation program for their offices adapted best to the program components and maintained an organized program throughout the study period.

Patient recruitment was conducted by specially trained research assistants. All patients were screened for eligibility for the study (see "Clinical Setting," above). Patients signed an informed consent form that indicated their smoking habit would be monitored at each regularly scheduled clinic visit, regardless of their decision to quit or to continue smoking. Patients were notified that they would be asked to provide a breath sample for carbon monoxide analysis at each regularly scheduled dental appointment and to answer questions immediately after seeing their dentist.

Nature of Training Program

Except for logistics, the training program for dentists was essentially identical to that provided for physicians. To accommodate the dentists from the practicing community, the lecture seminar was offered on four different dates: two afternoon sessions and two evening sessions. The first half of the program was intended to provide a common educational background on smoking. Because each assigned intervention method involved different procedures, the dentists went to one of four smaller group sessions during the second half of the seminar. Separate presentations were given to each group to review the appropriate procedures for each assigned intervention.

At the beginning of the general lecture, all dentists completed a two-page attitude and practice questionnaire concerning their personal smoking histories, their current smoking management practices for patients, and their current interests and beliefs in effectively helping patients stop smoking. The 1-hour general lecture presented evidence of the medical consequences of smoking, the benefits of quitting, the addictive nature of nicotine, and the effect of nicotine polacrilex on smoking cessation. Also discussed was the available evidence that dentists' advice could be effective in counseling patients. Dentists were encouraged to use a four-step counseling protocol developed at the National Heart, Lung, and Blood Institute for counseling smokers: (1) Ask your patients about smoking; (2) deliver a firm quit-smoking message; (3) mutually agree on a quit date; and (4) check your patients' progress at each regularly scheduled visit. Dentists were also given a copy of an NCI pamphlet, "Quit for Good," and were informed that copies would be provided to their offices for use with their patients who smoke.

The small group presentations centered on providing specifics for each intervention technique. Dentists in the control group were given a booklet containing the four-step protocol and were encouraged to counsel their patients who smoke. Dentists in the other three methods received the same instruction as the advice method plus additional instruction based on their assigned experimental condition. Information and handouts provided to the dentists were physician-based materials because dentist-based materials were not available at that time. The dentists had little resistance to using the materials and were able to adapt the physician-oriented information to their context.

Dentists in the nicotine polacrilex group were instructed on the use of fluorescent red stickers to flag charts of patients who were eligible to receive the nicotine replacement product at no cost. Dentists were told that research assistants would place the stickers and remove them after the patient had received the product. The uses, indications, contraindications, and side effects of nicotine polacrilex were discussed in detail. Offices were provided with product log books to record when nicotine gum was dispensed, and dentists were encouraged to record on the patient's chart when the product was dispensed. It was mandated that the product be stored in a safe, locked place.

In the reminder condition, dentists were instructed on the use of two fluorescent chart stickers to help remind them to follow the step-care protocol. A green sticker was used to remind them to ask the patient about smoking, and an orange sticker indicated that they should ask the patient to set a quit date. Dentists were informed that a feedback report issued to them bimonthly would provide the names of smoking patients they identified as well as the quit dates they had established with their patients. Unfortunately, it seemed that many feedback reports were not read or were ignored by the dentists. It is unlikely that the reports had any great impact on the dentists' behavior.

For the dentists in the combined condition (nicotine polacrilex plus reminder), instruction was given on the use of all three stickers and the dispensing and storing of nicotine polacrilex. For those dentists unable to attend any of the four seminars, a similar in-office presentation was given.

Approximately 1 week before the initiation of the intervention method in each office, a project director and research assistant assigned to that office (research assistants were assigned to an office on the basis of the office location—southwest, southeast, north) visited the office for a 1-hour meeting to review the record-keeping procedures and to answer any questions resulting from the general seminar. Initiation of offices was staggered for logistical purposes, to adequately train and monitor offices and to accommodate those offices that requested a delayed starting date. In-office training procedures began in October 1984, and all offices were initiated by April 1985. Three research assistants were employed to initiate and maintain the offices, allowing for each research assistant to be responsible for 14 to 17 offices throughout the study period. Of the 54 dentists trained, 50 actively participated in the program.

Results

The results of the study have been described in detail elsewhere (Cohen et al., 1987 and 1989b). The dentists' behavior under each intervention is shown in Table 17.

Because cigarette smokers often quit smoking and later relapse, the prevalence of smoking was estimated at two subsequent intervals. The first estimate (6 months) was defined as the smoking status determined at any visit that occurred at least 3 months after the initial appointment but not more than 9 months after it. The second estimate was at 1 year, which was defined as at least 9 months and 1 day after the initial visit and up to 15 months after the initial visit. If there was more than one visit during a time interval, the smoking status was determined by the status at the last visit during that interval. For patients who had a regularly scheduled appointment during

Table 17
Reported dentist counseling about cigarette smoking

	Percentage of Patients Reporting Actions		
	Asked About Smoking	Advised To Quit	Asked About Setting a Quit Date
Dentist Group			
Advice	31%	18%	3%
Gum	72	32	6
Reminder	59	29	14
Both	95	54	31

the critical period, their smoking status was confirmed through carbon monoxide assessment, the procedures for which are described elsewhere (Stookey et al., 1987). Patients who did not visit the dentist during the 6- or 12-month period were assumed to be smokers. Thus, the results are reported both for returnees, for whom biochemical validation was possible, and for all enrolled patients on the basis that a patient was a smoker unless there was biochemical evidence to the contrary.

A generalized linear model was used to analyze the results of the quit-smoking rates. The 6-month results are shown in Table 18. The generalized linear model for all enrollees produced borderline significant main effects for the gum group and for the reminder group. However, the coefficient for the reminder effect was negative. Statistically, this result is caused by the high cessation rates in the gum group coupled with the lower rate in the gum and reminder group. These rates for all returnees may not reflect the effectiveness of the intervention but may, in part, be artifacts of the number of patients who returned during the time window. Whereas those patients who did not return were classified as smokers, the cessation rate in both gum and reminder groups was depressed by a lower 6-month return rate (32.3 percent) than in the other groups (control 43.8 percent, reminder 43.3 percent, and gum 49.5 percent).

The results at 1 year are shown in Table 19. At 1 year, there was a significant effect of the gum for both those patients who returned during that time interval and for all patients. No other effects were significant.

Table 18
Confirmed success rates at the 6-month visit for each dentist intervention

	Percentage Who Quit	
	Returnees Only (n=428)	All Enrollees (n=1,027)
Dentist Group		
Control	7.1%	3.1%
Reminder	7.4	3.2
Gum	18.2	9.0
Both	9.4	3.0
	Generalized Linear Model Significant p Values	
Reminder	> 0.10	0.051
Gum	0.072	0.061

Table 19
Confirmed success rates at the 12-month visit for each dentist intervention

	Percentage Who Quit	
	Returnees Only (n=374)	All Enrollees (n=1,027)
Dentist Group		
Control	7.7%	3.1%
Reminder	8.6	2.8
Gum	16.3	7.7
Both	16.9	4.7
	Generalized Linear Model Significant p Values	
Gum	0.012	0.038

Special Resources Or Procedures

For a program of this size and intensity, special resources were necessary to achieve sufficient cooperation from the dental offices. Maintaining each office's motivation level and commitment to the program required constant attention from the research team.

In stage I, with program emphasis on the dentist rather than on the dental team, research assistants concentrated their efforts on implementing the program components, especially identifying patients who were smokers, and on providing open communication with the dentist. These two objectives proved difficult to achieve without the development of rapport between the research assistant and the office staff. Office staff members were often resistant to an outsider potentially disturbing their daily routine. Many were reluctant initially to include the research assistant as a working part of their program. It became apparent that the research assistants needed to find a way to integrate themselves and the program components into a regular part of the dental offices. This rapport development was crucial to the success of each office program.

The means to develop rapport varied with each office. In some offices, the research assistant would occasionally volunteer to assist the receptionist with clerical duties, such as filing or confirming patient appointments. This work not only relieved the receptionist of these tedious tasks but also provided the research assistant with an opportunity to blend the program functions into the regular office routine. While filing, the research assistant added stickers to the charts of newly recruited patients; while confirming appointments, the assistant obtained patients' smoking status. The working relationship that developed between the receptionist and the research assistant, and the subsequent routine implementation of the program components by the receptionist, soon led to a well-maintained smoking cessation program.

Personnel in some offices were not comfortable with having the research assistant help with clerical duties. In those offices, the research assistant tried to establish rapport with a specific staff member. Taking the time to make light conversation and to show an interest in the staff member gradually contributed to the development of trust between the two parties.

In other offices, the research assistant found a means to intercede with a solution to a current office problem. For example, one office was preparing to move and was struggling to find time to purchase file boxes to pack patient records. The research assistant surprised the office one afternoon by delivering a case of file boxes. This one simple gesture created a rapport with the office and prompted a newfound interest in the program. For the research assistant, finding a way to develop an essential positive rapport with the office was the most efficient way to assure smooth implementation of the program.

Barriers or Problems Overcome

Implementing a program of this nature led to the identification of a series of barriers or problems that needed to be overcome. Approaches initially anticipated to work often had to be adjusted to meet the demands of a given situation. For example, the logistics of covering offices from such a wide geographic area was anticipated to cause some difficulty with the requirement for research assistants to conduct an exit interview with every smoker to determine their status and the nature of the counseling they received. Initially, this problem was managed through reduction of the number of office sites; only group offices of two or more dentists each were recruited. When initial interest by some group practices decreased, single practitioner offices were then invited to participate. To help offset the increased site locations and provide a more even recruitment and followup schedule, dates for initiation of the program were staggered, and research assistants were assigned to a territory of Indianapolis to reduce travel time between sites as much as possible. Research assistants also carried voice pagers to relay messages from the research institute and eliminate the need for unnecessary travel to offices where a patient had failed to arrive or had canceled an appointment.

Another problem involved the slower than anticipated rate for identifying smokers in each dental practice and then subsequently recruiting them into the study. In stage I, dental offices were expected to identify and recruit 30 to 100 patients (an average of 40 patients per office) in an 8-month period. At 7 months into the program, only 471 of the anticipated 1,000 patients had been recruited in offices involved in the study. For those offices having difficulty in identifying patients who smoked, the research assistant and dentist met to discuss alternative ideas.

Originally, it was presumed most offices would have the smoking status indicated on the patients' charts. For those that did not, office staff members were expected to ask patients their smoking status over the phone when they confirmed recall appointments. However, in more than half the offices involved, smoking status was not available through the patients' records and the receptionists did not want to risk antagonizing patients by asking their smoking status over the telephone. The following suggestions were given to the dentist as alternatives for obtaining smoking status: (1) update each patient's medical history through the use of a new medical history form that included smoking status; (2) keep a running list of names in the operatory of patients who smoke as they were identified (hygienists had the best means for identifying smokers, through visible tar and nicotine stains at the time of the teeth cleaning); (3) have the dentist or hygienist check the appointment book each week to identify patients they recognized as smokers; and (4) have the research assistant stationed in the waiting room on a given afternoon each week to ask patients their smoking status as they arrived (given as a last choice because of constraints on the research assistant's time).

For those offices having difficulty with adjusting to the routine of a smoking cessation program and with overcoming their hesitancy to address patients about their smoking habit, a meeting was arranged among the dentist, research assistant, and project coordinator. An attempt was made to better tailor the program to each office's specific needs and to provide further ideas on approaching the patient about smoking.

In many cases these procedures, singly or in combination, catalyzed renewed interest in the program and resulted in an increase in the number of patients recruited. For those offices where a rapport was difficult or impossible to achieve, patient recruitment continued to be difficult.

Once the program had been initiated, a system was needed to identify followup appointments and to assess the smoking status of patients at 6 and 12 months after their recruitment date. The use of a 6-month preappointment recall system was presumed to be the means for obtaining followup interviews. The objective was to establish the patient's recall visit at the completion of the initial appointment. However, a wide range of office recall systems was used in the different offices. The following two systems were recommended: (1) the research assistant provided the receptionist with a list of patients due each month and the office staff, in turn, notified the research assistant when a patient scheduled an appointment (this was the weaker of the two systems because it mandated the cooperation of the receptionist in recognizing the participant and notifying the research assistant); and (2) the research assistant checked the appointment book weekly to determine if anyone in the study was scheduled for a recall appointment. The second method was preferred to the first but was not always permitted by the office staff. The second method also did not account for patients scheduling last-minute appointments. The best approach, still, was to develop a good rapport with the office staff to ensure cooperation with recall appointments. If a patient missed a recall appointment and the research assistant was notified about it within 24 hours, a followup interview over the phone was obtained.

The training of new office personnel also presented some problems. In stage I, the dentists were expected to educate their new staff members on the components of the program, but they often relied on the research assistant to do so. Not only were new staff members not trained for their responsibilities in the program, but also many were not informed of the program upon accepting their positions. A well-run recruitment and followup program could quickly be devastated by the arrival of an unwilling new employee. Research assistants took great pains to establish a rapport with new staff members. Treating the new employee to lunch to discuss participation in the program and carefully following progress each week helped to gradually reinstate the program to its original operation. Turnover in participating dental offices was high, and the retraining of new personnel was a continual responsibility of the research assistant.

Stage II Components

Recruitment Procedures

As previously stated, stage II was initiated 1 year before the completion of stage I. In August 1986, 354 dentists listed in the American Dental Association Directory and not currently participating in stage I were contacted by mail with a similar letter of introduction. Followup telephone calls found 53 dentists interested in meeting to further discuss the program. During meetings in the dentists' offices, the project coordinator explained the project goals, objectives, and procedures. Unlike the meetings in stage I, the level of team commitment required from the dental office was emphasized. The 42 dentists who agreed to participate were strongly encouraged to bring their staff members to the seminar.

Nature of Training Program

Dentists and their office staffs participating in the stage II program attended a seminar offered on one of four dates. This educational seminar used a format similar to the stage I training session. A general orientation seminar on the background of smoking opened the meeting and was followed by a breakout into three smaller groups for intervention training. Dentists also completed an attitude and practice questionnaire at the beginning of the meeting. Throughout the seminar, the dentists and office staffs were trained as a unit to emphasize team collaboration and commitment.

The first half of the program included the same information as the stage I general seminar but emphasized the team approach to a successful program. In stage I, it was observed that the hygienist often took the primary role of counselor, with the dentist providing reinforcement counseling and prescribing nicotine polacrilex when indicated. The team approach presented in the stage II seminar emphasized the involvement of staff members, in particular the hygienist, and encouraged the dentist to tailor the smoking cessation program to maximize the resources, skills, and interests of the dental team. The dentists were asked to assign an office coordinator to be responsible for maintaining the program and providing communication between the office and research personnel.

Experience in stage I showed that the mechanics of addressing the patient were a major concern for office personnel. The dentists and staff members were hesitant about addressing smoking with their patients. They were concerned about offending the patients and subsequently losing them from the practice. Therefore, during the stage II general seminar, specific techniques were illustrated for dentists to use when counseling the patients who smoke. A videotape developed at the University of California, San Francisco, was used to show physicians talking to patients about smoking. Shown is an interaction to assess a patient's interest in quitting, establishing a quit date, and receiving educational materials and encouragement. Also shown is an interaction between a physician and a patient who had made a quit attempt and then relapsed before the office visit. One segment depicts a conversation with a patient who is interested in discussing exercise but not smoking.

The videotape is very adaptable for the dental setting, and the taped interactions illustrate a positive, nonthreatening approach to smoking counseling. For example, rather than lecturing patients and emphasizing the health consequences of smoking, the physician role models ask questions such as, "Have you thought about quitting?" and "Are you ready to make another quit-smoking attempt?" The vignettes illustrate how to tailor the counseling for patients who have varying degrees of interest in stopping smoking. Dental teams were encouraged to use these skills with their patients who smoke.

After viewing the videotape, dental teams were encouraged to practice the techniques demonstrated on the tape. Despite the fact that the role models were physicians, the dental teams reported that the information was of great value to them.

At the conclusion of the general seminar, dentists and their office staffs were given copies of the "Quit for Good" pamphlet. They were informed that copies would be provided at no charge to their offices for patients who smoke.

During the second half of the seminar program, specific techniques pertaining to each intervention condition were outlined and discussed with the offices randomly assigned to those interventions. Dental practices in the control group were given the same booklet that the stage I group was given and were encouraged to follow the step-care protocol for counseling their patients who smoke. Dental practices in the other two interventions received the same instruction as the control group plus additional instruction based on their assigned condition.

Those persons in the free nicotine polacrilex method supported by research staff were instructed in basically the same manner as their counterparts in the stage I method. They were informed that red fluorescent stickers would be placed by research assistants on the charts of patients who were eligible to receive the nicotine replacement product. The dental teams were made aware that the stickers would be permanently removed once the product had been prescribed. The uses, indications, contraindications, and side effects of nicotine polacrilex were discussed in detail. The requirements for storing the product were also reviewed. Offices were provided with log books for recording when the product was dispensed, and participants were encouraged to enter on the patients' charts the date that the product was dispensed.

Offices assigned to the nicotine polacrilex prescription method supported by office staff were instructed on the use, indications, contraindications, side effects, and record-keeping procedures for nicotine polacrilex in a manner identical to the free-product group. However, because the purpose of this trial was to determine the feasibility of a dental team's carrying out the step-care protocol of a cessation program with only minimal support from the research team, this group of participants was taught how to perform the procedures needed to support the program on their own. This group was told that it was the responsibility of the office staff to take the provided stickers and label the charts of the patients listed on the enrollment roster. As stated in the results section, 77 percent of the charts were flagged by office staff as a result of the weekly roster of eligible patients.

Instead of offices being provided with free nicotine polacrilex to dispense to their patients, these offices were instructed on how to prescribe the product and were given a carbon-copy, prestamped prescription pad. The carbon copy allowed research personnel to periodically check when the product had been prescribed. Office personnel were instructed on the method for flagging the charts of eligible patients. They were informed that the research assistant would provide a list of patients recruited that week who were eligible for a prescription and who should have a sticker placed on their chart. The research assistant periodically checked charts to determine if stickers had been placed. As with the second group, dentists and hygienists were encouraged to review the product usage instructions with the patient and to record in the chart when the product had been prescribed. Those dentists and staff unable to attend any of the scheduled seminars (about 10 percent) were given a similar in-office presentation.

One week before each office began the study, the study coordinator and research assistant assigned to that office visited the office to deliver program material and review the program again with the dental team. Initiation of dental offices in stage II was again staggered for optimum recruitment and followup procedures. Of the 42 offices initially trained, 35 completed the program.

Results

To determine the extent to which the office staffs performed the tasks requested of them, office charts of the patients enrolled in the study were examined. In comparison with the 100 percent of charts that were flagged in the research-support condition, 77 percent of the charts were flagged in the office-staff condition.

Not surprisingly, the behavior of the dentists in counseling smokers was affected by the intervention condition. Office exit interviews of patients showed that 16 percent of control group patients, 20 percent of office-staff patients, and 34 percent of research-support patients (p=0.07) reported that their dentist had talked to them that day about smoking. Also, the percentages of patients given or prescribed the nicotine substitute were 6 percent, 14 percent, and 46 percent, respectively, for the control, office-staff, and research-support conditions ($p < 0.0001$). Neither the 6-month nor 12-month smoking cessation results produced statistically significant differences among the three groups, although the rates for the 12-month point were 3.1 percent, 6.9 percent, and 9.2 percent (p=0.10) for the control, office-staff, and research-support conditions, respectively.

Special Resources Or Procedures

In stage II, the work of the dental office as a team was emphasized. Developing rapport with the entire office was a major priority. Research assistants worked at making staff members feel they were an integral part of the success of the program. Some new procedures were integrated into stage II to aid implementation of the program. One such procedure was the requirement that one member of the office staff serve as the office program coordinator. Communication on specific program details was relayed through the office coordinator. In return, any problems or concerns regarding the in-office mechanisms of the program were communicated to the research staff through the office coordinator. The use of this new position was vital for opening the lines of communication and avoiding misunderstandings that arose in some of the offices involved in stage I.

Another procedure involved a scheduled weekly visit by the research assistant to the office. Regardless of the number of patients interviewed in each office in a given week, the research assistant made a visit to each office on the same day and time each week. The day and time were established by the office staff and then worked into the research assistant's schedule as closely as possible. This established a routine for the program and allowed staff members to share questions, concerns, or ideas about the program and present them to the research assistant at one time. Also at this time, and depending on the conditions mandated by the intervention technique assigned, the research assistant verified that there were ample supplies, checked the log book with the nicotine polacrilex count to determine if all of the product dispensed had been recorded, checked prescription pads to see if the product had been prescribed, and reviewed charts to see if stickers had been placed. The research assistant became a routine part of the office through the use of these weekly visits and, in addition, met with staff members once a month to field questions from the group as a whole. This fostered an exchange of ideas and emphasized the team approach to the program. The meetings lasted 10 to 15 minutes and usually were made a part of the regular monthly staff meeting. For those offices that did not hold regular monthly meetings and were unwilling to assemble as a group, the research assistant continued to conduct a monthly meeting with the office coordinator to discuss the program.

Incentives were also used as a new special resource in stage II. At the beginning of the recruitment period, offices were informed that a free lunch at a local restaurant would be awarded to each office that reached its quota for the number of patients recruited (i.e., 50 patients per dentist during the first year). The number of patients recruited to date was also reviewed at each staff meeting to continually motivate the teams toward their goal. For offices that were particularly struggling but making progress, coffee and donuts were given as an incentive to keep up the good will among the staff.

These special resources provided a vital connection in propelling the dental team toward a successful implementation of the smoking cessation program.

Barriers or Problems Overcome

There were fewer barriers and problems in stage II. Problems that had occurred in stage I could be anticipated and solved before they progessed in stage II. Continued emphasis was given to developing a rapport with the dental team, and approaches for handling familiar problems were refined. Problems such as high staff turnover and finding a means for determining patients' smoking status still occurred, but experience from stage I aided in the adoption of procedures discussed previously. No new problems surfaced in stage II that had not been confronted in stage I.

What Worked And Why

In stage II, the focus of a team approach brought together a group of interested staff members who all felt involved and consequently were more willing to work toward their goal. Those offices in which the program was most successful integrated the smoking cessation program with their office routine (Cohen et al., 1990). Those offices that never allowed the research assistant to get involved with their office routine never really integrated their programs. In successful offices, the research assistant was perceived as part of the office team. Dental staff turnover was great in many participating offices, and this hampered the ability of the research assistant to form a rapport with the team. To best sum up the success of this program, stages I and II required a dedicated research team, an interested dental team, and a trusting relationship.

What Did Not Work and Why

During stage I, the target of the intervention and training was the dentist. In stage II, it was the entire practice. The initial assumption, that dentists in stage I would orient and organize their staffs, proved faulty. The dentists were simply too busy to concentrate on orienting their staffs. Many tried to delegate their duties to a staff member, but a lack of communication often led to misunderstandings, and interest declined. Without the team approach, other staff members felt slighted and made no effort to become involved in the program.

There were some dental offices where the dentist did very well and accepted primary responsibility for the program. In most of these cases, however, the office had previously developed a true commitment to the values of the program and were motivated to succeed. Some dentists signed up for reasons other than the desire to help their smoking patients quit. These offices rarely developed successful programs (unless a motivated staff member, such as the hygienist, had enough influence and interest to keep the program going). In some cases, dentists later admitted becoming involved only to look good in the dental community or because they hoped to receive a free product to hand out to their patients.

What Would Be Done Differently Now

Two areas should be emphasized in implementation of office-based smoking cessation programs. The first is the fostering of a team approach and team spirit when implementing the program. The second is the creation of the conditions so that the program not only is integrated into routine care but also is sustained after the project support system is no longer present. Were the program to be implemented again, the investigators not only would continue to emphasize the team approach but also would concentrate more on clearly defining each of the roles involved in the office-based system for smoking cessation and including them as part of the written job roles and responsibilities for appropriate office staff. Furthermore, one of the roles needed was that of instructor for new office staff in their program responsibilities. Ideally, the instructor's role would be the responsibility of the office coordinator.

One task that could have been performed better was the instruction of patients in the use of a nicotine substitute. To increase the likelihood of the patient's adherence to the proper use of a nicotine substitute, free, individually packaged samples (from the manufacturer) could be provided for trial use in the office. This would allow the dentist or other health professional to field questions about correct use of the product before the prescription is purchased.

Another task that could have been improved was the use of chart reminders. In both stages I and II, stickers were provided to flag the charts of patients who were smokers. When a chart did not have a sticker, it was not readily apparent whether the patient was a nonsmoker or had never been asked about smoking. Ideally, receptionists could be trained to use stickers that identify patients as smokers or nonsmokers. They could immediately distinguish smokers from nonsmokers and identify those patients whose smoking status has not yet been obtained. This type of reminder system requires commitment on the part of the receptionist and office team but is an appropriate measure of long-term commitment by the practice to a smoking cessation program.

Because the investigators were interested in having a sample size sufficient to test the hypotheses under investigation, they enrolled all practices interested in participation. Had this not been a research study, the investigators might have produced better results by establishing a certain number of prerequisites before allowing a practice to participate. Just as the time and effort to counsel smokers will produce maximal results with those most ready to change their behavior, so too, the time and effort needed to train practitioners may be best spent with those most amenable to making changes. In making such a determination, it may be best to avoid offices that have a high level of staff turnover.

In future cessation programs involving dentists, the nature of the training sessions could be modified to produce a more personalized training session. The office could be given a list of very specific job duties to be distributed to all staff members with the understanding that a commitment to each person's responsibilities is necessary to make the program work under a team approach. Specific emphasis would be placed on a team member accepting the role of trainer when new office personnel are hired. This list would go one step beyond telling the office to make it a team commitment by demonstrating how the tasks can be distributed. Also, group training at the office would be more effective than in a large group session held away from the clinic environment. The general background seminar could still be accomplished through a large group program, but individual intervention techniques might be better demonstrated in site visits with small groups to further personalize the program. Although these changes would increase considerably the time demands on the research team, the final payoff of increased team commitment would make the initial investment of time worthwhile.

DIFFERENCES BETWEEN DENTAL AND MEDICAL PROGRAMS

In some respects, a dental practice is an easier environment for establishing a smoking cessation program as part of routine care. First, the purpose for most visits is prophylaxis, so patients start with a prevention orientation and often are not there for acute care. Another important factor is the amount of time a patient spends in the office. Most dental visits last from 30 minutes to 1 hour, whereas medical visits are often scheduled at 15-minute intervals. Thus, the time for adequate counseling is more available in most dental settings than in most medical settings. On the other hand, physicians perceive counseling patients about smoking as part of their clinical responsibility, while many dentists still are not comfortable with the role of smoking cessation counselor. This is demonstrated by many dentists having much greater interest in continuing education about smokeless tobacco than in cigarette smoking cessation.

Progress is continuing through a number of excellent dental team training programs conducted through the National Cancer Institute. The availability of materials tailored for the dental team appears to facilitate the willingness of dentists and their staffs to be involved in the national effort to make counseling about smoking cessation a routine part of health care.

REFERENCES

Cohen, S.J., Christen, A.G., Katz, B.P., Drook, C.A., Davis, B.J., Smith, D.M., Stookey, G.K. Counseling medical and dental patients about cigarette smoking: The impact of nicotine gum and chart reminders. *American Journal of Public Health* 77: 313-316, 1987.

Cohen, S.J., Kelly, S.A., Eason, A.A. Establishing smoking cessation programs in dental offices. *Journal of the American Dental Association* 20 (Suppl.): 28S-31S, 1990.

Cohen, S.J., Stookey, G.K., Katz, B.P., Drook, C.A., Christen, A.G. Helping smokers quit: A randomized controlled trial with private-practice dentists. *Journal of the American Dental Association* 118: 41-45, 1989a.

Cohen, S.J., Stookey, G.K., Katz, B.P., Drook, C.A., Smith, D.M. Encouraging primary care physicians to help smokers quit: A randomized controlled trial. *Annals of Internal Medicine* 110(8): 648-652, 1989b.

Stookey, G.K., Katz, B.P., Olson, B.L., Drook, C.A., Cohen, S.J. Evaluation of biochemical validation measures in determination of smoking status. *Journal of Dental Research* 66: 1597-1601, 1987.

The Tobacco Reduction and Cancer Control (TRACC) Program: Team Approaches to Counseling In Medical and Dental Settings[5]

Jack F. Hollis, Thomas M. Vogt, Victor Stevens,
Anthony Biglan, Herbert Severson, and Edward Lichtenstein

INTRODUCTION Physicians and dentists are effective smoking interventionists (Cohen et al., 1989a and 1989b; Cummings et al., 1989; Janz et al., 1987; Li et al., 1984; Ockene, 1987a; Wilson et al., 1988). Although surveys of physicians indicate that about half report advising "most" of their patients to stop smoking (Fortmann et al., 1985; Wells et al., 1984), the consistent success of controlled physician intervention studies emphasizes the need for improvements in smoking interventions delivered through the medical care setting. Wells and colleagues (1984) presented a model that related physician practices used in counseling smokers to personal habits, the reimbursement system, clinical training, motivation, perceived risk of smoking, perceived skill in counseling, and perceived benefit. To this model should be added the time constraints faced by so many physicians, particularly those in prepaid group practice settings.

Physician-delivered smoking interventions have distinct advantages and disadvantages. The advantages include the credibility of the physician, the teachable moment created by the juxtaposition of that credibility with an illness experience, and the potential for reinforcement of the intervention over many years. Disadvantages of physician interventions include inconsistent compliance by physician interventionists, variable levels of counseling skills, lack of training, lack of time, lack of incentive, and competition from more acute medical problems.

The Tobacco Reduction and Cancer Control program was designed as a mechanism for using the strengths of physician interventions while overcoming the disadvantages (Vogt et al., 1989). The general approach of TRACC has three steps: (1) randomized efficacy trials of intervention approaches; (2) demonstration studies of large-scale implementation; and (3) evaluation of the demonstration programs and dissemination to large medical care systems. TRACC was initiated in 1987 as a group of five randomized studies designed to determine effective methods for integrating

[5] Work on the TRACC program is supported by National Cancer Institute grant no. CA-44648.

smoking counseling into the medical care setting. It addressed interventions in outpatient, inpatient, and dental settings and included direct outreach to adolescents. TRACC interventions were, in most situations, introduced by providers but conducted by other appropriately trained medical personnel. Centralized systems identify smokers and also keep track of quit dates so that supportive followup calls can be made by trained phone callers. These approaches are applicable to other aspects of cancer control and behavior change as well. Currently, TRACC is completing step 1 (randomized efficacy studies) and is moving into a large-scale demonstration program. The following section discusses the approaches used in TRACC interventions and their impact on smoking behavior of patients in the Northwest Region of Kaiser Permanente, the Nation's largest managed care health maintenance organization.

NURSE-ASSISTED COUNSELING

Medical office smoking interventions generally rely on physicians to assess patient smoking status, provide advice and materials, determine readiness to quit, deal with barriers to change, and encourage patients to set quit dates and develop effective strategies for coping with withdrawal symptoms. Although motivated physicians with an appropriate training program and a well-organized system for monitoring and reinforcing physician compliance can significantly enhance cessation rates among patients (see reviews by Kottke et al., 1988; Ockene, 1987a; Pederson, 1982), it is less clear that such programs can be widely disseminated and easily sustained, especially in medical settings that are not research oriented.

In many primary care settings, physicians may spend only 15 minutes with the average patient. That time must be used to diagnose, discuss, and treat the presenting complaint; arrange needed referrals or routine screening; and respond to a variety of other patient concerns. As important as it is, smoking counseling frequently gets short shrift or is avoided altogether because of the pressures of acute care delivery. Physician-centered counseling also makes little use of nurses and other intervention resources available in clinical settings. Kottke et al. (1988) have concluded that various and repeated messages from all staff members through a number of communication channels constitute the most effective way to enhance impact.

Our initial aim was to develop a smoking intervention in the medical care setting for Kaiser Permanente, Northwest Region. To be practical, it had to be not only effective but also relatively easy to implement and sustain within a large managed care setting. We concluded that the intervention should contain the following components: (1) assessment of smoking status; (2) firm advice to stop smoking; (3) cessation videos, manuals, and mailings; (4) encouragement to set a specific quit date; and (5) a followup phone contact to check on progress. Assessment of smoking status at each visit highlights the importance of cessation to patients and is needed to direct intervention to those who need it. A physician's firm advice to quit takes advantage of his or her credibility and authority and creates a teachable moment. To reduce the burden on staff, information on cessation strategies and how to overcome barriers can be provided effectively and economically in the form of videos, manuals, and followup mailings. Patients who are ready to quit should be encouraged by staff to make a commitment to a personal action plan and select a specific quit date. To enhance perceived support and accountability, a followup call should be scheduled for 1 or 2 days after the quit date. Although all of these components may be helpful, we thought it unrealistic to expect that most primary care providers would consistently carry out all of these steps with their smoking patients. Instead, we decided to minimize the burden on the provider and test a team approach involving physicians, nurses, and other clinic staff.

The team approach to counseling offered several advantages over a physician-centered model. This approach took advantage of the physician's prestige and credibility to initiate the intervention process. Physician time and effort were minimized, however, by having nurses or other clinic-based staff reinforce the stop-smoking message, provide stop-smoking videos and manuals, encourage patients to set quit dates, and provide followup phone contacts. To reduce the burden on support staff, most of the motivational and educational information was delivered through manuals and videos tailored to the needs of the local patient population. Periodically, newsletters and other cessation materials were mailed by centralized clerks using a computerized patient tracking system.

The purpose of this project was to assess the feasibility and effectiveness of nurse-assisted outpatient smoking intervention procedures. The primary outcome was a comparison of the impact of physician-nurse team approaches to smoking counseling to brief physician advice alone. The study methods and findings are described below, and a more detailed presentation is available elsewhere (Hollis et al., 1991; Lichtenstein and Hollis, 1992).

Intervention Setting And Methods

Procedure

A phase III randomized clinical trial was carried out within two large Kaiser Permanente medical offices. All 60 internal medicine and family practice providers in the two medical offices were invited, and all participated in the intervention. The physician's role was simple; it included 30 seconds of clear advice to quit plus a referral to a nurse smoking counselor for additional intervention. Physician training was carried out in a single 1-hour meeting with some individual clinic followup. Training emphasized how to deliver brief cessation advice and refer patients to the clinic-based smoking counselor (e.g., a nurse). Role-playing, questions, and discussion were encouraged.

The nurse-delivered components were provided by several project staff members, headed by a lead counselor who was a nurse with no previous smoking cessation experience. Each counselor could handle the smoking patients of 16 to 20 physicians. The training for the counselors included role-playing from an intervention outline, observing a stop-smoking class, and several weeks of pilot testing. Others of the clinic staff were oriented to their roles during regular weekly staff meetings with some individual followup.

Receptionists asked all primary care patients to complete a brief health habits questionnaire while waiting for their appointments. Regular clinic nurses or clinical assistants collected the questionnaires as the patients were taken to exam rooms and attached a colored form to the medical chart of smokers to alert physicians to deliver the cessation advice and referral message.

Physicians delivered a 30-second stop-smoking advice message that was designed to minimize defensiveness and create a teachable moment. The form on the chart included the following script, but physicians were free to deliver the message in their own words:

> The best thing you can do for your health is to stop smoking, and I want to advise you to stop as soon as possible. I know it can be hard, and many try several times before they finally make it. You may or may not want to stop now, but I want you to talk briefly with our smoking specialist who has some tips to make stopping easier when you decide the time is right.

At the end of the visit, patients saw the on-site smoking counselor (i.e., a trained nurse). Two random digits in the patient's health record number were used to assign patients randomly to one of the following four conditions: advice only, self-quit training, group recruitment, or a combination treatment. Advice-only control subjects received the physician advice message and the brief National Cancer Institute pamphlet, "Why Do You Smoke?" Although little information on how to stop smoking was offered, clear and systematic physician advice was expected to be more effective than no treatment or usual care.

Self-quit subjects received physician's advice, and the nurse tested them for carbon monoxide. Patients were then left alone to watch a 9-minute video on how to quit on their own. The video was produced by Independent Video Services and Anthony Biglan, Ph.D., at the Oregon Research Institute, and it is available from Dr. Biglan. The video focuses on the steps other patients had used to quit successfully, the frequent need for repeated efforts, and the importance of setting a quit date and using substitutes for smoking. Patients were given a stop-smoking kit (e.g., gum, toothpicks, cinnamon sticks, quit tips) and a choice of one of three stop-smoking manuals (provided by the National Cancer Institute and the American Lung Association). Patients could also call a local stop-smoking hotline or attend a free 90-minute session on how to stop smoking, although those resources were almost never used. The counseling nurse also encouraged patients to set a specific quit date and a followup call was planned, usually within 2 to 4 weeks, to check on progress toward cessation. Finally, patients were mailed a set of stop-smoking tip s heets and, on request, a series of six attractive bimonthly newsletters devoted to smoking cessation.

Group-recruitment subjects also received physician advice, the carbon monoxide assessment, and a video. In this condition, the video encouraged patients to join the HMO's intensive nine-session stop-smoking program known as Freedom From Cigarettes (Stevens and Hollis, 1989). Patients were provided a brochure, a group schedule, and a time-limited coupon to waive the program fee. Patients were then invited to sign up for an upcoming group, and reminder postcards were sent 1 week prior to the scheduled meeting. The counseling nurse also called patients several days after the meeting to provide support for any progress.

Combination-treatment subjects also received advice, the carbon monoxide test, and a third video, which describes both self-directed cessation techniques and the pros and cons of joining a professionally run program. The self-help manual, stop-smoking kit, and the group materials and coupons were all provided. Subjects were encouraged to set a quit date or sign up for an upcoming group, and a phone call was arranged to check on progress. Tip sheets and the bimonthly newsletters also were provided.

Results

Recruitment

About 24 percent of this outpatient population reported smoking, and a total of 3,161 eligible smokers were identified over the year-long recruitment period. Of these, 2,707 (86 percent) received brief stop-smoking advice from a medical care provider. In this intent-to-treat design, all smokers who received physician advice were considered randomized subjects even if they failed to see the nurse for additional intervention. Fortunately, the vast majority of advised patients (87 percent) agreed to see the clinic counselor (Table 20). This rate was similar across the four groups. The four treatment conditions were similar also in terms of baseline age, sex, race, education, occupation, cigarettes per day, contemplation status, confidence in ability to quit, perception of weight status, and subjective health status.

Table 20
Cessation activities, by treatment condition

	Percentage in Treatment Condition				
	Advice Only	Self-Help	Group Recruitment	Combination Treatment	p <
Saw Counseling Nurse	89%	88%	85%	87%	0.06
Set a Quit Date	0	28	3	22	0.001
Attended Group Program	1	0	11	8	0.001

Acceptance of Intervention

Two-thirds of all randomized self-quit (69 percent), group-recruitment (68 percent), and combination-treatment (67 percent) patients completed a baseline carbon monoxide test as part of the intervention, and some what fewer saw the stop-smoking videos (63 percent, 57 percent, and 62 percent, espectively). Manuals and small, inexpensive "quit kits" were provided by hand (or mailed) to a majority of self-quit (91 percent) and combination-treatment (90 percent) patients. A brochure and fee waiver coupon for the group cessation program were accepted by 82 percent of group-recruitment patients, but only 60 percent of combination-treatment patients accepted. Table 20 also shows that 28 percent of all self-quit subjects agreed to set quit dates, usually within 2 to 4 weeks of the initial visit. It was our sense that encouraging patients gently to set quit dates was an important part of the process, and those who agreed to a specific quit date were significantly more likely to achieve abstinence than those who did not (16 percent vs. 11 percent, $p < 0.02$). About 11 percent of group-recruitment subjects attended at least one session of the HMO's intensive cessation program, but only 1 percent in the advice-only condition attended. Combination subjects chose a mix of cessation strategies.

Three months after the visit, subjects were mailed a brief survey and a subsequent reminder. Those who did not respond were contacted by phone and the survey was administered as a structured interview. The followup rates (88 percent) were similar across conditions.

At 3 months (Table 21), subjects in all three nurse-assisted conditions were significantly more likely to report one or more serious quit attempts than were those who received only physician advice. The three nurse-assisted conditions had similar abstinence rates (i.e., no cigarettes in the preceding week, with nonrespondents counted as smokers), and all three nurse-assisted interventions led to significantly higher quit rates (about 80 percent) than the rate for brief physician advice alone. Similar outcomes were noted when abstinence was defined as no tobacco use of any kind.

Table 21
Outcomes at 3-month followup

	Percentage in Treatment Condition				
	Advice Only	Self-Help	Group Recruitment	Combination Treatment	p <
Recalled Advice To Quit	56.4%	57.8%	60.8%	60.0%	NS
A Serious Quit Attempt	39.0	50.2	44.8	46.3	0.001
No Cigarettes in 7 Days[a]	7.6	12.9	14.1	13.0	0.001
No Current Tobacco Use[a]	6.2	11.0	12.0	10.6	0.002

[a] *Survey nonrespondents counted as smokers.*

Patients were asked on the baseline questionnaire if they were seriously interested in quitting in the next 6 months. Logistic regression analyses indicated that those contemplating quitting prior to intervention were significantly more likely to quit than were precontemplators, i.e., those not considering quitting (odds ratio=2.82, 95-percent confidence interval=1.95-4.08). However, contrary to our predictions, contemplation status did not interact with any of the three nurse-assisted treatment conditions. This indicates that the nurse-assisted interventions enhanced cessation equally for precontemplators and contemplators alike.

Discussion

About 3 to 5 minutes of physician counseling is an effective stop-smoking intervention, but many physicians find it difficult to consistently spend this amount of time in counseling. Team intervention approaches involving physicians, nurses, and other clinic staff offer two important advantages over traditional physician-centered approaches. First, they shift the time-consuming components of the intervention to other staff and to videos, thus facilitating physician participation in training and implementation. In this way, the approach minimizes what has been a major barrier to widespread dissemination of clinic-based smoking interventions. Furthermore, this shift does not produce a large burden for the nurse. With an organized system of information collection, physician referral, and use of videos, nurses can deliver the intervention in approximately 2 to 3 minutes of additional time per smoker. Second, relative to brief physician advice alone, the additional attention, support, and cessation tools provided by the clinic-based smoking counselor significantly enhanced both quit attempts and successful short-term abstinence. Preliminary analyses of 1-year followup data suggest that these positive effects are being maintained.

This study was unique in that it tested both a self-quit intervention and an approach designed to recruit smokers into an intensive stop-smoking class of the type that normally only a small minority of smokers (< 2 percent) are willing to use (Epstein et al., 1989; Ockene, 1987a and 1987b). In this intent-to-treat design, the abstinence rate for the group-recruitment condition included all subjects randomized to this treatment, whether they elected to attend the intensive program or not. Though actual attendance was modest (11 percent), it was 10 times greater than that for the advice-alone (1 percent) condition. Combination-treatment subjects received all intervention components. They chose a mix of cessation strategies but did no better than self-quit and group-recruitment subjects. Because all three nurse-assisted approaches similarly boosted the quit rates over physician advice alone, the most economical approach would seem most attractive. Analyses of cost-effectiveness are currently under way, but it is probable that training patients to quit on their own will be the easiest and least expensive to implement in most settings. However, heavier smokers may do better if referred to intensive stop-smoking programs, and some referral lists should be available.

As would be expected, patients who were seriously contemplating quitting prior to intervention were more likely than precontemplators to be abstinent 3 months later. We also expected that the nurse-assisted interventions would be more effective for contemplators than for precontemplators. There was no evidence that treatment interacted with contemplation status, however, and the nurse-delivered components increased quit rates roughly 80 percent for both contemplators and precontemplators alike. Still, because precontemplators were much less likely to quit, it may be worthwhile to tailor the intervention to the patient's level of readiness and to focus limited intervention resources on those who are seriously considering quitting in the near future.

Special features of this intervention that appeared to work well included the clinic team concept and the brief physician message that was so essential in gaining physician cooperation and consistency. Although it would certainly be useful for physicians with time and interest to do more of the smoking counseling themselves, even a minimal 30-second advice and referral message can be effective if a nurse can carry through with brief counseling immediately after the visit. The videos were also well received by staff as they reduced the time needed to motivate and teach patients how to quit. It was not possible to determine the separate impact of the videos on quit rates, but by reducing staff burden they may increase the chances of success. Another key element was the face-to-face contact with a trained and supportive nurse who provided strong encouragement to set a specific quit date in the near future.

Some aspects of the intervention did not work well. Receptionists did not hand out the lifestyle questionnaires consistently, and some patients did not complete the instrument. A better approach would be to have the nurse simply ask for smoking status when placing the patient in the exam room. Very few patients called the heavily promoted stop-smoking telephone hotline (Glasgow et al., 1991a). Even fewer chose to attend the well-publicized single-session stop-smoking programs (i.e., one 90-minute class).

In replicating this approach, we would (1) eliminate the baseline survey and have nurses or physicians assess smoking status; (2) simplify the nurse intervention by dropping the carbon monoxide assessment; (3) have the nurse assess readiness to quit after showing the video; (4) tailor the nurse intervention to each patient's stage of change; and (5) see that smoking status is reassessed and that stage-appropriate followup counseling is repeated at every subsequent visit.

Intervention can be tailored to the patient's level of readiness to quit in a variety of ways. First, the video that all smokers see should contain different segments relevant to smokers at the precontemplation, contemplation, and action stages of change. After the video, patients who are ready to quit should be encouraged to set a specific quit date in the near future and review strategies for cessation in a stop-smoking manual. Arrangements should be made for a followup call 1 or 2 days after the quit date. Patients who are contemplating quitting but who are not ready to set a quit date should be asked about their perceived barriers to cessation (e.g., fear of failure or weight gain) and should be encouraged to read relevant sections of a self-help manual. The staff should also express confidence in the patient's ability to quit and look for other ways to enhance self-efficacy. Contemplators can then be asked to consider the benefits of quitting between now and their next visit. We recommend that the counseling staff devote less time to precontemplators, who have little or no interest in quitting. There is little to be gained from lecturing such individuals. They should simply be encouraged to look over a manual and consider the benefits of quitting. The staff members should let these patients know that they are there to help when the patient decides the time is right.

Perhaps the most important findings to date are the attractiveness of this team approach to physicians and nurses and the relative ease with which it was implemented and maintained within a busy outpatient medical care delivery setting. After long-term effectiveness is confirmed, the effectiveness of nurse-assisted counseling within entire health plan populations will be evaluated and disseminated. This will require some additional training for nurses and a modest readjustment of their traditional role in outpatient settings. Fortunately, many nurses are eager to play a more active role in counseling patients about health-related behaviors and disease prevention. Though this study was conducted in an HMO, we believe a physician and nurse team approach to counseling smokers would be well suited to any medical office with personnel interested in seriously addressing the tobacco problem.

INTERVENTION WITH HOSPITAL PATIENTS

The most powerful smoking intervention strategy may be to identify situations in which smokers are most likely to quit on their own and then tailor interventions to take advantage of those teachable moments. Because patients' concerns about health are among the most frequently cited reasons for wanting to stop smoking (Pederson, 1982), interactions with health care providers provide some of the best opportunities for smoking intervention. In particular, health crises associated with hospitalization dramatically increase patients' concerns about smoking and provide a strong stimulus to stop. The purpose of the study reported here was to develop and evaluate a brief, inexpensive smoking cessation and relapse prevention program for hospitalized smokers.

Although relatively little is known about smoking cessation attempts and success among hospitalized patients, what is known is encouraging. Studies of patients with cardiovascular and pulmonary diseases (Daughton et al., 1980; Ockene et al., 1985) have produced relatively high but widely varying estimates of cessation rates, ranging from 20 to 51 percent among patients with pulmonary disease and from 22 to 62 percent among survivors of myocardial infarction (Burling et al., 1984; Ockene, 1987a). Outside of these special population studies, there have been very few studies of smoking cessation in the general population of hospitalized patients.

Effects of Hospitalization on Smoking

Survey of Hospitalized Smokers

In the Northwest Region of Kaiser Permanente, inpatient medical care is provided in two hospitals—the 220-bed Bess Kaiser Medical Center and the 236-bed Sunnyside Medical Center. A preliminary study that was conducted prior to implementation of a smoke-free hospital policy assessed the natural history of smoking cessation associated with hospitalization (Glasgow et al., 1991b). The purpose of the study was to determine the frequency of various cessation-related behaviors of patients during and after hospitalization and to identify variables associated with those behaviors. A heterogeneous sample of 526 HMO members who smoked prior to hospitalization and were hospitalized for nonterminal and not pregnancy-related conditions was surveyed 12 to 18 months later. Three events were studied: not smoking while hospitalized, attempting to quit after hospitalization, and smoking status 1 year after hospitalization. Similar factors were associated with not smoking in the hospital and quit attempts; for example, older persons and patients admitted with circulatory or respiratory problems were less likely to smoke in the hospital and more likely to try to quit. Self-reported abstinence from smoking for 1 month or longer at the time of follow-up included 16 percent of the former hospital patients. Overall, this initial study suggested that the hospital can be an effective setting for smoking cessation programs, especially those aimed at heavy smokers.

Smoke-Free Hospitals

Both of the HMO's hospitals adopted a strict no-smoking policy in mid-1988. This policy prohibits smoking by staff, visitors, and patients inside the buildings. As a result, most hospitalized smokers do not smoke during their stay, although a few do leave their beds to smoke outside. This policy results in an enforced period of abstinence from smoking at a time when patients are highly motivated to take health-protective actions. Initial results from subjects hospitalized subsequent to the hospital smoking ban are consistent with the earlier results. Approximately the same proportion of patients (18 percent) reported cessation after the policy was in effect as did those hospitalized before the ban. These results and conclusions of reviews of other smoking interventions (Glasgow and Lichtenstein, 1987; Schwartz, 1987) suggest that a smoke-free policy, by itself, is unlikely to result in permanent cessation for many patients.

Although the smoke-free hospital setting may not increase long-term smoking cessation by itself, it does provide an opportunity to reach patients with stop-smoking advice, counseling, and support. Typically, the immediate effects of nicotine withdrawal are surprisingly mild when patients are hospitalized, possibly because of other medical, surgical, and pharmacological interventions; the unique environment; and the fact that patients may attribute their discomfort to other sources. In any case, a stay in a smoke-free hospital provides a period of not smoking, often the longest period of abstinence since the patient started to smoke, and thereby provides an excellent opportunity for health care professionals to counsel patients in relapse prevention strategies (e.g., Curry et al., 1988; Marlatt and Gordon, 1985; Stevens and Hollis, 1989) before they return home.

Design and Intervention Methods

Study Design

The study was designed as a test of the efficacy of smoking cessation services provided to the general population of hospitalized smokers. Because of our interest in developing interventions applicable to the broadest possible population, we included virtually all of the nonobstetric adult patients, regardless of diagnosis or motivation to quit smoking. The only patients excluded were those whose hospital stay was less than 36 hours, postpartum patients, the terminally ill, and those who were hospitalized for alcoholism, drug abuse, or mental illness.

Smoking status and research consent were assessed by questionnaire at hospital admission. Those who reported smoking regularly any time during the preceding 3 months and who did not object to being contacted again in the next year were eligible for the study. To maximize the participation rate, the intervention was not mentioned in the explanatory portion of the initial questionnaire. Consent to participate in the intervention portion of the project was requested in person by the interventionist.

Randomization

Assignment of smokers to either the intervention condition or the usual-care control condition presented considerable logistic difficulties. Because most hospital rooms were doubles, simply randomly assigning patients to a condition might result in control participants' watching and listening to their roommates receiving the intervention. Therefore, randomization was accomplished by having the intervention team move back and forth between the two hospitals. During the first month, all research subjects in the first hospital received the smoking cessation intervention, whereas those in the second hospital received usual care. In the second month, the intervention team moved to the second hospital, and all of the participants in that hospital received the intervention while those in the first hospital received usual care. By alternating between the hospitals, the intervention team was able to minimize contamination between groups while dividing their efforts equally between the two hospitals. Subjects assigned to the control condition were not identified to the hospital staff or other health care providers and therefore received usual care. Usual care undoubtedly included advice to quit smoking in some cases.

While controlling for contamination between conditions, this research design had the disadvantage of not involving the nurses and other hospital staff members in the intervention effort. Our concern was that, once sensitized and trained in smoking cessation techniques, most hospital staff members would not be willing to limit their counseling efforts to intervention patients and not provide the smoking intervention to the control group patients. This conservative design provides a clean test of the effectiveness of the intervention without the addition of supportive efforts from nurses, an adjunct that would be expected to increase intervention effectiveness.

Intervention

Hospital-based intervention components included a bedside counseling session, a 12-minute videotape, an array of printed self-help material, chewing gum and other cigarette substitutes, and access to a free telephone advice service. Attempts were made to provide all of these components to each intervention patient, although logistic difficulties and patient requests sometimes interfered. After leaving the hospital, subjects received a 1-week followup call from the smoking counselor, a monthly series of followup mailings, and continued access to the telephone advice service. These intervention components are described below.

Experienced smoking counselors with master's degrees attempted to contact all intervention patients prior to their discharge from the hospital. Although some patients were seen in an intermediate care unit, most were seen in the general medical and surgical wards. Counseling began with asking the patients if they would be willing to talk to a smoking counselor. Only 4 percent declined to see the counselor. After obtaining consent, counselors assessed readiness to quit by asking patients whether they had smoked since entering the hospital and whether they planned to resume smoking after leaving the hospital. Because of the hospital smoking ban, only 20 percent reported leaving their beds to smoke (typically 1 to 2 cigarettes per day), and more than half of the intervention patients indicated a desire to remain nonsmokers after leaving the hospital. Patients were then asked if they would be willing to watch a 12-minute videotape produced for hospital patients. Those who agreed were shown the tape, but counselors had the option of not showing the tape if the patients were heavily drugged and likely to fall asleep while watching the tape. The videotape included discussion of advantages of quitting smoking during hospitalization, interviews with ex-smokers who stopped smoking as a result of hospitalization, advice about what to expect on returning home (for example, strong urges to smoke), and tips on how to deal with urges to smoke while in the hospital and after going home. Of the 78 percent of intervention subjects who saw a counselor, 44 percent viewed the videotape.

In addition to showing the videotape, the counselors spent about 15 minutes with each patient discussing smoking cessation methods. Patients who were not considering quitting (precontemplators) were urged to consider the hospital stay as a golden opportunity to quit. It was pointed out to patients that, in spite of their not having had much control over their health, one positive thing they could do was to plan to quit smoking.

Those who were already contemplating quitting were encouraged to consider themselves ex-smokers from this point on and to make a resolution to not smoke when they returned home. Those who had resolved to not start smoking again (recent quitters) were encouraged to anticipate upcoming difficult situations and to develop specific plans of action to deal with those situations. The focus of this part of the intervention was to carefully prepare for dealing with urges to smoke that were likely to occur after the return home.

At the end of the counseling session, the interventionist scheduled a followup phone call with the patient. The purpose of this call, made about 1 week after discharge, was to provide the patient with continued support and provide an opportunity for the counselor to give further advice regarding relapse prevention. A second call was attempted a few weeks later to all of those who reported not smoking 1 week after discharge.

Additional self-help materials and six issues of a bimonthly newsletter were mailed to participants after their discharge from the hospital. The purpose of the mailings was to reinforce the efforts of those who had stopped smoking and to trigger renewed efforts to quit for those who were still smoking. Newsletters included testimonials from those who had stopped smoking, tips on how to quit on your own, and phone numbers to call to obtain further self-help information. Each issue included a reminder that TRACC participants had access to a special 24-hour advice line.

Smoking Cessation Followup

All intervention and control participants were surveyed approximately 3 months after hospital admission. Those we were unable to contact between 60 and 120 days after hospitalization were considered lost to followup. The questionnaire response rate was excellent, with 49 percent returned by mail, 39 percent completed as an interview, 5 percent refused, and 6 percent lost to followup. Return rates did not differ between the intervention and control groups.

Results from the 3-month assessments of 1,114 patients are encouraging, with 13.6 percent of the control subjects and 20.4 percent of the intervention subjects reporting no smoking in the previous 7 days (χ^2=8.7, p=0.003), and 9.5 percent of the controls and 14.6 percent of the intervention subjects reporting no smoking for 2 months or more (χ^2=6.59, p=0.01). Subjects who refused assessment or were lost to followup were considered smokers. Table 22 presents the 3-month outcome data, by hospital.

Implementing a Hospital-Based Intervention

The essential elements of this intervention could be readily implemented by most acute-care hospitals. Probably the most important component of the intervention was the bedside counseling session. This portion of the intervention could be delivered by nurses, respiratory therapists, health educators, or other qualified staff after they received training in smoking cessation counseling techniques. Such training is now available in most American cities. Potential counselors will be much more effective with 30 to 40 hours of training. They will be most effective if they can quickly assess a patient's readiness to change, and if they have some experience dealing with denial, overconfidence and, most important, relapse prevention techniques. A skilled smoking counselor will be more effective than an inexperienced one in the hospital setting. This is in contrast to the outpatient setting, where minimal training and skills are sufficient.

The written self-help materials used in this project were obtained either directly from the National Cancer Institute, the American Lung Association,

Table 22
Participants from hospitals reporting no smoking for at least 7 days at 3-month followup

	Percentage in Each Treatment Condition		
	Usual Care	Intervention	p Value
Bess Kaiser Medical Center (n=601)	14.4%	21.1%	0.032
Sunnyside Medical Center (n=513)	13.4	21.0	0.022

and the American Cancer Society or adapted from materials obtained from those sources. New written materials are probably unnecessary, except for special populations for which there are no available materials.

The video developed for our program would be appropriate for the Pacific Northwest, but developing new videos for use outside this area, with regionally appropriate scenes and with local ex-smokers as role models, is recommended. Tapes for the current study were produced for about $1,000 per minute. Quality tapes can be produced for $500 to $1,500 per minute or less if other, prepared tapes are used as a source. The relatively low cost of modern videotape production allows for the customizing of materials for the intended audience. In the future, this research team hopes to expand the audience by using interactive videodiscs to assure that the models in each segment match the viewer in age, sex, and ethnic identity.

After hospital discharge, a followup phone call about 1 week later is an important relapse prevention tool. One week after leaving the hospital, most patients who stopped smoking in the hospital had not yet relapsed and reported that a followup call was helpful. Perhaps a call from a centralized source, that is, someone other than the original counselor, would be as helpful as it was in the outpatient study. As in the outpatient study, very few persons called the advice line, and unless such a telephone resource is available from local agencies at no cost, we do not recommend it as a prerequisite for the intervention. Followup mailings may have been of some help, but we have no way to evaluate their impact.

ST INTERVENTION FOR DENTAL PATIENTS

Although the proportion of the American population that smokes has been steadily declining over the past 25 years (US DHHS, 1986), consumption of chewing tobacco and moist snuff (smokeless tobacco, ST) has been increasing (Marcus et al., 1989). Although less research has been done on the health effects of smokeless tobacco, there is a clear association between ST use and oral cancer as well as cancer of the esophagus, larynx, and stomach (US DHHS, 1986). The growing body of evidence about the harmful effects of smokeless tobacco has led to an increasing interest in intervention programs for ST users.

There have been few published reports of smokeless tobacco intervention effects. There are published reports of ST cessation programs with adolescents (Eakin et al., 1989) and adults (DiLorenzo et al., 1991) that have used smoking cessation methods with smokeless tobacco users in small-group treatment. The results of those interventions have been encouraging, but a more cost-effective program is needed to affect large numbers of ST users. The study described here evaluated routine dental clinic visits as an opportunity to intervene in the use of smokeless tobacco. Because a large proportion of the population receives some dental care annually (Cohen et al., 1989a) and because the oral health effects of ST use are often obvious during an oral examination, the dental office is an ideal setting in which to conduct an ST cessation program.

Building on the success of smoking cessation programs delivered in medical offices (Cohen et al., 1989b; Secker-Walker et al., 1987), the investigators developed an ST cessation program suitable for the dental care setting. The intervention program was designed for delivery by dental hygienists and dentists in the context of regular oral health care. The dental care providers used this opportunity to assess any oral health effects of each patient's use of smokeless tobacco and then give the patient unequivocal advice to stop. It was hypothesized that this is a time when ST users would be most receptive to advice to quit. A regularly scheduled oral health visit to the dentist could provide a unique teachable moment for counseling the ST user.

Survey of Dentists, Hygienists, and Patients

Prior to the project intervention, a survey was conducted to determine the receptivity of both patients and dental office staffs to ST interventions (Severson et al., 1990). Overall, 42 dentists, 44 hygienists, and 1,506 age-eligible male patients completed the survey. The survey of patients indicated that 4.7 percent used smokeless tobacco and 39.0 percent of the ST users were interested in receiving cessation advice. One-third of the ST users reported that they would consider such advice.

Dentists were more comfortable giving advice to ST users than to smokers. The relevance of chew and snuff to oral health is the most obvious explanation for this. Dentists and hygienists reported that they customarily discussed health hazards of ST use (77 percent) and sometimes advised smokeless tobacco users to quit or cut down (23 percent).

Results of the dental office survey were encouraging. Patients reported being receptive to cessation advice (41 percent) and, in fact, expect it from dental professionals. That receptivity to advice from dentists and hygienists is supported by data from in-depth interviews with smokeless tobacco users (Severson et al., 1990). Dentists and hygienists were interested in having specific materials on smokeless tobacco and receiving training in giving cessation advice, and they felt more comfortable and effective in giving advice to ST users than to smokers.

Intervention Setting and Methods

Setting

This project was conducted in the Kaiser Permanente Dental Care Program, a prepaid, managed-care, group-practice, HMO program that currently provides comprehensive dental care to more than 160,000 members in the Pacific Northwest. The project was a randomized clinical trial in which patients were assigned to either usual care (control) or the smokeless tobacco intervention condition. Patients were identified as ST users via a tobacco use survey that they completed when coming for a routine dental hygiene visit. Emergency patients and those appearing for surgery or orthodontic care were excluded.

Intervention

When they arrived at the clinics, patients aged 15 or older were asked by the receptionist to complete a one-page questionnaire on tobacco use. Those who agreed to complete the survey and reported current use of smokeless tobacco became participants in the study. Eligibility was assessed by the clinic receptionists, who then assigned the patient to a usual-care or an intervention group. Although most patients complied with the request to complete the tobacco use survey, the member assistant (receptionist) often neglected to give out the survey, and approximately 60 percent of eligible members actually completed the questionnaire. Despite frequent prompts by the research project staff, most noncompletion was because of the receptionist's failure to pass out the survey instrument.

After completing the tobacco use survey, patients assigned to the control condition did not receive special attention from the dental clinic staff. No mention of their involvement in the study was made in the patients' dental care charts, and their status as ST users was not revealed to the hygienists and dentists. Depending on the individual practice habits of the dental care providers, patients receiving usual care may or may not have been advised to stop using tobacco. For patients assigned to the intervention condition, an envelope was put into each dental chart identifying them to the hygienist and dentist as ST users and intervention participants. The envelope included special data collection forms as well as self-help intervention materials.

Intervention activities were designed to fit comfortably into the usual routine of any dental office. Typically, the visits begin with the hygienist making a complete oral exam and then providing prophylactic treatment. This routine includes feedback on oral health status and advice on how to improve oral self-care procedures. When seeing an intervention patient, the hygienist recorded plaque and inflammation data on a special research data form and made a thorough examination of soft tissues, looking for keratotic lesions (leukoplakia). Although a soft tissue exam is routine, the research protocol called for a more detailed report of all lesions and their precise location in the mouth. The hygienist also asked the patient to show where he kept tobacco in his mouth. After assessment and dental treatment, the hygienist gave the patient direct advice to quit using all tobacco products.

Routine clinic procedures call for the dentist to examine patients after they have seen the hygienist. The dentists also discussed keratotic lesions with patients, discussed the harmful effects of smokeless tobacco, and gave their own brief message to stop using tobacco. It was emphasized that care providers must deliver an unambiguous message to ST users: All tobacco products are harmful to health and they should stop now. This constituted the counseling component of the special intervention.

As part of the intervention, the patient was asked to view a 10-minute videotape at the end of the visit. The video produced for this project begins with a humorous segment designed to help the patient relax and includes an interview with a dentist discussing the health consequences of ST use. The video also includes a series of interviews with former users describing the benefits of quitting and the methods they used to quit. After viewing the video, the hygienist encouraged the patient to use a self-help booklet, "Enough Snuff," provided to them and to call a 24-hour advice line for further assistance. The hygienist also attempted to get the patient to set a specific quit date and noted whether he was willing to do so. At the end of this brief counseling session, the subject was given a quit kit containing chewing gum, toothpicks, a nontobacco mint-leaf tobacco substitute, and a set of tip sheets with advice on how to quit.

Followup Phone Calls

About a week after the dental clinic intervention, subjects were called by a project staff member to reinforce the clinic-based intervention activities and to offer further advice and support for quitting efforts.

Additional support activities after the clinic visit included bimonthly mailings of tip sheets and a newsletter.

Followup Data Collection

To assess the effects of intervention, all intervention, control, and comparison-site participants were surveyed approximately 2 to 3 months after being seen at the dental office. Sixty days after entering the study, all subjects were sent a followup questionnaire about their tobacco use since their dental office visit. If they did not return the questionnaire within 14 days, they were sent a second copy, and if a questionnaire was not returned after another 14 days, they were called and asked to complete the questionnaire as a telephone interview. Those not contacted within 120 days after their dental visit were considered lost to followup.

Results

A total of 245 intervention subjects and 272 usual-care controls were recruited for the study. As expected, the use of smokeless tobacco was highest in the younger age groups (15- to 19-year-olds and 20- to 29-year-olds). The portion of ST users who did not also smoke was also highest in the youngest groups. Thirty-five percent of the chew-only group was in the 20 to 29 age range.

Acceptability of Intervention

The hygienists and dentists provided excellent cooperation in this study. Most were enthusiastic about delivering the intervention, and they failed to do so only on rare occasions. However, the clinic receptionists sometimes neglected to administer the tobacco use survey. The busy nature of the clinic and demands on staff time made the administration of a separate tobacco survey problematic. It is recommended that those implementing similar programs include smoking questions as part of a routine intake form or use other identification methods that do not make additional time demands on receptionists.

Somewhat surprisingly, the intervention was acceptable to the vast majority of patients. Fewer than 5 percent of the intervention subjects refused intervention completely, and an additional 10 percent refused to watch the video.

Three-Month Followup

The followup questionnaire response rate was excellent, with 47 percent returned by mail and 43 percent completed as telephone interviews. Of the remainder, 7 percent of the participants declined to complete the interview and 3 percent were lost to followup. The overall followup rate for the intervention group was 91 percent, and for the usual-care group 89 percent.

Self-reported abstinence from all tobacco use at 3 months included 22 percent of the intervention subjects and 14 percent of the control subjects. Table 23 shows a breakdown of tobacco use at 3 months according to tobacco use at baseline. The success of the intervention appears higher for patients who report using only smokeless tobacco at baseline (26 percent abstinent at followup) than for men who used both cigarettes and chew (12 percent abstinent at followup). This was true for both intervention and control subjects. Of additional interest is the fact that very few of the ST-only subjects reported cigarette use only at followup (1 percent and 4 percent for intervention and control subjects, respectively), so we have some confidence that quitting smokeless tobacco use did not prompt the use of cigarettes as an alternative.

Discussion

The 3-month followup data of the dental office intervention for smokeless tobacco cessation support the efficacy of the intervention. Twenty-two percent of the ST-using patients randomly assigned to the brief intervention reported they had quit the use of all tobacco, whereas only 14 percent of the usual-care subjects reported quitting. This significantly higher rate of self-reported quitting is strong support for the use of office visits for oral health care as teachable moments for advising patients to quit using smokeless tobacco.

The results of this study are similar to other tobacco-use interventions in outpatient settings that have also reported a significant effect of having dentists (Cohen et al., 1989a) and medical office staff provide direct advice to quit (Glynn, 1988). Glynn reports that most physician advice and minimal

Table 23
Three-month followup tobacco use, by baseline tobacco use

	Followup Tobacco Status										
	No Tobacco		Chew Only		Chew and Smoke		Smoke Only		No Followup		Total
	%	(n)	%	(n)	%	(n)	%	(n)	%	(n)	(n)
Intervention Participants, Baseline Use											
Chew only	26	(45)	57	(97)	3	(5)	1	(2)	12	(21)	170
Chew and smoke	12	(9)	12	(9)	27	(20)	32	(24)	17	(13)	75
Total	22	(54)	43	(106)	10	(25)	11	(26)	14	(34)	245
Control Participants, Baseline Use											
Chew only	17	(33)	67	(128)	3	(5)	4	(7)	9	(18)	191
Chew and smoke	6	(5)	19	(15)	46	(37)	17	(14)	12	(10)	81
Total	14	(38)	53	(143)	15	(42)	8	(21)	10	(28)	272

interventions offered in medical settings report average quit rates of 10 to 12 percent at 1 year. It is likely that the 3-month self-reported quit rates for smokeless tobacco will decline over the year as many patients relapse. However, even if 50 percent of the patients in both study conditions relapse between the 3-month and 1-year evaluations, the ST quit rates would still appear to be consistent with previous research using a 1-year biochemically confirmed quit assessment.

For the intervention group, men who reported using only smokeless tobacco reported a 25-percent quit rate, whereas men who reported at baseline that they used both cigarettes and chew had only a 17-percent quit rate. The two quit rates are significantly different ($p < 0.01$). It appears that men who use both cigarettes and smokeless tobacco find it more difficult to quit.

This intervention was implemented by the dentist and hygienist in the context of routine oral health care. Although the demands on receptionists should be minimized, dentists and hygienists reported that brief, direct advice to quit using smokeless tobacco fit well within the time allotted for the regular oral health exam. In practice, this intervention would require even less time, since the research protocol required extra data collection forms. Hygienists played the key role by pointing out the smokeless tobacco-related oral health effects to the patient, showing the video, providing a self-help manual, and encouraging the patient to set a quit date. This brief interaction was critical, and most of the patients were willing to take the extra time to be briefly counseled. Dental hygienists were comfortable pointing out oral lesions and relating them to ST use but less comfortable in asking the patient to watch a video or providing counseling advice. The video viewing was sometimes a problem because of lack of privacy.

Previous studies have confirmed that smokeless tobacco users expect to receive a message to quit from their physician or dentist and are receptive to it. In a recent interview of ST users, 54 percent reported wanting to quit in the next year and 69 percent reported recent attempts to quit (Severson et al., 1990). Dentists and hygienists have an opportunity to advise users of smokeless tobacco to quit, and the context of an oral health care office visit provides a unique teachable moment in which the user may be most receptive to cessation advice. Although the long-term cessation rates are not yet known, these early results suggest that dentists and hygienists can have a significant impact on smokeless tobacco use and thus on public health.

SMOKING CESSATION AMONG ADOLESCENTS

Purpose and Target Group

Any comprehensive effort to reduce the prevalence of smoking among members of an HMO should include a program to prompt cessation among adolescents. Adolescence is the time when most smokers begin smoking. Many novice smokers are not yet addicted, so cessation could prove easier than it is for adults. Moreover, it would seem appropriate to have a program that is uniquely tailored to the needs and interests of adolescent smokers, rather than offering them the same program that is provided to adults.

On the other hand, the efficacy of a smoking cessation program for adolescents cannot be assumed. A number of programs that have been evaluated have not produced significant quitting among adolescents (Diguisto, personal communication, August 1990). Therefore, the authors developed and evaluated a smoking cessation program for adolescent members of Northwest Kaiser Permanente.

Methods

Intervention

The program was designed to provide continuing contacts with adolescent smokers in an effort to increase their willingness to quit, prompt them to make quit attempts, and provide skills and social reinforcement for quitting. The centerpiece of the program was an office visit with a nurse practitioner at a convenient Kaiser Permanente clinic.

Adolescents were invited to attend these visits during in-home assessments that were made in the course of a survey of adolescent health behavior. However, the majority of visits (70 percent) were actually scheduled through phone contacts. These recruitment methods were dictated by the need for experimental evaluation of the program. It is unlikely that they would be used by a clinic in normal circumstances. Rather, contact with adolescent smokers would most likely occur in the course of their coming to the clinic for treatment of other problems.

Sessions typically lasted 60 minutes. They began with a brief discussion of family history of cancer and the provision of information about breast self-exam to girls and testicular self-exam to boys. The family smoking history and the young person's smoking history and current behavior were then discussed. Reasons for quitting and barriers for quitting were discussed next. Most patients reported having tried quitting and failed.

Carbon monoxide testing was done initially, but it was later dropped because of the low CO levels resulting from the relatively low level of smoking by the young people (Biglan et al., 1985). Giving the adolescents feedback about their carbon monoxide levels thus tended to suggest that their smoking was not a problem.

A key component of the program was a videotape that was made especially for this program. It was designed to make smoking cessation seem like a popular option for teens and to provide information from attractive young people about how to quit. After the video, the nurse practitioner discussed its contents with the teenager and provided information about quitting. The discussion centered on the situations in which smoking occurred and the barriers to quitting. With light smokers, two questions that helped get at the need to quit were, "Do you have cravings?" and "When do you have your first cigarette?" These opened up discussion of getting hooked and the value of trying to quit. The adolescent was then given a "quit kit" that contained the same materials that were given to adults (a cinnamon stick, sugarless chewing gum, a rubber band, and a refrigerator magnet with the number of our quit-smoking hotline).

Most teens indicated a desire to quit smoking, and they were assisted in developing a plan for quitting. It included specific things to do in situations where smoking was most likely, a plan to talk to friends and family members who were likely to be helpful, and ideas for self-rewards for accomplishing small goals such as a day without cigarettes. In the initial work, an explicit quit date was elicited from each teen; however, very few actually quit on their quit date. The practice was subsequently discontinued, because failure to quit on the targeted date seemed likely to undermine commitments to the other features of the plan.

In an additional effort to reinforce quitting, a lottery was developed. Teens received chances for a $100 gift certificate. They had to be abstinent to win.

Followup phone calls were routinely made. The investigators tried to contact each adolescent 1 week after the office visit. This sometimes proved very difficult, because many teens were hard to reach by phone. In the event that young patients did not want to attempt to quit at the time of the office visit, they were asked if they could be called a month later. Repeated contacts by phone were common. They occurred over a period of 2 to 3 months and only when the adolescent expressed continued interest in quitting and in having phone contacts.

Experimental Evaluation

The evaluation of this program was designed to reveal whether the program reduced the prevalence of smoking among adolescents aged 14 to 17 whose families were members of Northwest Kaiser Permanente and who were identified as smokers at the outset of the program. For the assessment, 16,399 teens were sent a questionnaire on a variety of health habits. Of these teens, 8,126 returned the questionnaire. The 1,155 teens (14.2 percent) who reported having smoked a cigarette in the prior 7 days (as well as a small sample of nonsmoking comparison adolescents) were asked to participate in an extensive assessment of teen health that was conducted in their homes. Among the girls, 325 (46.0 percent) agreed to participate, whereas 168 boys (37.2 percent) agreed to participate. This difference was statistically significant.

In the home assessment, adolescents were asked about their smoking behavior and asked to provide samples of expired air CO (Biglan et al., 1985) and saliva, which were analyzed for cotinine (Jacob et al., 1981). They also answered extensive questions about their engagement in other forms of problem behavior. A parent—typically the mother—was also asked to complete a questionnaire about the adolescents' behavior, family interactions, and parental health behavior. Subjects completing the home assessment were randomly assigned to either a smoking cessation program or a no-treatment control group. There were 229 smokers and 61 nonsmokers in the cessation condition, and 257 smokers and 52 nonsmokers in the control condition.

These same home assessment procedures were repeated 12 months and approximately 18 months later. Data from the 1-year assessment are currently available.

Results

There was simply no evidence that the intervention program prompted the adolescents to stop smoking. Table 24 presents means and tests of differences between treatment and control subjects who reported smoking at the time of the screening questionnaire. The groups do not differ on any self-report or physiological measure of smoking behavior. The subjects in the treatment program reported more quit attempts, but the difference was only significant at $p=0.06$.

Can Adolescents Be Prompted To Quit?

Our results, thus far, cast doubt on the utility of smoking cessation programs for adolescents. It can, of course, be argued that a different program—perhaps one that involved more extensive contacts—could be successful. However, the nurse practitioners who conducted this program would point out that it was very difficult to achieve the small amount of contact that was achieved with these young people. An effort to increase contact might be very costly in practitioners' time.

It might also be argued that a program that worked only with those adolescents who volunteered that they wanted to quit might prove efficacious. However, our contacts with this sample of young people make us skeptical. Although most said they wanted to quit, when asked, it was extremely rare

Table 24
Effects of the program on adolescent smoking

	Treatment	Control	F	p
Variable				
Cigarettes in past month	194.83	228.24	0.02	0.89
Percentage who smoked in past 7 days	36.00	34.00	30.00	0.59
Percentage who smoked in last 30 days	27.00	25.00	3.00	0.87
Cigarettes in past 24 hours	6.02	7.11	0.00	0.98
Current smoking	6.59	6.98	2.31	0.13
Carbon monoxide	5.91	6.34	0.02	0.90
Cotinine	93.14	117.09	0.27	0.61
Index of smoking	-0.15	-0.08	0.04	0.96
Attempts to quit in past year	2.78	2.30	3.45	0.06

for a young person to contact us in response to our mailed advertising about the cessation program; most contacts were prompted by our phone calls or invitations delivered at the first home assessment.

Some hints as to why it is hard to get these young people to stop smoking are provided by analysis of the correlates of their smoking behavior. The multiple correlation between an index smoking behavior and measures of seven other problem behaviors (alcohol consumption, high-risk sexual behavior, poor grades, lack of prosocial behavior, antisocial behavior, use of illicit drugs other than marijuana, and use of marijuana) was 0.60, accounting for 36 percent of the variance in smoking. The multiple correlation predicting smoking from measures of five aspects of family interaction and six aspects of peer influence was also 0.60. Thus, cigarette smoking occurs in the context of many other problems and in the context of a problematic social environment. It may be impossible to excise this behavior from such a context. Instead, it may be necessary to develop programs that comprehensively address the social conditions that produce the above-mentioned problem behaviors.

It may be premature to conclude that programs focused solely on smoking cessation among adolescents will not work. However, given the evidence thus far, it seems probable that some radically different approach to prompting quitting among adolescents will be needed.

SUMMARY AND IMPLICATIONS

The implementation and outcome data presented for the four TRACC interventions provide consistent support for the team approach. Not only was it possible to enlist clinic assistants, nurses, physicians, dental hygienists, dentists, and counselors to provide brief cessation advice and counseling augmented by written materials and videos, but also, once under way, the program received strong support from providers and their staffs. Some receptionists found the patient screening, recruitment, and consent process burdensome, but these problems could be minimized or avoided in a nonresearch environment. With this exception, staff and providers found the "required" activities to be feasible and convenient. Providers had positive feelings about the interventions because they perceived that they were addressing an important, previously neglected health issue in a nonburdensome manner.

The data also consistently show that patients—who were being seen for typical medical or dental problems—both accepted and responded to the interventions. Most patients agreed to receive the interventions, and the short-term data for adult patients show significant treatment effects. Providers need not worry about patients' negative reactions to raising the smoking issue.

The three projects aimed at adult tobacco use all yielded significant reductions in tobacco use, indicating that the team approach is at least as effective as sometimes more intensive physician or dentist interventions (Cohen et al., 1989b; Cummings et al., 1989; Janz et al., 1987; Li et al., 1984; Ockene, 1987a; Wilson et al., 1988). One-year followup data are needed before assessment of the long-term impact of these interventions is made. The preliminary 1-year results are consistent with the data presented here.

The single, and unfortunate, exception is the failure of the trial intervention to affect adolescent tobacco use. Whether health care settings can affect adolescent tobacco use remains an open question. Certainly, adolescent motives for smoking and patterns of use (as well as adolescent health and psychology) suggest that interventions in the medical care setting are unlikely to have a major short-term impact on adolescent smoking. School and peer-group approaches are more promising.

The investigators are already moving toward institutionalizing the adult tobacco use interventions in outpatient and hospital settings by turning them over to provider staff, as was done originally in the dental clinic intervention. For example, nurses—again assisted by videos—can provide most of the outpatient intervention with respiratory therapists leading the inpatient program.

There is the potential for applying this team approach in many settings, including the private sector. Nurses are typically interested in expanding their treatment and educational responsibilities. Video interventions are feasible in many health care settings, and video materials can reduce the instructional burden on staff. The exciting potential of interactive video is being explored also. This new technology permits patients to select change strategies suitable to their particular needs and can even further reduce staff counseling time.

A key role remains for the physicians: They must initiate or sanction the introduction of the smoking issue. Moving the interventions out of a research context will permit better use of repeated prompts and messages, for example, outpatient followup of hospitalized patients.

The interventions all were enhanced by a sophisticated, computerized tracking system that triggered the delivery of telephone and mail prompts (and data collection). Other large health care systems would also have such systems available. They can also be conscripted to yield other information relevant to cancer control, such as that pertaining to cervical or breast screening.

The TRACC projects illustrate the potential for low-cost, population-based cancer control interventions that exploit the teachable moments in medical settings. The keys to successful implementation and maintenance included promoting change at the organization or system level, applying available technology (computerized tracking, tailored videos), and using support staff to assist primary care providers in counseling patients. This approach appealed to providers and patients, and it overcame many of the barriers to implementation of cessation advice in medical settings.

ACKNOWLEDGMENTS We gratefully acknowledge the high level of cooperation received from the management and medical care staff of the Northwest Region of Kaiser Permanente. We also thank the staff of the Oregon Research Institute and Independent Video Services for their key roles in producing the instructional videos used in this project.

REFERENCES

Biglan, A., Gallison, C., Ary, D.V., Thompson, R. Expired air carbon monoxide and saliva thiocyanate: Relationships to self-reports of marijuana and cigarette smoking. *Addictive Behaviors* 10: 137-144, 1985.

Burling, T.A., Singleton, E.G., Bigelow, G.E., Baile, W.F., Gottlieb, S.H. Smoking following myocardial infarction: A critical review of the literature. *Health Psychology* 3(1): 83-96, 1984.

Cohen, S.J., Stookey, G.K., Katz, B.P., Drook, C.A., Christen, A.G. Helping smokers quit: A randomized controlled trial with private-practice dentists. *Journal of the American Dental Association* 118: 41-45, 1989a.

Cohen, S.J., Stookey, G.K., Katz, B.P., Drook, C.A., Smith, D.M. Encouraging primary care physicians to help smokers quit: A randomized controlled trial. *Annals of Internal Medicine* 110(8): 648-652, 1989b.

Cummings, S.R., Richard, R.J., Duncan, C.L., Hansen, B., Vander Martin, R., Gerbert, B., Coates, T.J. Training physicians about smoking cessation: A controlled trial in private practices. *Journal of General Internal Medicine* 4(6): 482-489, 1989.

Curry, S.J., Marlatt, G.A., Gordon, J., Baer, J.S. A comparison of alternative theoretical approaches to smoking cessation and relapse. *Health Psychology* 7: 545-556, 1988.

Daughton, D.M., Fix, A.J., Kass, I., Patil, K.D. Smoking cessation among patients with chronic obstructive pulmonary disease (COPD). *Addictive Behaviors* 5: 125-128, 1980.

DiLorenzo, T.M., Kern, T.G., Pieper, R.M. Treatment of smokeless tobacco use through a formalized cessation program. *Behavior Therapy* 22: 41-46, 1991.

Eakin, E., Severson, H., Glasgow, R.E. Development and evaluation of a smokeless tobacco cessation program: A pilot study. *National Cancer Institute Monographs* 8: 95-100, 1989.

Epstein, L.H., Grunberg, N.E., Lichtenstein, E., Evans, R. Smoking research: Basic research, intervention, prevention, and new trends. *New Health* 8: 705-721, 1989.

Fagerstrom, K.O. Effect of nicotine chewing gum and followup appointments in physician-based smoking cessation. *Preventive Medicine* 13: 517-527, 1984.

Fortmann, S.P., Sallis, J.F., Magnus, P.M., Farquhar, J.W. Attitudes and practices of physicians regarding hypertension and smoking: The Stanford Five-City Project. *Preventive Medicine* 14: 70-80, 1985.

Glasgow, R.E., Hollis, J.F., McCrae, S., Lando, H., LaChance, P.A. Providing an integrated program of low intensity tobacco cessation services in an HMO. *Health Education Research* 6(1): 87-89, 1991a.

Glasgow, R.E., Lichtenstein, E.L. Long-term effects of behavioral smoking cessation interventions. *Behavioral Therapy* 18: 297-324, 1987.

Glasgow, R.E., Stevens, V.J., Vogt, T.M., Mullooly, J.P., Lichtenstein, E. Changes in smoking associated with hospitalization: Quit rates, predictive variables, and intervention implications. *American Journal of Health Promotion*, 6(1): 24-29, 1991b.

Glynn, T.J. Relative effectiveness of physician-initiated smoking cessation programs. *Cancer Bulletin* 40: 359-364, 1988.

Hollis, J.F., Lichtenstein, E., Mount, K.M., Vogt, T.M., Stevens, V.J. Nurse-assisted smoking counseling for medical settings: Minimizing demands on physicians. *Preventive Medicine* 20: 497-507, 1991.

Jacob, P. III, Wilson, M., Benowitz, N.L. Improved gas chromatographic method for the determination of nicotine and cotinine in biologic fluids. *Journal of Chromatography* 222: 61-70, 1981.

Janz, N.K., Becker, M.H., Kirscht, J.P., Eraker, S.A., Billi, J.E., Woolliscroft, J.O. Evaluation of a minimal-contact smoking cessation intervention in an outpatient setting. *American Journal of Public Health* 77(7): 805-809, 1987.

Kottke, T.E., Battista, R.N., DeFriese, G.H., Brekke, M.L. Attributes of successful smoking cessation interventions in medical practice: A meta-analysis of 39 controlled trials. *Journal of the American Medical Association* 259: 2882-2889, 1988.

Li, V.C., Coates, T.J., Spielberg, L.A., Ewart, C.K., Dorfman, S., Huster, W.J. Smoking cessation with young women in public family planning clinics: The impact of physician messages and waiting room media. *Preventive Medicine* 13: 477-489, 1984.

Lichtenstein, E., Hollis, J.F. Patient referral to a smoking cessation program: Who follows through? *Journal of Family Practice* 34: 739-744, 1992.

Marcus, A.C., Crane, L.A., Shopland, D.R., Lynn, W.L. Use of smokeless tobacco in the United States: Recent estimates from the Current Population Survey. *National Cancer Institute Monographs* 8: 17-23, 1989.

Marlatt, G.A., Gordon, J.R. *Relapse Prevention: Maintenance Strategies in the Treatment of Addictive Behaviors*. New York: Guilford Press, 1985.

Ockene, J.K. Physician-delivered interventions for smoking cessation: Strategies for increasing effectiveness. *Preventive Medicine* 16: 723-737, 1987a.

Ockene, J.K. Smoking intervention: The expanding role of the physician. *American Journal of Public Health* 77: 782-783, 1987b.

Ockene, J.K. Trends in smoking intervention. In: *Smoking and Health: A National Status Report.* U.S. Department of Health and Human Services, Centers for Disease Control, Office on Smoking and Health. DHHS Publication No. (CDC) 87-8396, 1987c.

Ockene, J.K., Hosmer, D., Rippe, J., Williams, J., Goldberg, R.J., DeCosimo, D., Maher, P.M., Dalen, J.E. Factors affecting cigarette smoking status in patients with ischemic heart disease. *Journal of Chronic Disease* 38: 985-994, 1985.

Pederson, L.L. Compliance with physician advice to quit smoking: A review of the literature. *Preventive Medicine* 11: 71-84, 1982.

Schwartz, J.L. *Review and Evaluation of Smoking Cessation Methods: The United States and Canada, 1978-1985.* U.S. Department of Health and Human Services, Public Health Service, National Institutes of Health, National Cancer Institute, Division of Cancer Prevention and Control. NIH Publication No. 87-2940, 1987.

Secker-Walker, R.H., Hill, H.C., Solomon, L.J., Flynn, B.S. Smoking cessation practices in dental offices. *Journal of Public Health Dentistry* 47: 10-15, 1987.

Severson, H.H., Eakin, E.G., Lichtenstein, E., Stevens, V.J. The inside scoop on the stuff called snuff: An interview study of 94 adult male smokeless tobacco users. *Journal of Substance Abuse* 2: 77-85, 1990.

Stevens, V.J., Hollis, J.F. Preventing smoking relapse, using an individually tailored skills-training technique. *Journal of Consulting and Clinical Psychology* 57: 420-424, 1989.

U.S. Department of Health and Human Services. *The Health Consequences of Using Smokeless Tobacco: A Report of the Advisory Committee to the Surgeon General.* U.S. Department of Health and Human Services, Public Health Service, National Institutes of Health, National Cancer Institute. DHHS Publication No. (NIH) 86-2874, 1986.

Vogt, T.M., Lichtenstein, E., Ary, D., Danielson, R., Glasgow, R.E., Hollis, J.F., Hornbrook, M.C., Mullooly, J., Severson, H., Stevens, V. Integrating tobacco intervention into a health maintenance organization: The TRACC program. *Health Education Research* 4(1): 125-135, 1989.

Wells, K.B., Ware, J.E., Jr., Lewis, C.E. Physicians' attitudes in counseling patients about smoking. *Medical Care* 22(4): 360-365, 1984.

Wilson, D.M., Taylor, D.W., Gilbert, J.R., Best, J.A., Lindsay, E.A., Willms, D.G., Singer, J. A randomized trial of a family physician intervention for smoking cessation. *Journal of the American Medical Association* 260(11): 1570-1574, 1988.

APPENDIX A
Screening Form for Study on Assessing Patient's Health Risks

Date ____________________

Subject No. ________________

The health center thanks you for considering being in our study.

We are assessing health risks to patients in our practice. If you decide to enter the study, you will benefit by having your physician discuss one of your risks in depth and provide you with free health information.

Before you decide whether to enter our study, we would like you to answer the following questions to determine whether you are eligible for the study.

1. Your age: _______
2. Your sex: male female (please circle one)
3. Do you exercise regularly? Yes No
4. Do you smoke cigarettes daily? Yes No
5. Do you consider yourself overweight? Yes No
6. Do you use safety belts regularly? Yes No
7. Do you drink alcohol? Yes No

Please return this screening form to the practice research coordinator to determine if you are eligible for the study. The coordinator will inform you of your eligibility and provide you with further information if you are interested.

APPENDIX B
Study on Physician Advice for Smoking Cessation

You are invited to be in a study on physician advice about smoking. The study only requires you to stay a few minutes longer so your physician can talk to you about smoking. In addition, based on chance, you may receive a prescription for nicotine gum. A follow-up visit to further discuss smoking will be offered to you. You and a spouse or friend will be asked to fill out a one-page questionnaire 2 weeks and 6 months from now. If at 6 months you are not smoking, you will be asked to return to the clinic to give a breath sample. For this inconvenience you will receive $10.

The only risk of this study will be possible withdrawal symptoms and side effects from nicotine gum. Serious side effects from the gum are rare. Minor side effects such as irritated throat, nausea, upset stomach, hiccups, jaw ache, and dependence on the gum occur in less than 25 percent of smokers. These side effects can be controlled by how vigorously you chew the gum.

Although we can foresee no significant risk for this research, in the event that this research activity results in a physical injury, medical treatment will be available, including first aid, emergency treatment, and followup care [as] needed. Payment for any such treatment must be provided by you and your third-party payor, if any (such as health insurance, Medicare, and so forth).

If you should decide not to participate, or to withdraw from this study, your decision will not prejudice your future medical care.

If you have any questions about this study, please contact Dr. William Wadland at the University of Vermont [phone number]. You may contact Caryn Gronvold at the University of Vermont [room number, phone number] for more information about your rights as a research subject or for more information about how to proceed should you believe that you have been injured as a result of your participation in this study.

- -

You are making a decision whether or not to participate. Your signature indicates that you have read the information provided and have decided to participate.

______________________________________ ____________________

signature date

____

signature of research coordinator

APPENDIX C
Entry Questionnaire

Entry Date ________
Subject No. ________

1. Give the full name of your cigarettes:

   ____

   Check the blanks which describe your cigarette:

   Filtered ______
   King Size ______
   120mm ______
   100mm ______
   85mm ______
   Regular ______
   Menthol ______
   Hard pack ______
   Lights ______
   Ultralights ______

2. The average number of cigarettes you smoke per day _____ (only one number please).
3. Your age when you started smoking on a regular basis. _____
4. Do you use cigars, pipes, or smokeless tobacco?

   ____ Yes ____ No

5. Do you inhale? Always Sometimes Never (circle one)
6. Do you smoke more during the morning than during the rest of the day?

   ____ Yes ____ No

7. How soon after you wake up do you smoke your first cigarette? _____ minutes _____ hours
8. Which cigarette would you hate to give up? ______________________________
9. Do you find it difficult to refrain from smoking in places where it is forbidden, e.g., in church, at the library, cinema, etc.? Yes ____ No ____
10. Do you smoke if you are so ill that you are in bed most of the day? Yes ____ No ____
11. Circle the highest grade you have completed:

    0 1 2 3 4 5 6 7 8 9 10 11 12 13 14 15 16 16+

12. What is your major present occupation? (Describe fully, including student, housewife, unemployed, or retired. Also describe your business as small, medium, or large.)

    ____

13. Are you married? Yes ____ No ____

14. Does insurance pay for any part of your prescriptions?

    ____ Yes ____ No

15. How many of the people who live with you smoke cigarettes? _____

16. For the purposes of the study, we need to know your total family yearly income. (This will be kept confidential.)

    Less than $15,000 _____

    $15,000 to $29,000 _____

    $30,000 to $44,999 _____

    More than $45,000 _____

17. Most people have mixed feelings for and against their smoking, with a part of them wanting to stop and a part of them wanting to go on smoking.

    a. How much would you say that you want to *stop* smoking?

    _____ not at all _____ a little _____ some _____ a lot _____ don't know

    b. And how much does a part of you want to *go on* smoking?

    _____ not at all _____ a little _____ some _____ a lot _____ don't know

18. Do you intend to quit smoking in the next month or so?

    ___ definitely not ___ probably not ___ possibly ___ probably ___ definitely ___ don't know

19. If you decided to give up smoking within the next month, do you think you would succeed?

    ___ definitely not ___ probably not ___ possibly ___ probably ___ definitely ___ don't know

We need to collect identification data from you so that we can find you 6 months from now:

20. What is your full name? ______________________________

21. Give your full home address.

    Street: ______________________________

    City, Zip: ______________________________

    Phone: ______________________________

22. Give your work address.

    Company: ______________________________

    Immediate supervisor: ______________________________

    Street: ______________________________

    City, Zip: ______________________________

    Phone: ______________________________

23. Give name and address of spouse/friend who can act as your observer. This person will verify your smoking status.

Name: ____________________

Street: ____________________

City, Zip: ____________________

Phone: ____________________

APPENDIX D
Medical Screening Form

Name ______________________________

Subject No. ______________________________

Date ______________________________

Physician ______________________________

Heart attack in the last 6 months	Yes	No
Irregular heart or arrhythmia	Yes	No
Active temporomandibular joint disease	Yes	No
Worsening or unstable angina	Yes	No
Pregnant or planning to be	Yes	No
Breast-feeding	Yes	No
Able to chew gum	Yes	No

Other ______________________________

OK for patient to be on nicotine gum:

____

Physician's signature

APPENDIX E
Generic Reminder Sheet

1. Ask if ever thought about quitting and reason. If none, volunteer one.
2. State reversibility of symptom (2 weeks), disease (1 year), or risk (10 years).
3. Recommend cessation (use word "I").
4. Describe "Quit and Win":
    a. It's for habit part of smoking.
    b. Tips from successful ex-smokers.
    c. Use as menu. Choose 3 to 5 strategies that are do-able.
5. Open assignment envelope.

APPENDIX F
Reminder Sheet for Gum Group

6. Instructions on gum.

   Give rationale: to decrease withdrawal.

   It works.

   Stop smoking abruptly.

   Chew PRN early in craving.

   Chew slowly to control side effects. Side effects decrease in first week.

   Use till no craving, and then decrease gradually.

   Biggest mistakes: use too little for too short a time.

   Keep gum with you.

   Read booklet.

   The Rx is good for 6 months in case you decide to quit later.

7. Ask for questions.
8. Ask for commitment to quit.
9. Ask for quit date.
10. Offer followup by appointment or phone.

APPENDIX G
Reminder Sheet for No-Gum Group

6. Ask biggest fear:
    a. Generic responses

        Withdrawal symptoms are transient.

        Distract yourself by keeping busy.

        Decrease demands on yourself.

        Avoid tempting situations for a while.

        Use time-outs or remember reason for cessation for urges.

        Increase activity (not necessarily exercise).

        Read booklet.

    b. Specific responses for weight:

        Weight gain doesn't necessarily occur or last.

        To counteract loss of anorectic and oral behavior, watch snacks and sweets but don't change meal sizes.

        To counteract decreased BMR, increase activity.

7. Ask for questions.
8. Ask for commitment to quit.
9. Ask for quit date.
10. Offer followup by appointment or phone.

APPENDIX H
Physician Data: Initial Visit

Subject No. ____________________

Date ____________________

Physician ____________________

Did you obtain a commitment to quit? Yes No

Did you obtain a quit date? Yes No

If so, what is the date? ________ ________ ________
Month Day Year

APPENDIX I
Exit Questionnaire #1
(All Patients)

Subject No. ____________________

Did your physician:

1. Ask you a reason to stop smoking?

    _____ Yes _____ No

2. Tell you that the effects of smoking are reversible?

    _____ Yes _____ No

3. Tell you about the booklet to aid the habit part of smoking cessation?

    _____ Yes _____ No

4. Ask you to try to quit?

    _____ Yes _____ No

5. Ask you for a quit date?

    _____ Yes _____ No

6. Offer to see you 1 to 2 weeks after your quit date?

    _____ Yes _____ No

Please answer the following questions. Some are the same questions you answered prior to receiving physician's advice.

7. Most people have mixed feelings for and against their smoking, with a part of them wanting to stop and a part of them wanting to go on smoking.

    a. How much would you say that you want to *stop* smoking?

    ____ not at all ____ a little ____ some ____ a lot ____ don't know

    b. And how much does a part of you want to *go on* smoking?

    ____ not at all ____ a little ____ some ____ a lot ____ don't know

8. Do you intend to quit smoking in the next month or so?

    ___ definitely not ___ probably not ___ possibly ___ probably ___ definitely ___ don't know

9. If you decided to give up smoking within the next month, do you think you would succeed?

    ___ definitely not ___ probably not ___ possibly ___ probably ___ definitely ___ don't know

10. Rate how much your physician convinced you to stop smoking.

    0=Not at all

    1=A little

    2=Somewhat

    3=Very much

11. Rate how confident your physician was in giving you advice to stop smoking.

    0=Not at all

    1=A little

    2=Somewhat

    3=Very much

APPENDIX J
Exit Questionnaire #2
(No-Gum Group)

Subject No. ____________________

Did your physician:

1. Ask your biggest fear about cessation?

   ____ Yes ____ No

2. Give you a way to combat your feared problem with cessation?

   ____ Yes ____ No

APPENDIX K
Exit Questionnaire #3
(Nicotine Gum Group)

Subject No.__________________________

Did your physician:

1. Tell you about nicotine gum to aid the withdrawal part of smoking cessation?

   ____ Yes ____ No

2. Tell you that if you use the gum you should:

   Stop abruptly?

   ____ Yes ____ No

   Use the gum when you have an urge for a cigarette?

   ____ Yes ____ No

   Chew the gum slowly to avoid side effects?

   ____ Yes ____ No

   Chew the gum till you have no craving for cigarettes, and then taper off the gum?

   ____ Yes ____ No

   Read a booklet about the gum when you get it at the pharmacy?

   ____ Yes ____ No

APPENDIX L
One- to Two-Week Followup for Smoking Cessation Study

Subject No. ________________

Date ________________

Please fill out this form and return in the self-addressed envelope as soon as possible. If we do not receive the form within 1 week, we will need to call you at home.

1. Have you tried to stop smoking since you entered the study?

   ____ Yes ____ No

   IF YES, ANSWER QUESTIONS 2-6.

   IF NO, YOU ARE FINISHED. THANK YOU.

2. How many times have you tried to stop since you entered the study? _____
3. When was the first time you tried to stop after seeing your physician?

______	______	______
Month	Date	Year
(1-12)	(1-31)	(19--)

4. Are you smoking cigarettes now? ____ Yes ____ No
5. Rate how helpful your physician's advice was in stopping smoking.

0	1	2	3
not at all	somewhat	moderately helpful	most helpful

6. Rate how helpful the "Quit and Win" booklet was in stopping smoking.

0	1	2	3
not at all	somewhat	moderately helpful	most helpful

APPENDIX M
Six-Month Followup for Smoking Cessation Study

Subject No. ____________________

Date ____________________

Please fill out this form and return in the self-addressed envelope as soon as possible. If we do not receive the form within 1 week, we will need to call you at home.

1. Have you tried to stop smoking since you entered the study?

   ___ Yes ___ No

   IF YES, ANSWER QUESTIONS 2-4.

   IF NO, YOU ARE FINISHED. THANK YOU.

2. How many times have you tried to stop since you entered the study? ___

   2a. When was the first time you tried to quit after you entered the study?

______	______	______
Month	Date	Year
(1-12)	(1-31)	(19--)

3. Are you smoking now? ___ Yes ___ No

   3a. If you are not smoking, when did you last have a cigarette?

______	______	______
Month	Date	Year
(1-12)	(1-31)	(19--)

4. Are you using cigars, a pipe, or smokeless tobacco?

   ___ Yes ___ No

APPENDIX N
Followup Questionnaire on the Use of Nicotine Gum

Subject No.______________________

Date __________________________

You received a prescription for nicotine gum from your physician. Please answer the following questions and return in the self-addressed envelope.

1. Did you fill the prescription?

   ____ Yes ____ No

2. Rate how helpful you found the nicotine gum in quitting smoking:

0	1	2	3	4
not at all	somewhat	moderately	most helpful	didn't use

If you answered yes to question #1, please complete the following questions.

Please name the pharmacy that you used to obtain nicotine gum.

____

(pharmacy name)

____

____

(address of pharmacy)

____

(telephone of pharmacy)

We will contact your pharmacy to verify your use of the nicotine gum. We appreciate your assistance.

THANK YOU.

Chapter 3
Training of Physicians in Training

CONTENTS

Introduction
Thomas E. Kottke 189

Interventions for Smoking Prevention and Cessation
Robert Goldberg, Judith K. Ockene, Katherine Kalan,
and Jean Kristeller 191
Purpose of the Project 191
Rationale and Special Requirements 191
Target Audience 192
Recruitment Procedures 193
Nature of the Program 194
Smoking Intervention Approaches 196
Special Resources and Procedures 198
Products of the Project 198
Study Results 199
Questions To Resolve 203
What Might Be Done Differently 205
References 205

Effects of Two Realistic Interventions To Teach Smoking Cessation Counseling to Primary Care Residents: A Randomized Trial
Victor J. Strecher, Michael S. O'Malley, Victor G. Villagra,
Elizabeth E. Campbell, Jorge J. Gonzalez, Thomas G. Irons,
Richard D. Kenney, Robert C. Turner, C. Stewart Rogers,
Mary F. Lyles, Susanne T. White, Clare J. Sanchez,
Frank T. Stritter, and Suzanne W. Fletcher 207
Purpose of the Study 207
Training Program 208
Evaluation 210
Results 215
Discussion 220
References 222

Appendixes
A. Smoking Intervention Communication Grid 223
B. Outline of the Advice and Counseling Smoking Intervention Approaches 224
C. Physician Responses to Patients' Concerns 226

Training of Physicians in Training

Editor: Thomas E. Kottke

INTRODUCTION If physicians in training, particularly residents, are to become effective smoking cessation interventionists, the following questions must be answered:

- Can smoking cessation experts train residents to deliver effective smoking cessation advice?
- Can residents be trained in smoking cessation techniques effectively by nonspecialists?
- What sort of environment is required if residents are to be trained in smoking cessation techniques?

The two papers in Chapter 3 focus on these issues. In the first paper, Goldberg and colleagues demonstrate that after just a few hours of training, residents can successfully help their patients stop smoking. These residents were in the training programs of the Department of Internal Medicine and Department of Family Practice at the University of Massachusetts. Their training consisted of a 1-hour small-group session and a brief period for residents to receive feedback on individual performance. The residents were trained to use one of three interventions with each patient: advice only, counseling, or counseling plus prescription of nicotine-containing gum. According to data collected from 1,224 trial participants, the 6-month rates for smoking cessation increased significantly in proportion to the intensity of the intervention the residents delivered. Counseling plus prescription of nicotine-containing gum was more effective than was counseling alone; and both of those interventions were more effective than was advice alone.

In the second paper, Strecher and colleagues describe how medical education generalists can successfully transfer smoking intervention skills to residents. They also demonstrate that prompting residents to intervene is not enough if the residents do not know what the intervention should be. Recognizing that most residency programs would devote only minimal time to training physicians in the delivery of smoking interventions, Strecher and coworkers tested two interventions—a prompt on the medical record and a two-session tutorial for the resident—in a design that compared the effects of a control group, a group that received the prompt alone, a group that received the training alone, and a group that received both the prompt and the training. The ability of the interventions to increase both the frequency of counseling and the number of techniques used to help the patient was tested in 11 primary care training programs.

While frequency of counseling was increased by both the tutorials and the prompts, the increase in counseling associated with the prompts alone (5 percentage points) was not statistically significant. In addition to increasing the frequency of counseling, the tutorial doubled the number of intervention techniques used by the residents.

Both papers demonstrate that residents can be trained to give successful smoking intervention advice only if adequate resources and priority are devoted to the task. Even though the chief of medicine and the training program directors supported the program at the University of Massachusetts, educating the 196 residents was, in the words of Goldberg and colleagues, "a formidable and demanding organizational task." A full-time project coordinator was needed both to recruit residents to the training sessions and to reschedule the sessions when the residents did not attend. Goldberg and coworkers also found that it was "essential" for a research assistant to be present in each clinic to assure that the interventions were delivered as indicated. Likewise, support by all individuals, from the department chairs to the clinic staff, was considered essential for success.

Strecher and colleagues shared these experiences: Arranging for followup of the initial tutorial session required a concerted effort, and integration of the prompt form into the medical record proved difficult. They concluded that without the commitment of a faculty member at each site, the program would have failed.

The message from these two papers is clear and consistent: While resident physicians need prompting, they need more than prompting alone if they are to help their patients stop smoking. However, the necessary skills can be acquired in as little as 2 hours. Furthermore, the training can be provided by faculty generalists; experts in smoking cessation are not required. It is very clear, however, that neither training in smoking cessation nor the interventions that result from such training will diffuse into training programs spontaneously because serious attention to smoking is not currently on the medical agenda. If doctors are to be trained in the skills to deliver smoking cessation counseling, and if they are to believe that dealing with smoking is not an optional activity, adequate time, along with the necessary human and fiscal resources, must be devoted to the task.

Interventions for Smoking Prevention and Cessation

Robert Goldberg, Judith K. Ockene, Katherine Kalan, and Jean Kristeller

PURPOSE OF THE PROJECT The goals of the randomized clinical trial reported here were (1) to develop and evaluate a structured educational program for training medical residents (and, secondarily, attending physicians) to intervene with their patients who smoke cigarettes and (2) to evaluate, using a randomized clinical trial design, the effect of three physician-delivered smoking intervention approaches (advice only, counseling, and counseling plus nicotine-containing gum) in combination with two followup approaches (minimal, maximal) on the 6-month smoking cessation rates of an ambulatory outpatient population. In addition, the investigators examined the effect of these intervention approaches on patients' long-term smoking behavior at 12, 18, and 24 months after randomization.

RATIONALE AND SPECIAL REQUIREMENTS Physicians have contact with at least two-thirds of all smokers annually. Therefore, the majority of the 50 million current adult smokers in the United States could potentially be reached by physicians during the course of ongoing medical care. This high patient-physician contact rate, even if coupled with only a small absolute effect on smoking prevalence, could produce substantial changes in smoking behavior in the general population of smokers.

A number of earlier clinical trials demonstrated that physicians' provision of simple advice to stop smoking could increase the quit rates of patients seen in a general medical population (Ewart et al., 1983; Handel, 1973; Li et al., 1984; Porter and McCullough, 1972; Russell et al., 1979; Wells et al., 1984; Wilson et al., 1982). Recent randomized clinical trials have consistently demonstrated that physicians who are prompted to intervene, or who receive special training to assist smokers during the course of regular medical encounters, have a greater effect on the smoking behavior of their patients than that of physicians not so trained or prompted (Cohen et al., 1987; Cummings et al., 1989; Kottke et al., 1988; Ockene et al., 1991; Wilson et al., 1988).

Physicians indicate that their willingness to intervene with smokers in their practice would be enhanced if they felt confident of their ability to have a positive effect on patients' smoking habits. Medical school and residency training programs, however, do little to foster the development or maintenance of skills in this area. Residency programs in particular offer little or no opportunity for training in communication skills and behavioral intervention for problems such as unhealthy lifestyle behaviors.

Given that physicians can have a potentially substantial impact on a large group of smokers, questions remain as to whether there is yet more that the physician can offer the smoker within the context and constraints of usual medical care. In particular, little investigative work has been carried out to adapt the successful behavioral counseling approaches of psychologists and health educators to the physician-patient encounter. Questions also remain as to whether the physician's role in smoking cessation could be augmented with additional counseling by health counselors who are not physicians. The present trial was carried out among resident physicians in training to address these concerns and others.

TARGET AUDIENCE

Residents

Medical residents in training, from the Departments of Internal Medicine and Family Practice affiliated with the University of Massachusetts Medical School, were targeted as the physician study sample during each of their postgraduate years. These residents were selected for the following reasons:

- The physicians were at a stage in their careers where training is a natural accompaniment to their career and practice aspirations. Residents expect to be taught novel approaches to lifestyle and lifestyle-related problems that could be incorporated into their eventual clinical practices. As this is a logical training point, any positive findings drawn from this study in the training of physicians in smoking cessation techniques and of their effective use of such techniques could be assimilated easily into other training programs and medical practice settings.
- Physicians in training are young and energetic, and typically they welcome participation in research projects, provided that their involvement does not consume too much time and does not detract from other areas of their training and from patient care responsibilities.
- The structured environment of ambulatory care teaching clinics, which are organized under the aegis of a medical school, provides an ideal setting for the conduct of such a randomized trial and for data collection and monitoring.

Patients

Patients attending five ambulatory clinics (two internal medicine and three family practice) affiliated with the University of Massachusetts Medical Center were recruited for this study. Each of the clinics was located within a 25-mile radius of the University of Massachusetts Medical Center. Participating patients averaged 35 years of age; slightly more than half (57 percent) were female; 91 percent were white; their average level of education was 12.5 years; and they smoked, on average, slightly more than one pack of cigarettes per day.

RECRUITMENT PROCEDURES

Medical Residents

The time slot for training residents in internal medicine was taken from their daily noon educational sessions, which are carried out on a regular basis throughout the academic year. Originally, letters were sent by the Chief of Medicine from the Department of Internal Medicine to reinforce the importance of the study and the key role of participation by residents. Further support for the residents' participation in the study was provided by the director of the residency training program, who, on a number of occasions, discussed the importance of training in smoking intervention and of the overall study. The director provided members of the study staff with the time needed for training sessions. In addition, each of the directors from the clinics where the study took place supported the training activities of the study and allocated clinic time for residents to be trained as needed.

Residents in the Department of Family and Community Medicine were recruited through the directors of their training program and trained in a relatively similar fashion. An appropriate amount of time was allocated from their clinical responsibilities for attending the group training sessions and the individual feedback session. Reflecting the success of the training program and genuine interest and commitment to learning new smoking intervention techniques, a large proportion of the attending physicians in the participating primary care clinics requested and received training in smoking intervention.

Despite the support of key persons involved in the educational training of the internal medicine and family practice residents, recruitment and training of the 196 house officers over the 4 years of the project turned out to be a formidable and demanding organizational task. A full-time project coordinator spent a considerable portion of her time in the first years of the project writing letters to residents who missed the training sessions to inform them of the future training dates and times; placing telephone calls to all eligible residents to encourage them to attend the training sessions; and coordinating the pretraining assessments, group training, and individual tutorial sessions. Although it was impossible to examine systematically the extent of time spent by the project staff in recruiting residents to the smoking intervention training sessions, it was estimated that the project coordinator spent approximately half of her time on such activities. Residents who were unable to attend the group training sessions were provided individual teaching sessions. The important structural elements in facilitating resident attendance were (1) keeping the training sessions relatively brief (less than 1 hour at a time) and task oriented and (2) providing a free lunch as an incentive for residents to attend the training sessions. Later sections of this paper describe approaches to recruitment that were particularly helpful, as well as those approaches that might have been modified in light of the experience from this trial.

Patients

To facilitate the recruitment of patients to this study, as well as monitor the delivery of the various smoking interventions by the residents, a research assistant was placed at each of the participating clinics. Each of the respective research clinic assistants was placed in a highly visible and accessible area of the clinic to enhance recruitment activities. This person determined the eligibility of potential study participants, obtained informed consent, and randomized each eligible and consenting subject to the study.

NATURE OF THE PROGRAM

The entire training and research protocol of the Physician-Delivered Smoking Intervention Project was approximately 3 hours in length (Ockene et al., 1988 and 1991; Quirk et al., 1990). One-half hour was devoted to pretraining assessments of residents' baseline knowledge, attitudes, and skills. Two hours were devoted to formal group training, which included some discussion of the research protocol, and one-half hour to individual posttraining assessment and protocol review with members of the study staff. Thus, the actual resident training took approximately 2 hours.

A total of 196 internal medicine and family practice residents affiliated with the University of Massachusetts Medical School participated in the study and attended the training sessions, held about 2 weeks apart during regularly scheduled teaching times. Generally, residents were trained in groups of 10; however, because of their schedules, it sometimes became necessary to conduct the training sessions in smaller groups. In the first 2 years of the study, 66 residents were trained each year; in the final 2 years, only new incoming interns, 32 each year, were trained. It was necessary to conduct 18 training sessions to completely train the 66 eligible residents during the first year of the study. In the second year, after determining that residents were generally available during the scheduled noon conference hour, the investigators reduced the number of training sessions to 14. In subsequent study years, after the training protocol was well established in the curriculum, there was an average of eight training sessions annually.

Sessions typically were offered during the residents' regularly scheduled noon conference teaching hour, during which the residents are exposed to daily lectures from all clinical departments. Lunch was provided free to the participating residents. Two weeks prior to the training sessions, each resident received a letter from the residency director and study investigators to inform them of the upcoming training and the importance of their participation. To encourage the residents' participation in the trial, several reminders of the training session were sent close to the time of actual training; on the day prior to training, notes were placed in the residents' mailboxes; and on the morning of the training session, study staff members telephoned residents to confirm the meeting time and place and further encourage them to attend.

During the project's training sessions, residents were trained in three physician-delivered interventions: provision of personalized advice to assist patients in stopping smoking; use of brief, patient-centered behavioral counseling; and use of the behavioral counseling approach plus the prescription of nicotine-containing chewing gum. The educational methods used in the residents' training included the following: a slide presentation reviewing epidemiological findings on the risks associated with smoking; discussion of the benefits of cessation in both healthy persons and those with chronic disease; and discussion of smoking as an addictive behavior. In addition, the residents observed each of the smoking interventions via a videotaped, simulated interaction that demonstrated the smoking cessation techniques. The residents then practiced each quit-smoking approach by first critiquing a simulated encounter between two residents and then through role-playing, with each resident playing the role of physician or patient. The videotape and role-playing exercises were used in both sessions. At the second training session, evaluation of nicotine dependency and appropriate prescribing practices for nicotine gum were discussed. Residents were also informed of the importance of followup contacts in the counseling and the counseling-plus-nicotine-gum interventions and the need to keep within the intervention protocol to which the patients were randomly assigned.

The final half-hour training session was completed with each resident individually. During this session, the resident was videotaped using the counseling approach with a surrogate patient and the videotape was reviewed and feedback given by a project instructor. At this final session, a member of the study staff reviewed the study protocol with each resident and addressed questions concerning the project and the resident's role in it.

The patient-centered counseling intervention emphasized the use of guided questioning of patients by residents, as related to the following content areas (see Appendix A):

- Desire and motivation to change smoking behavior;
- Past experience with smoking cessation;
- Factors that inhibit smoking behavior change (barriers or problems);
- Resources for change (strengths) and methods for dealing with factors that may interfere with the smoking cessation or reduction plan; and
- A plan for change.

In each of the content areas of the counseling protocol, the counseling skills of the residents were assessed in the areas of eliciting and providing information as well as in eliciting and responding to patients' feelings.

At the completion of the individual training session, each resident was provided with a $25 gift certificate to use toward the purchase of books or other educational materials at the university bookstore. In addition, each resident's name was placed into an annual lottery from which one resident was eventually chosen and given a further financial incentive.

SMOKING INTERVENTION APPROACHES

The three physician-delivered interventions consisted of the conditions described in the following sections (Ockene et al., 1988 and 1991; Quirk et al., 1990).

Advice Only

Patients assigned to the advice-only condition received a brief smoking cessation message from the resident physician that personalized each patient's risk of smoking and encouraged each patient to stop smoking. For example, the resident might say to the patient, "Stopping smoking is particularly important for you because you have high blood pressure and an elevated cholesterol level, and stopping smoking could help reduce your risk of heart disease." Interested patients were also offered a list of available smoking cessation resources in the community. Although participating physicians were asked not to extend further smoking interventions or counseling to patients randomly allocated to this condition, if the patient initiated questions about how to stop smoking or requested specific help, such as a prescription for nicotine-containing gum, the residents were free to respond as they believed was clinically appropriate. A sample of the script recommended for use by residents for patients randomized to the advice-only intervention and the particular aspects of this intervention are presented in Appendix B.

Counseling

In addition to receiving the minimal advice-only intervention, each patient randomized to the counseling condition received behavioral counseling. As previously described, this intervention approach explored a number of patient-centered areas related to behavior change. Through open-ended questions, the resident elicited information about the patient's desire and motivation to change smoking behavior, past experiences with stopping, problems that might inhibit the change, current concerns, resources available for changing smoking behavior, and interest in developing a personalized plan for cessation and followup. Trained residents were taught to structure the counseling approach around these specific behavior-related content areas and were provided with model questions, such as "How do you feel about your smoking?", "Have you ever stopped smoking before?", and "How were you able to stop smoking in the past?" A sample script for the counseling intervention and guidelines for its use are shown in Appendix B.

The sequence of questioning developed for use by the residents has a cognitive and behavioral theoretical basis with the principal focus on the development of positive self-efficacy in the patient. In other words, the counseling intervention helps patients to identify the personal skills and resources necessary to stop smoking and to feel confident of their ability to stop smoking and their commitment to do so. This approach was chosen because previous studies of smoking behavior change have shown that when an individual believes it is possible to make the desired change, there is greater likelihood that such change will occur. Residents were also trained to provide simple behavioral self-management recommendations (such as taking a walk after dinner instead of smoking a cigarette) and to be supportive of the patient's cessation and/or tapering efforts. A written agreement or a plan for change in the patient's smoking behavior was formulated between the patient and physician as a form of contracting between the two parties. The plan for change included a quit date, if deemed appropriate, and other changes in smoking behavior such as changing brands or tapering the number of cigarettes smoked each day. A copy of the agreement was given to the patient along with a list of community resources and an NCI-produced self-help booklet, "Quit for Good."

Patients were requested to schedule a followup appointment with the resident within 2 weeks or a followup telephone call if a visit was not possible. At that time, the physician was to address changes in the patient's smoking behavior and intervene appropriately. Trained residents were also provided with a single page of suggested responses to patients' concerns about stopping or reducing smoking (Appendix C). The responses were important because physicians often reported feeling at a loss when patients expressed feelings or concerns that the physicians were not prepared to address. The recommended responses helped to increase the physician's own feelings of efficacy. Although it was impossible to assess systematically the amount of time residents spent in each of the intervention approaches, the interventions were designed to be relatively brief and to be incorporated into a regular medical care encounter.

Counseling Plus Prescription Gum

Patients randomly assigned to the counseling-plus-gum condition received the basic patient-centered counseling intervention and also were offered nicotine-containing chewing gum as a resource to aid in the cessation process. Patients interested in using the gum and willing to set a specific quit date were provided with a prescription for up to three boxes of the gum at no charge. Patients who were not ready to stop smoking were informed that they could request the gum at any time during the course of the project once they agreed to stop smoking. As part of the training program, residents were taught about how to instruct patients in the proper use of the gum and how best to respond to concerns that patients might raise about using the gum. After seeing their physicians, patients were seen for several minutes by a clinic assistant associated with the study, who instructed them more fully in the use of the gum.

Followup to Intervention

In addition to the three physician-delivered intervention approaches, patients were further randomized to two followup conditions, as described below.

Maximal Followup

Patients randomized to the maximal-followup condition received telephone calls from trained counselors (master's-level psychologists or health educators) at approximately 1, 2, and 3 months after the initial physician contact and randomization. The same counselor made all three telephone calls to a single study participant. Personalized letters followed each counseling call and were keyed to the patient's smoking status as determined by the previous call. Patients were congratulated for any changes they had made in their smoking behavior and encouraged to continue to work toward complete cessation. The calls were somewhat structured and were keyed to information from the baseline questionnaire and to changes in smoking status. The counselor used a series of open-ended questions similar to those the physicians used in the patient-centered counseling approach, provided behavioral recommendations, and negotiated a smoking cessation or maintenance plan with the patient, as appropriate.

Minimal Followup

When patients were assigned to the minimal-followup condition, no further counseling contact was provided. All patients, whether in the maximal- or minimal-followup group, were informed of the initial 6-month telephone monitoring calls at the time of their initial physician visit. They were informed also that they would be called to determine changes in their smoking status at 12, 18, and 24 months after randomization.

SPECIAL RESOURCES AND PROCEDURES

As noted previously, a research assistant was placed at each of the participating clinic sites to facilitate the recruitment of patients and oversee the physician-delivered interventions. These assistants were essential because they reminded the clinic staff, physicians and nurses, that they were participating in the study. The research assistant delivered a sealed intervention packet to the resident who would be intervening with the enrolled and randomized patient. The resident then broke the seal of the intervention package, which contained a brief suggested script that could be tailored for use with each randomized patient. This script reduced the need for recall on the part of the intervening physician and standardized the delivery of the assigned intervention. The packet also contained all appropriate support materials, such as the list of available community resources and self-help materials to be used with each randomized patient.

To further support the participation of residents in this study, and to emphasize the importance of the counseling techniques and their relevance for use with other lifestyle-related problems, interested attending physicians at the respective clinics were also informed of the goals and objectives of the study and were trained in the various quit-smoking intervention approaches.

PRODUCTS OF THE PROJECT

Samples of the counseling intervention approach used in this study and sample scripts of the intervention protocols are provided in Appendixes A and B, respectively. In addition, physician responses to patients' concerns that might be commonly raised when they are asked to stop or reduce the number of cigarettes they are presently smoking are outlined in Appendix C. The responses that could be used by the trained residents were developed so that the residents would feel more secure and comfortable in replying to the most typical concerns that patients had in terms of stopping or reducing the number of cigarettes they were currently smoking. During the initial role-playing exercises involving residents, members of the research staff became aware of the need to emphasize that the residents did not have to be experts about all factors that would assist patients in making the behavioral changes necessary to stop smoking.

However, the residents clearly felt more comfortable with delivery of the various smoking interventions once they had several responses that they could draw upon to allay patients' concerns.

This study developed a training package that includes a facilitator's manual, 47 slides, a 35-minute videotape, structured role-plays, and training materials that integrate the physician-delivered smoking intervention approaches of advice, counseling, and prescription of nicotine polacrilex (Nicorette) into a unified intervention algorithm. An office practice management kit also was developed as part of the study and is included in the training package.

STUDY RESULTS

What Worked And Why

Physician Changes

Pretreatment and posttreatment measurements showed that residents exhibited significant positive change in the three skill areas of providing information, eliciting information, and eliciting and responding to feelings expressed by patients with respect to smoking cessation (Ockene et al., 1988; Quirk et al., 1990). Overall scores, based on a point scale from 0 (no evidence of the skill) to 3 (highly appropriate use of the skill), showed significant changes after training in providing information (1.23 to 1.48), eliciting information (0.95 to 1.74), and eliciting and responding to feelings (0.47 to 1.03) (all $p < 0.001$). Significant differences also were observed in the application of these skills to a number of content areas. In the complete pretraining and posttraining resident data, residents showed improvements after training in assessing patients' desire and motivation to change their smoking behavior, in questioning patients about their previous experiences with smoking changes, in identifying factors that might inhibit any changes in their patients' smoking status, and in helping patients identify and use available resources for changing their smoking behavior. Residents also showed significant improvements after training in formulating specific plans for change with their smoking patients. Baseline measurements conducted at the commencement of the trial indicated that participating residents thought that in general it was very important to help both healthy and sick patients to stop smoking and that formal training in smoking cessation was very important (mean=4.3 on a 1- to 5-point scale). Favorable changes in residents' knowledge of the risks of smoking cigarettes and attitudes toward smoking and smoking cessation also were observed over the course of the study.

From the patients' perspective, those in the behavioral counseling and counseling-plus-nicotine-gum conditions were significantly more likely to report that their physician had been very helpful in their efforts to alter their smoking behavior than were those individuals assigned to the advice-only group. These differences were seen regardless of the patients' success or lack thereof in quitting smoking.

For assessing maintenance of counseling skills, a subsample of residents was selected to examine changes in residents' long-term counseling behavior (Quirk et al., 1990). Although the findings from this small and select sample of residents call for cautious interpretation, the surveyed residents continued to exhibit positive and measurable changes in the three general skill areas at 1 year after training completion. In spite of the inherent difficulties in identifying particular aspects of the training sessions that may have facilitated the effective training of residents (given the different staff involved, training conditions, group dynamics, and other factors), the use of role-playing seemed to be particularly effective in opening up residents and in giving them experience in administering the program interventions.

Although the investigators had some initial trepidation about the use of role-playing with residents and the likelihood of getting residents actively involved in such exercises, it became readily apparent that, in an appropriate context, residents were receptive to role-playing. They enjoyed the interactive exchange of playing patient and provider, and they became demonstrably more comfortable in the delivery of the various smoking intervention approaches. Role-playing became a highly informative educational approach in that, by observing the study staff as well as other residents and then delivering the intervention themselves, residents were able to provide and receive feedback on those approaches and techniques that could assist their patients with smoking cessation.

Patient Smoking Cessation

According to data from 1,224 trial participants, 6-month cessation rates increased significantly as the intensity of the physician-delivered intervention increased ($p < 0.005$) (Ockene et al., 1988). Among patients randomized to the advice-only condition, 9.1 percent reported cessation for at least 1 week at the time of the 6-month telephone contact. Patients receiving the behavioral-counseling and counseling-plus-gum interventions reported 1-week cessation rates of 11.9 percent and 17.4 percent, respectively. Comparable differences in adjusted cessation rates were seen when multiple regression analysis was used to control for a variety of potentially confounding baseline characteristics. The adjusted findings revealed that patients in the counseling-plus-gum group demonstrated almost twice the likelihood of quitting (95-percent confidence intervals=1.2, 3.2) as those in the advice-only group; whereas patients in the counseling group demonstrated a likelihood of quitting 1.6 times that of patients in the advice-only group (95-percent confidence intervals=1.0, 2.6). However, no significant differences were observed in the 6-month cessation rates of randomized patients according to type of followup (minimal phone followup was 11.2 percent; maximal phone and letter followup, 13.9 percent).

A similar pattern of increasing quit rates with increasing levels of physician intervention was observed for continuous abstinence from smoking of greater than 3 months reported at the time of the 6-month followup contact. Of the advice-only patients, 5.9 percent had been completely off cigarettes for at least 3 months at the time of the 6-month monitoring calls; the rates were 9.2 and 13.2 percent for patients in the counseling and counseling-plus-nicotine-gum interventions, respectively ($p < 0.005$).

How soon patients stop smoking after contact with a physician provides additional information about the immediate impact that the physician can have on patients' smoking behavior. The length of time between the physician visit and initial successful cessation suggested that the more intensive the physician intervention, the greater the likelihood for early cessation. For example, approximately 15 percent of smokers in the counseling-plus-gum group reported having stopped smoking within a day of their initial physician visit, compared to 11 percent in the counseling group and 4 percent in the advice-only group ($p < 0.001$).

The length of time that patients abstain from cigarettes immediately after being seen by a physician is another measure of initial physician impact on patients' smoking behavior. The results of this trial suggest that the more intensive the physician-delivered intervention, the longer the period of abstinence after the initial contact.

A trend for an intervention effect was observed for the maintained self-reported abstinence rates at the time of the 12-month telephone followup. That is, 6.2 percent of patients who received physician advice only reported not smoking at both the 6- and 12-month contact points after baseline randomization. The proportion of patients who reported not smoking for at least 1 week prior to the telephone contact at each of these two followup assessment points was 8.1 percent for patients in the counseling group and 10.6 percent for those in the counseling-plus-nicotine-gum condition.

No significant differences were observed, however, for the 12-month, 1-week point prevalence cessation rates among the three physician-delivered intervention groups. Among patients randomized to the advice-only group, 15.2 percent reported being abstinent from cigarettes for at least 1 week; the corresponding percentages for patients in the counseling and counseling-plus-nicotine-gum groups were 12.9 and 16.7 percent, respectively. The absence of a main effect is attributable primarily to an increased number of "new stoppers" in the advice condition. It is highly probable that this higher prevalence of new cessation in the advice condition is a crossover effect rather than a result of the delayed impact of the brief advice-only intervention. "Crossover" means that patients in the advice-only group who continued to see their study physician probably ended up receiving more intensive counseling between the time of the 6- and 12-month followup contacts, resulting in higher rates of cessation.

After the residents saw their patients for the initial study contact, they were not restricted to their original intervention condition. With the exception of the project stickers that identified patients participating in the study, there were no identifiers placed on the patients' charts to indicate their original randomized condition. In spite of there being no observed trends in 1-year quit rates related to intensity of smoking intervention, and possible subsequent confounding between randomized groups in the subsequent use of the various smoking interventions, it was encouraging to note the high quit rates in the advice group, suggesting a clearly positive effect of physician advice on patients' long-term quit rates.

Integration of the Training Model

Although the integration of the physician-delivered smoking intervention training into the residency program was not a measured trial outcome, it was clearly necessary if the trial was to be successfully implemented. This report, especially the last section, indicates how such integration was facilitated. It is also of note that even after the study ended, the residency program directors strongly supported the continued teaching of the project protocol. All incoming medical residents at the University of Massachusetts Medical School have come to expect such training as part of their residency program.

What Did Not Work and Why

As is consistent with most population-based clinical trials, efforts to recruit the projected number of patients to the study fell behind the projected schedule. This was caused by operational factors as well as the unexpected low rate of current cigarette smoking among the populations surveyed. Also, early in the trial it became apparent to the investigators that they would need a multiplicity of institutional resources, recruitment techniques, and variations in the methods by which residents would be taught the various smoking intervention approaches. For example, the provision of training without lunch or refreshments did not work; nor did training sessions lasting more than an hour, as the training began to impinge on the residents' clinical responsibilities. In the early training aspects of the trial, residents may have suffered information overload as the investigators attempted to condense a lot of information into a limited timeframe. The investigators soon realized that they had to keep the resident training simple and understandable without presenting excessive didactic material, and they realized the need for considerable role-playing in the three quit-smoking intervention approaches. It is certainly likely that the cultural norms and milieu of the residents' environment are influential in the adoption of, or failure to adopt, training in smoking intervention or other lifestyle intervention techniques. It is clearly important not only to obtain the support and enthusiasm of those involved in the daily clinical training of medical residents, but also to create a receptive and open environment in which residents can be shown the importance of such training and foster its encouragement among peers.

Problems With Implementation

The results of this study confirm and extend current knowledge of the beneficial impact that physicians can have on the smoking behavior of their patients. The study demonstrated that patients who received brief, patient-centered, behavior-oriented counseling, with or without the prescription of nicotine gum, were considerably more likely to change their smoking behavior than were patients who were provided brief advice to stop smoking. The impact of these interventions on quit rates was seen immediately after intervention and at 6 months after randomization. It was also evident in terms of the length of time patients were able to continue abstaining from cigarettes.

One concern that physicians expressed about delivering smoking interventions was that they might offend and alienate patients who are not yet ready to quit, particularly if the physicians do more than offer brief advice. However, in this trial the patients rated physicians as substantially more helpful when they offered counseling or counseling plus nicotine gum than when they simply gave advice to stop smoking. This was true whether the patients went on to quit or not. As most smokers go through several stages of readiness to change their smoking status (Prochaska and DiClemente, 1983), it is important that physicians feel confident in exploring smoking issues with smokers who are not highly motivated to quit. Patient-centered counseling is designed to minimize defensiveness on the part of the smoker and it can be used repeatedly, thereby taking advantage of another characteristic of usual health care—intermittent contact over extended periods of time with a regular health care provider.

Conversely, the results of this study do not support the use of followup telephone counseling by ancillary staff to facilitate changes in patients' long-term smoking behavior. This result was surprising because it did not fit the pattern observed by Kottke and colleagues (1988). Although the telephone counselors were well-trained and skilled, no face-to-face contact had occurred between the study patients and the counselors, and patients may have perceived their calls as impersonal, intrusive, or unwarranted.

The results of the present study suggest also that resident physicians can be successfully trained in the delivery of patient-centered, behavioral counseling for smoking cessation. Residents demonstrated enhancement of not only their attitudes toward smoking cessation approaches, but also their ability to affect favorably their patients' smoking behavior. A further mark of success for the training program was that it was requested by, and extended to, attending physicians working in the clinics in which the study was carried out.

QUESTIONS TO RESOLVE

Despite the encouraging results of the present study (Ockene et al., 1988 and 1991; Quirk et al., 1990), a number of questions remain unanswered and warrant further investigation. Is the effectiveness of patient-centered counseling attributable to the greater amount of time spent by the physician or to the *manner* of counseling? Can the counseling techniques used in this study be taught readily in other settings and to physicians at other levels of professional development? There are also unanswered questions about how best to use the clinic environment to foster smoking prevention and cessation among patients attending the clinic and how best to prompt the resident physicians to deliver the smoking intervention.

Another major set of questions has to do with identifying the necessary and effective followup of patients who smoke. Perhaps telephone counseling followup would increase cessation efforts when offered by someone known to the patient, or if the patient were able to decide whether or not to receive such additional counseling.

Although no data are available to address this question, another important area for future research is whether this type of brief, patient-centered counseling can be used by physicians to intervene effectively with other behavioral risk factors such as physical exercise (Harris et al., 1989) and lowering cholesterol (Report of the National Cholesterol Education Program, 1988). Given that the authors have shown that residents can be trained to deliver effective quit-smoking messages to their patients, it is hypothesized that physicians in training and practicing physicians might also use such approaches in helping patients to modify their intake of saturated fat and total fat and to find effective ways to increase their energy expenditure on a long-term basis. Finally, the authors do not know how best to maintain the quit rates observed in this trial, given the minimal interaction that occurred between patient and physician.

There are a number of additional issues related to physician training. Support from the department chairs, directors of the residency training programs and clinics, and the staffs of clinics at which the study took place was considered essential in successfully training the residents, recruiting patients, and carrying the study to completion. Attending physicians in the clinics also were perceived as agents of support and sanction for the residents' activities.

There remain unanswered questions as to whether one can assess the stages of readiness for the adoption of training in smoking intervention in a physician sample, and whether efforts should be aimed specifically at residents who are seriously contemplating or eager to get such training. The receptivity to training is expected to be quite high among such physicians, whereas those physicians who are in a precontemplation stage for receiving and adopting such training might be initially bypassed. Such targeting of physicians might result in more effective and efficient recruitment, as well as training, of health care providers in smoking cessation techniques.

The optimal timing for the various training activities involved in educating residents in the use of such counseling techniques is unknown. Meals and additional incentives (e.g., gift certificates or possibly continuing medical education credits for attending physicians) should most definitely be provided as a means to recruit and retain the parties involved. Questions also remain as to when and if resident or attending physicians might need additional maintenance or booster training sessions to reinforce and bolster their smoking intervention efforts. At present, the authors' training program has been incorporated into the medical residents' curriculum, providing a further institutionalization of the program.

The most effective ways to train resident physicians remain to be determined. For example, should members of a study staff train key physicians who will in turn be responsible for training their residents (training the trainers)? Or, on the other hand, might self-training materials be used by targeted personnel and might use of these materials be considered adequate training?

WHAT MIGHT BE DONE DIFFERENTLY

Although, in general, it was thought that the recruitment and training of physicians for this trial were satisfactory, particularly as the study investigators accrued experience with methods that might or might not work for recruiting the physicians and study sample, the logistics were quite formidable. The principal investigator and project coordinator are key to the successful recruitment and retention of physicians, and these individuals must be highly visible and approachable. Early and continued involvement of the director of the residency training program and the chair of the medical department from which residents are recruited is also essential to the successful conduct of such a trial. In addition, it is extremely important to identify and involve key clinic staff from each of the participating clinics at which residents practice early on, so that the residents' role in the study will be fostered and obstacles minimized.

With regard to the structure of training sessions, the study showed that between 6 and 10 participants was the ideal number, so that each individual resident could successfully role-play each of the interventions to be used. In addition, within several months after the physician has become involved in such a trial, regardless of the number of patients treated with the intervention, booster training sessions should be developed to maintain a high degree of competency for the various smoking interventions. More attention should be directed also to the training of residents in smoking relapse prevention, as this was a problem that affected the study's 12-month findings.

REFERENCES

Cohen, S.J., Christen, A.G., Katz, B.P., Drook, C.A., Davis, B.J., Smith, D.M., Stookey, G.K. Counseling medical and dental patients about cigarette smoking: The impact of nicotine gum and chart reminders. *American Journal of Public Health* 77: 313-316, 1987.

Cummings, S.R., Coates, T.J., Richard, R.J., Hansen, B., Zahnd, E.G., Vander Martin, R., Duncan, C., Gerbert, B., Martin, A., Stein, M.J. Training physicians in counseling about smoking cessation: A randomized trial of the "Quit for Life" program. *Annals of Internal Medicine* 110(8): 640-647, 1989.

Ewart, C.K., Li, V.C., Coates, T.J. Increasing physicians' antismoking influence by applying an inexpensive feedback technique. *Journal of Medical Education* 58(6): 468-473, 1983.

Handel, S.P. Change in smoking habits in a general practice. *Graduate Medical Journal* 49: 679-681, 1973.

Harris, S.S., Caspersen, C.J., DeFriese, G.H., Estes, F.H., Jr. Physical activity counseling for healthy adults as a primary preventive intervention in the clinical setting. *Journal of the American Medical Association* 261: 3590-3598, 1989.

Kottke, T.E., Battista, R.N., DeFriese, G.H., Brekke, M.L. Attributes of successful smoking cessation interventions in medical practice: A meta-analysis of 39 controlled trials. *Journal of the American Medical Association* 259: 2882-2889, 1988.

Li, V.C., Kim, Y.J., Ewart, C.K., Terry, P.B., Cuthie, J.C., Wood, J., Emmet, E.A., Permutt, S. Effects of physician counseling on the smoking behavior of asbestos-exposed workers. *Preventive Medicine* 13: 462-476, 1984.

Ockene, J.K., Kristeller, J., Goldberg, R., Amick, T.L., Pekow, P.S., Hosmer, D., Quirk, M., Kalan, K. Increasing the efficacy of physician-delivered smoking intervention: A randomized clinical trial. *Journal of General Internal Medicine* 6: 1-8, 1991.

Ockene, J.K., Quirk, M.E., Goldberg, R.J., Kristeller, J.L., Donnelly, G., Kalan, K.L., Gould, B., Greene, H.L., Harrison-Atlas, R., Pease, J., Pickens, S., Williams, J.W. A residents' training program for the development of smoking intervention skills. *Archives of Internal Medicine* 148: 1039-1045, 1988.

Porter, A.M.W., McCullough, D.M. Counseling against cigarette smoking. *Practitioner* 209: 686-689, 1972.

Prochaska, J.O., DiClemente, C.C. Stages and processes of self-change of smoking: Toward an integrative model of change. *Journal of Consulting and Clinical Psychology* 51(3): 390-395, 1983.

Quirk, M., Ockene, J., Kristeller, J., Goldberg, R., Donnelly, G., Amick, T., Kalan, K. Training family practice and internal medicine residents to counsel patients who smoke: Improvement and retention of counseling skills. *Family Medicine* 23: 108-111, 1990.

Report of the National Cholesterol Education Program Expert Panel on Detection, Evaluation, and Treatment of High Cholesterol in Adults. *Archives of Internal Medicine* 148(1): 36-69, 1988.

Russell, M.A., Wilson, C., Taylor, C., Baker, C.D. The effect of general practitioners' advice against smoking. *British Medical Journal* 2: 231-235, 1979.

Wells, K.B., Ware, J.E., Jr., Lewis, C.E. Physicians' practices in counseling patients about health habits. *Medical Care* 22(3): 240-246, 1984.

Wilson, D., Wood, G., Johnston, N., Sicurella, J. Randomized clinical trial of supportive follow-up for cigarette smokers in a family practice. *Canadian Medical Association Journal* 126: 127-129, 1982.

Wilson, D.M., Taylor, D.W., Gilbert, J.R., Best, J.A., Lindsay, E.A., Willms, D.G., Singer, J. A randomized trial of a family physician intervention for smoking cessation. *Journal of the American Medical Association* 260(11): 1570-1574, 1988.

Effects of Two Realistic Interventions To Teach Smoking Cessation Counseling To Primary Care Residents: A Randomized Trial[1]

Victor J. Strecher, Michael S. O'Malley, Victor G. Villagra, Elizabeth E. Campbell, Jorge J. Gonzalez, Thomas G. Irons, Richard D. Kenney, Robert C. Turner, C. Stewart Rogers, Mary F. Lyles, Susanne T. White, Clare J. Sanchez, Frank T. Stritter, and Suzanne W. Fletcher

PURPOSE OF THE STUDY The NCI Smoking, Tobacco, and Cancer Program trials of smoking interventions by physicians have demonstrated that smoking cessation counseling by physicians can help smokers quit. How best to disseminate widely effective smoking cessation counseling and increase physicians' use of it remains an issue. Residency training programs offer a natural, though standard, opportunity to teach effective smoking cessation counseling to large numbers of physicians.

The authors developed two realistic, generalizable interventions to increase smoking cessation counseling by primary care resident physicians: the tutorial and the prompt. Both were based on the same minimal-contact smoking cessation counseling protocol, one similar to those used in the STCP Physician Smoking Trials. The tutorial used a "training of trainers" approach in conjunction with the familiar tutorial format to teach smoking cessation counseling to residents. The prompt used a chart-based reminder to teach residents smoking cessation counseling by prompting and guiding them to do counseling.

The investigators then used a randomized factorial design to determine changes in residents' counseling practices and their patients' cigarette smoking after the two interventions. The trial evaluated the effectiveness of the tutorial and the prompt across 11 residency training programs and 3 primary care specialties: internal medicine, family medicine, and pediatrics. This paper summarizes previously published results and examines the utility of

[1] Supported by the University of North Carolina Faculty Development Program in General Medicine and General Pediatrics (PE54004, Bureau of Health Professions, Washington, D.C.) and by grants from the National Cancer Institute (R03-CA43994), the North Carolina Chapter of the American Heart Association (1986-86-37-A), and the University of North Carolina Center for Health Promotion and Disease Prevention.

training in smoking cessation counseling as well as barriers that impede implementation of such training (Campbell et al., 1991; Kenney et al., 1988; Strecher et al., 1991).

TRAINING PROGRAM

Background: Defining Realistic Interventions

What constitutes a realistic intervention to increase the use of smoking cessation counseling by residents in primary care training programs? A realistic intervention should address two questions: (1) What is an effective and generalizable smoking cessation counseling protocol that physicians can use in a practice setting? and (2) What are the most effective and generalizable ways to teach, reinforce, and remind physicians to use the smoking cessation counseling protocol?

The smoking cessation counseling protocol that resident physicians use with their patients who smoke should reflect the realities of clinical practice. Busy physicians involved in ongoing patient care need simple, efficient, and effective counseling skills. A number of studies have shown that minimal-contact smoking cessation counseling programs can be effective (Cohen et al., 1987; Cummings et al., 1989; Janz et al., 1987; Kottke et al., 1989; Wilson et al., 1988).

Most residency training programs likely would provide only minimal time for residents to learn the protocol and develop their counseling skills. Given the extensive curricula of such programs, training in smoking cessation counseling would be provided most easily through already planned seminars or in another seminar format. Although interactive sessions would be better for teaching counseling skills, seminars are the method of choice in many residency programs.

An alternative to seminar teaching would be use of a prompting system that reminds physicians to perform routine clinical and preventive procedures. By enhancing the prompt, the system could guide counseling as well as remind physicians to perform the counseling, and physicians would learn smoking cessation counseling by doing. Such teaching would not impose on residency curricula. Because either manual or computer systems can be developed and maintained in most settings, the training would also be generalizable.

Given a seminar-based teaching intervention, it seems likely that a faculty physician associated with the residency program or the institution would have to do the teaching. Because the faculty physicians would probably have little or no formal training in smoking cessation counseling, a training-of-trainers approach would be appropriate and generalizable. Physician teachers would be centrally trained in the smoking cessation counseling protocol. Their training would be extensive, involving expertise in smoking cessation counseling, general behavior change and relapse prevention counseling, and medical education/adult learning strategies.

Finally, teaching resident physicians to do smoking cessation counseling presents unique challenges. Residents' pessimism about the effectiveness of smoking cessation counseling makes them reluctant to undertake counseling in their busy practices. Any training approach for smoking cessation counseling must attempt to convince residents of the importance and effects of smoking cessation counseling by physicians. Residents are also adult learners who receive instruction while actively caring for patients. Teaching must be succinct and relevant to their immediate experience.

Using these principles, the authors developed two interventions to promote minimal-contact smoking cessation counseling by physicians: a tutorial and a prompt. A detailed description of both interventions and their development is available elsewhere (Campbell et al., 1991).

Minimal-Contact Counseling

Both interventions taught physicians a minimal-contact smoking cessation counseling protocol based on work by Strecher, by investigators in the STCP Physician Smoking Trials, and by other researchers in the field (Cummings et al., 1986; Gritz, 1988; Kottke et al., 1988; Ockene, 1987; Strecher et al., 1985). According to the protocol, the physician first assessed the patient's motivation to quit smoking. If the patient did not express an interest in quitting, the protocol suggested that the physician attempt to motivate the patient to quit by discussing the health, social, and financial benefits of quitting smoking and by setting a goal toward quitting. If the patient was motivated to quit, the physician was to explore the patient's obstacles to quitting, consider the use of nicotine gum, set a quit date, write a prescription for a quit date, and give the patient self-help materials. Whether or not the patient was motivated to quit, the protocol had the physician follow up on the counseling.

The Tutorial

The tutorial consisted of two sessions in smoking cessation counseling that could be incorporated into ongoing residency training. The sessions were based on seven principles of adult education adapted from Gagne and Briggs (1979):

- Gaining the resident's attention,
- Making clear the objectives,
- Presenting material in varied ways,
- Providing guidance,
- Having the resident practice,
- Providing feedback on performance, and
- Assessing performance.

The initial 1-hour session included a 10-minute slide presentation/lecture on smoking and smoking cessation; a 10-minute presentation of the minimal-contact smoking cessation protocol, incorporating a handout flowsheet; a 10-minute videotape demonstrating two successful counseling interactions; and a 20-minute group discussion and evaluation. The videotape presented one interaction with a motivated patient and one with an unmotivated patient. Approximately 2 weeks after the initial session, residents attended individual or small group followup sessions to discuss their initial attempts to counsel patients.

In both sessions, the tutorial attempted to counter residents' pessimism about the effectiveness of smoking cessation counseling by emphasizing that a 10- to 15-percent quit rate among all smokers seeing a physician each year—a success rate difficult for the individual physician to discern—would generate nearly a half-million new nonsmokers each year and could save thousands of lives. The tutorial for pediatric residents was identical to that for internal medicine and family practice residents, except that pediatricians were taught to counsel the patient's parents rather than the patient.

A clinic director or a faculty member involved in the residency training program conducted the tutorial at each site. The trainers were fellows in the University of North Carolina Faculty Development Program. As part of the program, each of the fellows had received training in smoking cessation counseling, general behavior change, and medical education/adult learning. The fellows and the program faculty developed the smoking cessation protocol and the two interventions, designed the randomized trial to evaluate the interventions' effects, and authored this study. Thus, the current study approximates the training-of-trainers approach—although the physician trainers in this study were probably more involved and committed to the interventions than other faculty members would be.

The Prompt

The prompt provided chart-based reminders for physicians to counsel patients to stop smoking and to guide physicians in that counseling (Figure 1). At patient check-in, clinic nurses identified patients who were smokers. Nurses then attached a one-page flowsheet summarizing the minimal-contact counseling protocol to the front of the medical chart. The prompt was identical to the flowsheet used in the tutorial. In pediatric residency programs, nurses determined which parents smoked and placed the prompt on the charts of their children.

EVALUATION

The authors used a randomized factorial design to determine the effects of the two realistic teaching interventions, alone and in combination. To investigate the generalizability of the interventions, the investigators tested them in 11 residency training programs representing three primary care specialties.

Figure 1
Smoking cessation counseling flowchart

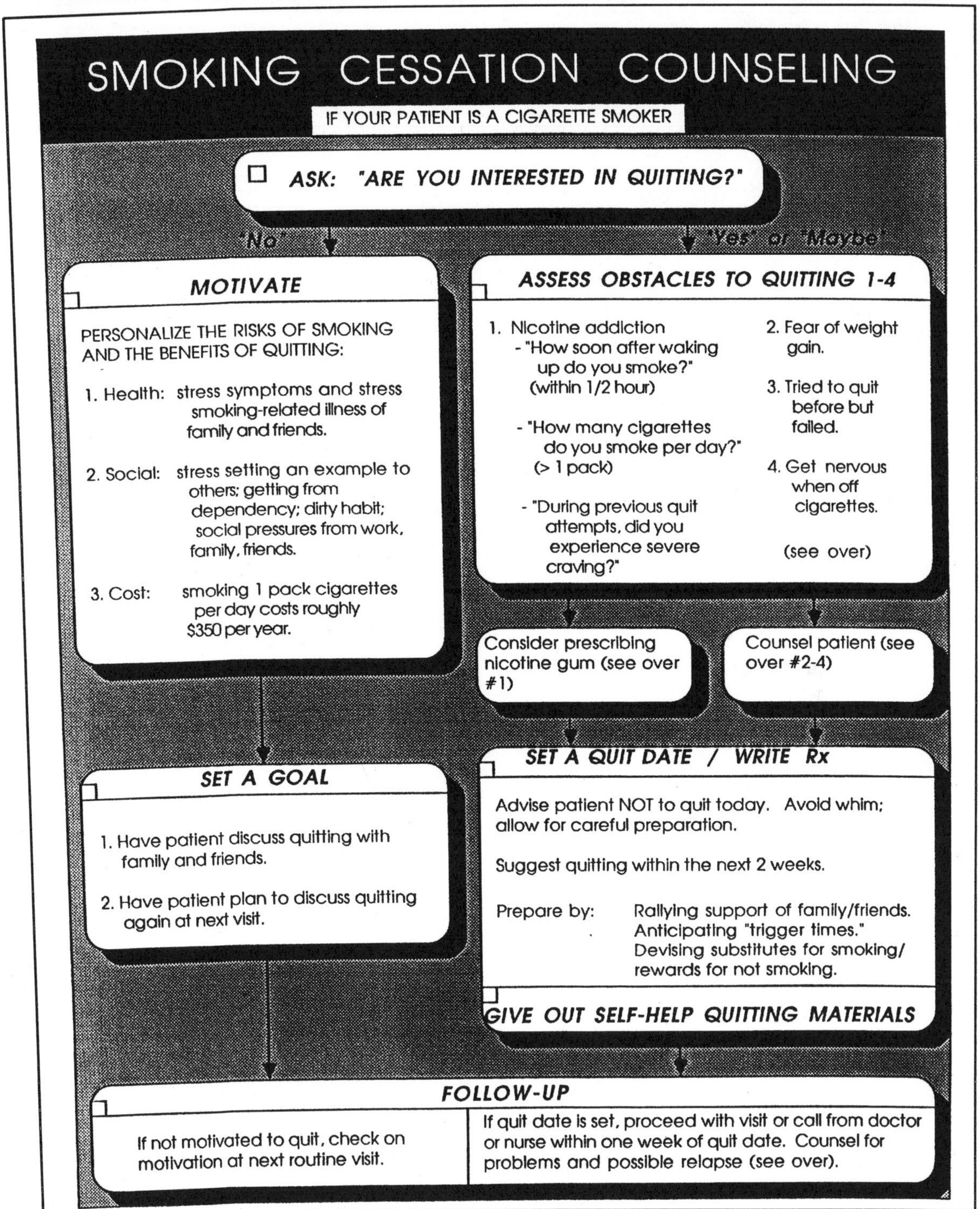

Source: UNC Faculty Development Program. Copyright University of North Carolina, Chapel Hill; used with permission.

Figure 1 (continued)

1: PRESCRIBING NICOTINE GUM

RATIONALE: Nicotine gum supplies nicotine (the possible basis of addiction) without carbon monoxide or carcinogenic tars. Nicotine from gum is released slowly (if gum is chewed slowly) without sharp nicotine boli produced through cigarette smoking.

GUIDELINES FOR USE OF GUM:

- Quit smoking before using gum.
- Chew gum slowly (about one chew for every normal puff interval), keeping taste and tingle at minimal level.
- Use for craving -- about 10-15 pieces per day.
- Taper from gum and stop using gum after 3 and 6 months (withdrawal from gum has been difficult for some patients).

2-4: OBSTACLES TO QUITTING

2. FEAR OF WEIGHT GAIN:

- 2/3 of quitters gain weight; only 1/3 gain weight and keep a significant amount of weight.
- Weight gain can be prevented by a modest diet and exercise.
- Patient may crave sweets -- warn about this.
- Compulsive eating may suggest nicotine withdrawal -- patient may respond to nicotine gum.

3. FAILED IN PRIOR ATTEMPTS TO QUIT:

- Most successful quitters require several tries.
- Circumstances of relapse should be studied to prepare for next try.

4. NERVOUSNESS:

- May be a sign of nicotine withdrawal (see #1).
- Tranquilizers are not effective in breaking smoking habit.

RELAPSE

Indicate that most successful quitters required several tries -- many people need to LEARN HOW TO QUIT.

Analyze relapse experience ("When and where did you smoke your cigarette?"). Have smoker develop strategy for coping with that experience.

Recycle smoker into new quit date and schedule follow-up.

Clinical Setting And Target Audience

The trial took place in 11 primary care training programs: 6 in internal medicine, 3 in family medicine, and 2 in pediatrics. The programs were distributed across three university medical centers (University of North Carolina at Chapel Hill, East Carolina University School of Medicine, and Bowman Gray School of Medicine) and four university-affiliated community hospitals (Charlotte Memorial Hospital, Charlotte, North Carolina; New Hanover Memorial Hospital, Wilmington, North Carolina; Moses Cone Memorial Hospital, Greensboro, North Carolina; and the Geisinger Medical Center, Danville, Pennsylvania).

All residents who saw patients in the ambulatory care setting at least one-half day per week throughout the study period were eligible for the trial. Those who did not complete a pretest questionnaire were dropped from the trial. Adult patients were people aged 17 to 75 who were making a return visit to a study physician and who reported smoking five or more cigarettes in the preceding 7 days. At the two pediatric sites, parents of patients, rather than the patients themselves, were eligible.

Trial Design

The authors used a randomized factorial design, alone and in combination, to test the two interventions (Figure 2). For the physician pretest, residents completed self-administered questionnaires to provide self-reports on smoking cessation counseling frequency and content, their attitudes, and their training. For pediatric residents, questions were adapted to address counseling of patients' parents.

After the pretest, residents were randomly assigned, by clinic half-day session, to one of four groups: tutorial only, prompt only, tutorial plus prompt, and control. The physician posttest was administered 6 months after completion of the tutorials and the start of the prompts.

During the 6 months between the physician pretests and posttests, research assistants at each site used a structured questionnaire to interview patients who smoked and who had just seen a study physician. Patients were asked about their smoking habits and physician advice to stop smoking. Up to 10 patients were interviewed for each physician.

Six months after the initial exit interview, telephone interviewers, who were blind to residents' and patients' group assignments, obtained patient reports on current smoking status. Patients who reported stopping smoking were offered $15 to return to their clinic site for a short interview during which a breath sample was obtained for biochemical verification of smoking cessation. Patients whose breath samples had carbon monoxide concentrations greater than 8 ppm were considered smokers (Jarvis et al., 1987).

Outcomes

The primary outcomes of the trial with respect to physicians were the frequency and content of counseling practices. Frequency was measured as the percentage of return smokers that residents counseled, and content was measured as the number and mix of five specific techniques residents reported using in counseling. The five techniques were setting a quit date, prescribing

Figure 2
Trial design and participation by physicians and patients

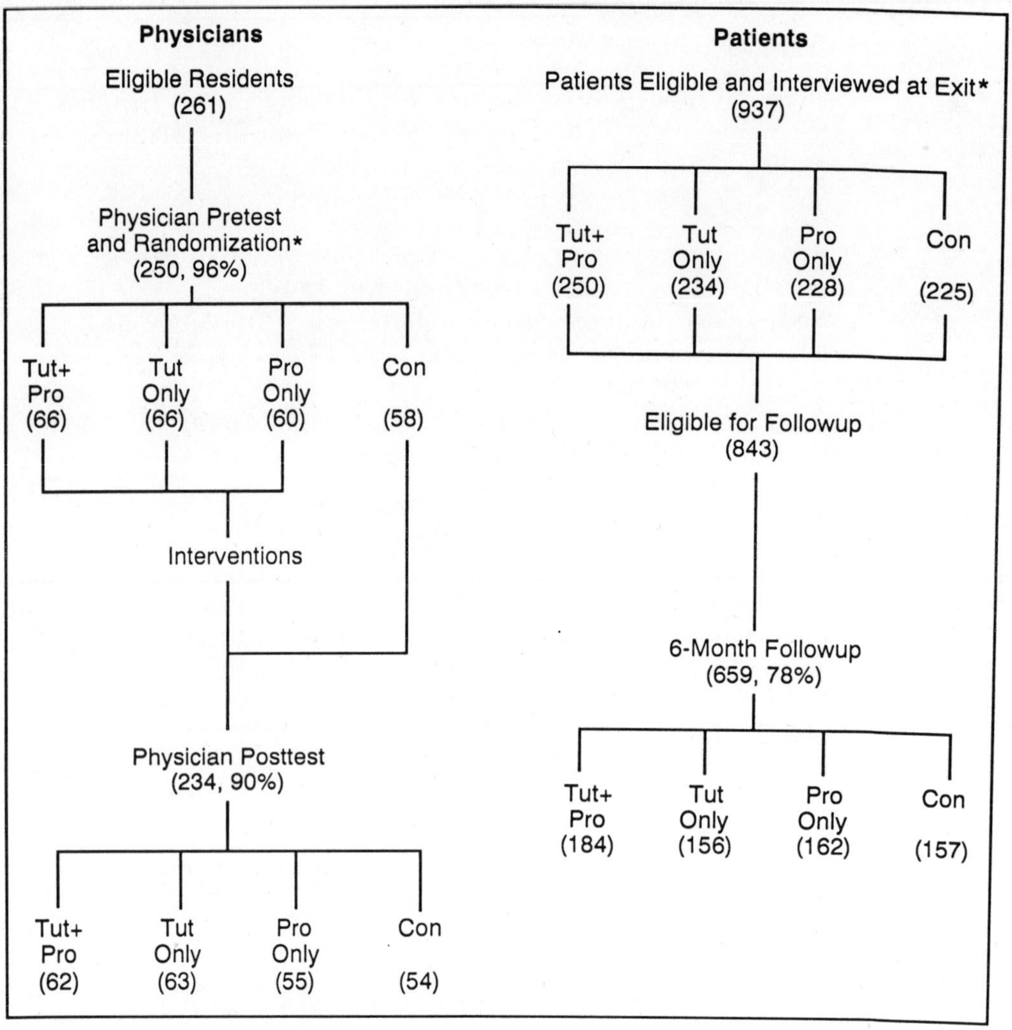

** Tut, tutorial; Pro, prompt; Con, control.*

Source: Strecher et al., 1991; used with permission of the authors.

a quit date, prescribing nicotine gum, giving the patient self-help material, and providing followup. Residents were considered to have used a technique if they said they used it often or always with their patients who smoked.

Both physician self-report and patient exit interview reports (aggregated by physician) were used for assessing resident counseling practices. Several secondary physician outcomes also were examined, including use of techniques to motivate patients to quit smoking and three attitudes toward smoking cessation counseling: confidence, perceived preparedness, and perceived success.

The primary patient-related outcome was the patient quit rate, measured by the percentage of each resident's patients who reported they had quit smoking within 6 months of the exit interview. Biochemical testing of expired carbon monoxide was used to verify the patients' self-reported status as ex-smokers. However, because the biochemical test verified the self-report in all but two cases, and because the percentage of patients with biochemical verification varied by patient group, self-reported status was used as the primary dependent variable.

RESULTS

Physician Self-Reports

Of the 261 residents eligible for the trial, 234 (90 percent) completed all phases of the trial, including 157 physicians in internal medicine (67 percent), 52 in family practice (22 percent), and 25 in pediatrics (11 percent). Participation did not differ by study group or site. Individual sites contributed a mean of 21 residents, with a range of 11 to 44.

Pretest Results

Prior to the interventions, all four groups were similar for study outcomes and other selected characteristics. Residents reported that they advised cessation for 63 percent to 70 percent of return patients who smoked cigarettes but used only 0.5 to 0.7 of five specific counseling techniques (Figure 3). About half of the residents reported that they had had smoking cessation training of some kind in the preceding 6 months. The groups did not differ in terms of resident specialty or year of training. Pretest results for trial participants plus residents from two additional pediatric programs have been published else where (Kenney et al., 1988).

Changes in Counseling Frequency

After the interventions, the self-reported frequency of smoking cessation counseling increased in the tutorial-plus-prompt and tutorial-only groups (Figure 3). Analysis of covariance (ANCOVA) to compare the two interventions showed that only the tutorial produced significantly greater posttest counseling frequency. After adjustment for pretest scores and specialty, the posttest mean frequency for physicians receiving the tutorial was significantly higher than that for nontutorial physicians (76 vs. 69 percent, $p < 0.05$). Counseling frequency also tended to be higher for those receiving the prompt than for those who did not (75 vs. 70 percent), but the difference was not statistically significant. There was no significant interaction between the tutorial and the prompt. Nor was there any significant interaction between either intervention and physician specialty.

Changes in Counseling Content

Self-reported counseling content followed a pattern similar to that for counseling frequency (Figure 3). The use of ANCOVA to control for pretest scores and specialty showed that the mean number of techniques reported by tutorial physicians was double that reported by nontutorial physicians (1.5 vs. 0.7, $p < 0.001$). The number of techniques reported by those receiving the prompt was only slightly higher than those who did not (1.2 vs. 1.0, $p > 0.05$). Again, there was no interaction effect for the two

Figure 3
Physicians' self-reported counseling practices*

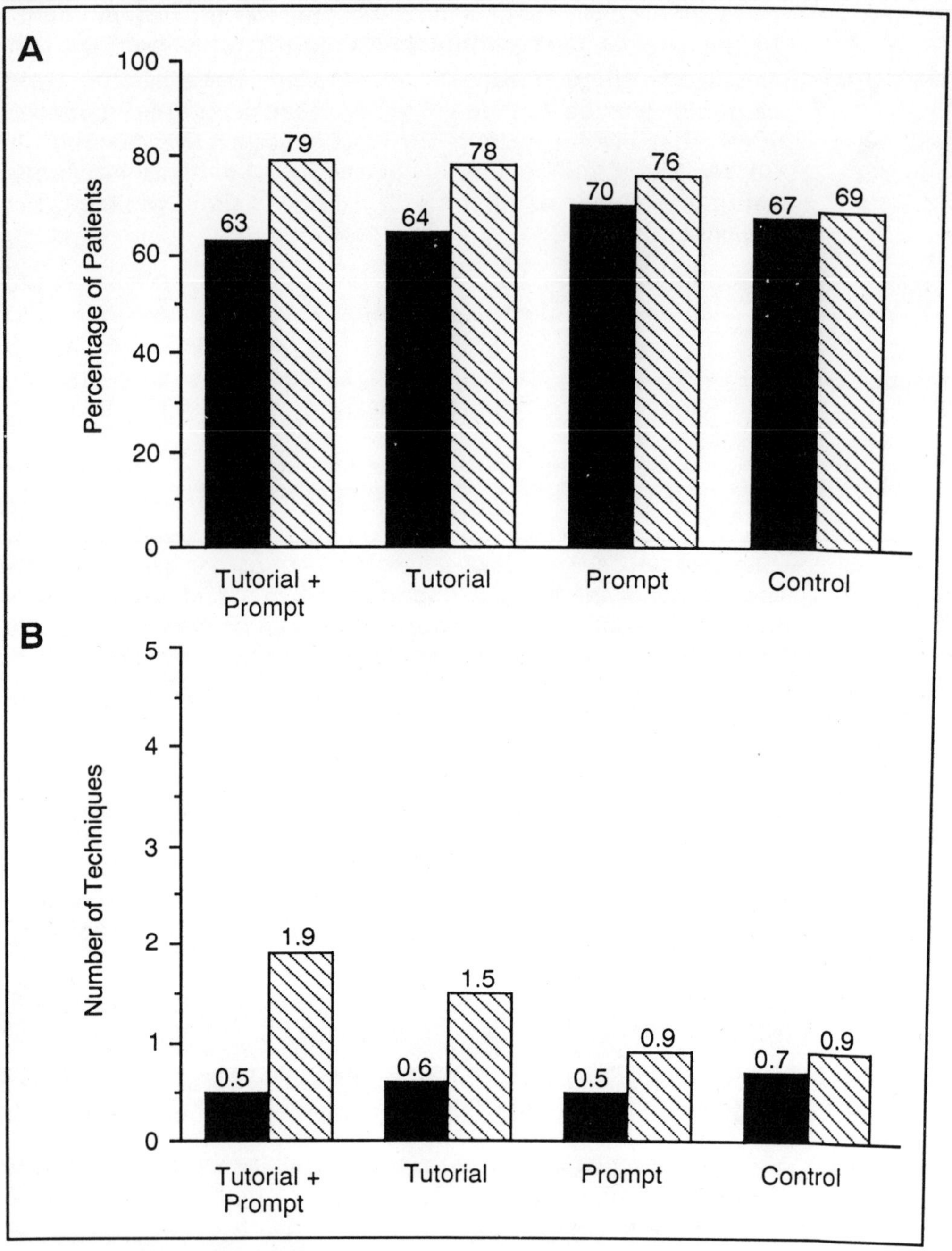

** A, frequency: percentage of patients advised to quit. B, content: number of five techniques used. Black bars, pretest; striped bars, posttest.*

Source: Strecher et al., 1991; used with permission of the authors.

interventions combined and no interaction between either intervention and physician specialty.

Patient Reports

Participation

During the 6-month period between the start of the interventions and the physician posttest, 937 exit interviews were conducted with patients at 10 sites, representing 203 of the 250 randomized physicians in the trial. One family medicine site with 24 physicians was unable to participate, and 23 of the 226 remaining physicians did not have any patients interviewed. The mean number of interviews completed per physician was 4.1. There were no significant differences in pretest counseling frequency, content, or attitudes between the 203 physicians with exit interview patients and the 23 without.

The 937 patients included 736 internal medicine patients, 80 family medicine patients, and 121 parents of pediatric patients; their mean age was 45 years. The majority of the patients were female (63 percent), and most patients had less than a high school education (59 percent). About half were nonwhite, and about half were married. One-third of the patients reported they had no insurance coverage. The mean number of cigarettes they smoked per day was 19. Most (69 percent) reported a previous attempt to stop smoking, and 71 percent reported that they smoke a cigarette within 30 minutes of waking. The patients represented approximately 66 percent of the smokers who could have participated in the study. Only 6 percent of the eligible smokers refused to participate. The remaining 28 percent could not be contacted at exit or by telephone within 3 days of the clinic visit.

Frequency and Content

Patient exit interviews corroborated the changes indicated by physicians (Table 1). The use of ANCOVA to control for physician specialty showed that the percentage of patients reporting physician advice was significantly higher ($p < 0.05$) for tutorial (62 percent) than for nontutorial physicians (53 percent) and for prompt (62 percent) than for nonprompt physicians (57 percent).

Patient reports also indicated changes in counseling content in the same direction reported by physicians (Table 1). With adjustment for physician specialty, patients reported significantly more counseling techniques used by tutorial physicians than by nontutorial physicians (mean of 0.6 vs. 0.3, $p < 0.05$). Physicians in the prompt group used slightly more techniques than did nonprompt physicians (mean of 0.5 vs. 0.4), but the difference was not significant. More tutorial physicians than nontutorial physicians used each of the five techniques, but the differences were significant ($p < 0.05$) only for prescribing a quit date and scheduling followup. Differences between physicians receiving the prompt and those who did not were small and not statistically significant.

Patient vs. Physician Reports

Though patients corroborated the physician reports to a great extent, physicians reported more frequency and content of smoking cessation counseling than did patients. Across all groups, physicians reported giving significantly ($p < 0.05$) more advice (76 percent) than patients

Table 1
Patient reports of physician counseling practices, by study group[a]

	Tutorial + Prompt, Percentage (n=55)	Tutorial Only, Percentage (n=51)	Prompt Only, Percentage (n=50)	Control, Percentage (n=47)
Counseling Frequency:				
Return Patients Advised To Quit[b]	74%	73%	71%	58%
Counseling Content				
(Mean number of five techniques used per patient)[c]	(0.9)	(0.7)	(0.6)	(0.5)
Sets quitting date	12	9	7	6
Writes quitting-date prescription[b]	9	6	1	2
Prescribes nicotine-containing gum	20	17	15	13
Gives self-help materials	15	10	11	13
Schedules followup visit	51	53	42	37

[a] *All percentages are mean percentages.*
[b] *ANOVA, $p < 0.05$.*
[c] *ANOVA, $p < 0.10$.*
Source: Strecher et al., 1991; used with permission of the authors.

reported receiving (69 percent). Physicians also reported using significantly more techniques than the patients remembered (1.3 vs. 0.7, $p < 0.01$). Because physicians were asked about the counseling they generally provided and patients were asked about counseling received during one specific visit, physician reports would likely be higher than patient reports.

Six-Month Patient Followup

Participation

Patients without a home telephone (n=78) and patients who died, were institutionalized, or moved out of state (n=16) were excluded from the 6-month followup. Of the remaining 843 patients, 659 (78 percent) were interviewed by phone 6 months after their exit interview, with no differences in followup rate between study groups. According to exit interview data, excluded patients and patients lost to followup were no different from those who remained in the trial with respect to physician counseling frequency, the number of cigarettes smoked per day, or report of a previous quit attempt. However, they were more likely to report that they smoked a cigarette within 30 minutes of waking.

Patient Quit Rates

The rates of patients' smoking cessation in the intervention groups were generally higher than those in the control group, although study group differences were not statistically significant (Figure 4). According to self-reports, quit rates in the intervention groups ranged from 5.3 percent (tuto rial only) to 8.2 percent (tutorial plus prompt), compared with 5.2 percent

Figure 4
Six-month rates for patients' smoking cessation*

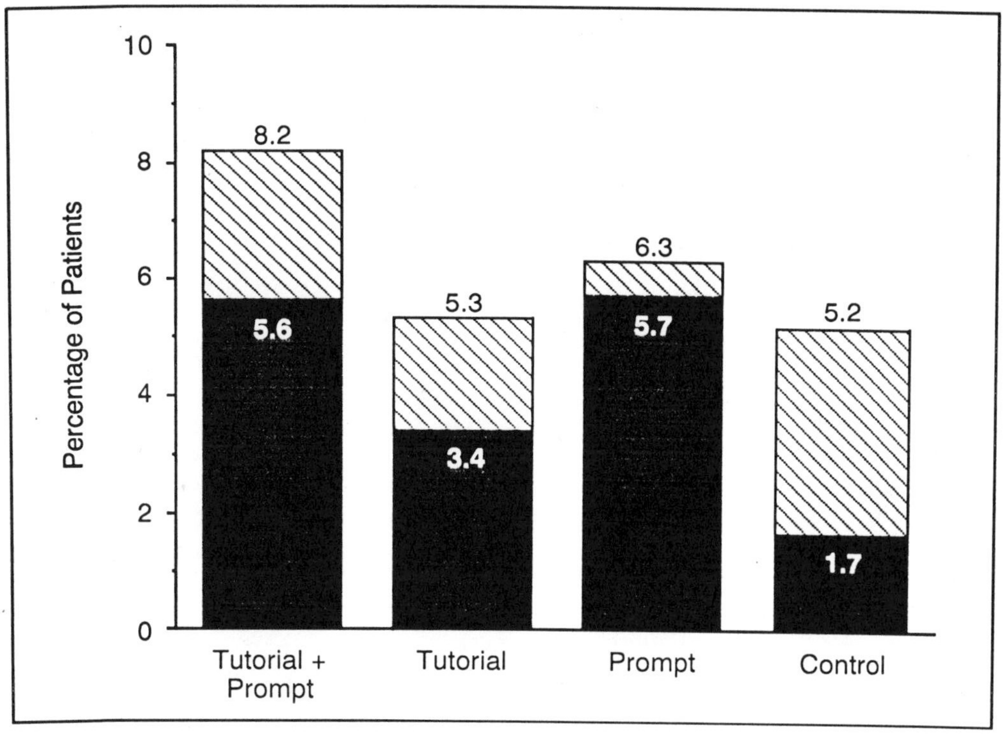

** Shaded bars, self-reported; black bars, biochemically verified.*
Source: Strecher et al., 1991; used with permission of the authors.

for the control group. According to the biochemically verified quit rates, intervention group rates of smoking cessation ranged from 3.4 percent (tutorial only) to 5.7 percent (prompt only), compared with 1.7 percent for the control group.

Self-reported patient quit rates for tutorial physicians, when adjusted for physician specialty, were higher than those for nontutorial physicians (4.9 vs. 3.7 percent), though the difference was not significant. For physicians in the prompt group, self-reported patient quit rates were also higher than those for the control physicians (5.2 vs. 3.4 percent) and were not statistically significant. Biochemically verified cessation rates followed a similar pattern, and there were no statistically significant differences among groups.

Patients undertook smoking cessation in spite of limited contact with physicians. Only 45 percent of all the patients in followup reported having seen their physician during the 6 months after the exit interview, with 67 percent of those patients reporting that the physician gave advice to quit smoking.

Quit Attempt Rates Patient quit attempt rates, the percentage of each resident's patients reporting at least one quit attempt during the 6-month followup period, ranged from 58 percent (tutorial plus prompt) to 50 percent (tutorial only) to 44 percent (prompt only); the rate for the control group was 49 percent. Adjusted for physician specialty, quit attempt rates for patients of the tutorial physicians were higher than those for patients of nontutorial physicians (47 vs. 40 percent), though the differences were not significant. For physicians in the prompt group, quit attempt rates were lower than those for nonprompt physicians (40 vs. 47 percent), but the difference was not statistically significant.

DISCUSSION Results from the authors' randomized trial involving 234 residents from 11 training programs and three specialties demonstrated that a training-of-trainers program can be effective in enhancing residents' practices with respect to smoking cessation counseling. Whether used alone or in combination with the tutorial, the prompt—a second intervention that employed a chart-based reminder—had less effect on residents' counseling practices. Although reporting a lower level of activity, patients tended to corroborate physicians' smoking cessation counseling reports; however, only small changes in patients' smoking behavior were found, and differences among experimental groups were not significant.

The trial examined the effects of a preventive health care intervention under conditions generalizable to most residency training programs in North America. A training program faculty member, not smoking cessation experts, conducted the tutorial at each site, and in-place nursing staffs administered the prompt. Residents in the study represented 3 primary care specialties, 4 community hospitals, 3 university medical centers, 82 U.S. medical schools, and 6 foreign medical schools. Because only 10 percent of residents did not complete the trial, it was unlikely that self-selection by physicians affected the results.

As far as the authors know, no previous study of training in smoking cessation counseling has included pediatric residents. The effects of parents' smoking on children's health and subsequent smoking behavior make parental counseling increasingly important (American Academy of Pediatrics, 1986). Although pediatric residents reported counseling frequency and content at lower levels than those reported by the internal medicine and family medicine residents prior to intervention, the pediatric residents' response to the interventions did not differ from that of other residents (Kenney et al., 1988).

Two barriers were encountered in implementation of the intervention. First, arranging for delivery of followup of the tutorial was difficult and required a concerted effort from the faculty. Second, integration of the prompt form into the medical record often proved difficult. A number of sites had stringent policies that tended to restrict the incorporation of new information into the record. The investigators found that both of these barriers could be overcome through the efforts of the on-site faculty member. Organizational change is often found to result from efforts by a champion for change in the existing system (Orlandi, 1987). Use of on-site faculty also appeared to have a positive influence on participation by residents. Having a faculty member who is the designated smoking counseling "expert" on site allowed residents to easily refer to this person when they encountered interesting counseling experiences.

A number of explanations for low rates of smoking cessation found among patients in the experimental groups are possible. First, the patients included in the study may have been less likely to quit smoking after 6 months than were patients in other settings. Study patients were predominantly black, female, and less educated. Smoking cessation among these patients is less frequent (Novotny et al., 1988). Second, fewer than half of the patients saw their physicians during the 6-month followup period; there was little opportunity for residents to reinforce previous counseling. The total amount of time spent on smoking cessation counseling is exceedingly small in comparison to the time spent in more formal cessation programs and is far outweighed by the number of social reinforcements to continue smoking. Third, because interventions were incorporated into ongoing training programs and residents at each site worked closely with one another, some contamination occurred. Almost two-thirds of the residents who did not receive the tutorial reported awareness of it, although most claimed that such awareness did not change their counseling practices.

Another factor accounting for low cessation rates could have been the intervention itself. Although the intervention was based on commonly recommended smoking cessation strategies, it also was developed so as to minimize expenditure of counseling time. This required minimizing open-ended probes and prolonged discussion about reasons for quitting, past quitting history, or the involvement of significant others in quitting. In other words, efforts to make the counseling strategy convenient for the physician may have also diminished the effectiveness of the strategy.

The authors recommend that future cessation efforts based in physician office practices include more attention to the role of other office staff members and to changes in the office system. Concerted, coordinated efforts from intake nurses, physicians' assistants, family nurse practitioners, and other health professionals in addition to the physician should minimize time constraints on all office staff while maximizing counseling effectiveness. These efforts may require systematic changes in the way candidates for smoking cessation counseling are identified, approached, and followed. Examples of such systematic efforts have been provided by Cohen and colleagues (1987) as well as Kottke and coworkers (1989).

ACKNOWLEDGMENTS The authors thank the patients, parents, and physicians who participated in the trial; the nursing staffs at participating institutions for assistance with the prompting system; Keith Cochran, Julie Curry, Rebecca Denson, Elizabeth Dickman, Gina Flemming-Maget, Sam Hart, Mary Angela Lee, Terry Loomis, Stephen McLoughlin, Deborah Moser, Jane Raney, Ph.D., Scott Robson, Sharon Sugarawa, Deborah Traugh, R.N., and Zoe Wood for providing research assistance and data management; Cynthia France, Ph.D., of the Office of Research and Education in the Health Professions, University of North Carolina at Chapel Hill, for assistance in developing the tutorial; Stan Alexander and the Television Section of the Medical Sciences Teaching Labs at the University of North Carolina at Chapel Hill for producing the tutorial videotape; Margaret Pennypacker, Jane Silver, and the staff of Social Research Associates, Research Triangle Park, North Carolina, for conducting the followup telephone survey of patients; and David Siscovick, M.D., Department of Medicine, University of Washington, for providing valuable suggestions and ideas for the study.

REFERENCES

American Academy of Pediatrics. Report of the committee on environmental hazards: Involuntary smoking a hazard to children. *Pediatrics* 77: 755-757, 1986.

Campbell, E.E., Villagra, V.G., Rogers, C.S., et al. Teaching and promoting smoking cessation counseling in primary care residencies: Description of a method. *Teaching and Learning in Medicine* 3(1): 20-27, 1991.

Cohen, S.J., Christen, A.G., Katz, B.P., Drook, C.A., Davis, B.J., Smith, D.M., Stookey, G.K. Counseling medical and dental patients about cigarette smoking: The impact of nicotine gum and chart reminders. *American Journal of Public Health* 77: 313-316, 1987.

Cummings, K.M., Giovino, G., Emont, S.L., Sciandra, R., Koenigsberg, M. Factors influencing success in counseling patients to stop smoking. *Patient Education and Counseling* 8: 189-200, 1986.

Cummings, S.R., Richard, R.J., Duncan, C.L., Hansen, B., Vander Martin, R., Gerbert, B., Coates, T.J. Training physicians about smoking cessation: A controlled trial in private practice. *Journal of General Internal Medicine* 4(6): 482-489, 1989.

Gagne, R.M., Briggs, L.J. *Principles of Instructional Design* (2nd edition). New York: Holt Rinehart and Winston, 1979.

Gritz, E.R. Cigarette smoking: The need for action by health professionals. *CA—A Cancer Journal for Clinicians* 38: 194-212, 1988.

Janz, N.K., Becker, M.H., Kirscht, J.P., Eraker, S.A., Billi, J.E., Woolliscroft, J.O. Evaluation of a minimal-contact smoking cessation intervention in an outpatient setting. *American Journal of Public Health* 77(7): 805-809, 1987.

Jarvis, M.J., Tunstall-Pedoe, H., Feyerabend, C., Vesey, C., Saloojee, Y. Comparison of tests used to distinguish smokers from nonsmokers. *American Journal of Public Health* 77: 1435-1438, 1987.

Kenney, R.D., Lyles, M.F., Turner, R.C., White, T.S., Gonzalez, J.J., Irons, T.G., Sanchez, C.J., Rogers, C.S., Campbell, E.E., Villagra, V.G., Strecher, V.J., O'Malley, M.S., Stritter, F.T., Fletcher, S.W. Smoking cessation counseling by resident physicians in internal medicine, family practice, and pediatrics. *Archives of Internal Medicine* 148: 2469-2473, 1988.

Kottke, T.E., Battista, R.N., DeFriese, G.H., Brekke, M.L. Attributes of successful smoking cessation interventions in medical practice: A meta-analysis of 39 controlled trials. *Journal of the American Medical Association* 259: 2882-2889, 1988.

Kottke, T.E., Brekke, M.L., Solberg, L.I., Hughes, J.R. A randomized trial to increase smoking intervention by physicians: Doctors Helping Smokers, round I. *Journal of the American Medical Association* 261: 2101-2106, 1989.

Novotny, T., Warner, K.E., Kendrick, J.E., Remington, P.L. Socioeconomic factors and racial smoking differences in the United States. *American Journal of Public Health* 78: 1187-1189, 1988.

Ockene, J.K. Physician-delivered interventions for smoking cessation: Strategies for increasing effectiveness. *Preventive Medicine* 16: 723-737, 1987.

Orlandi, M.A. Promoting health and preventing disease in health care settings: An analysis of barriers. *Preventive Medicine* 16: 119-130, 1987.

Strecher, V.J., Becker, M.H., Kirscht, J.P., Eraker, S.A., Graham-Tomasi, R.P. Evaluation of a minimal-contact smoking cessation program in a health care setting. *Patient Education and Counseling* 7: 395-407, 1985.

Strecher, V.J., O'Malley, M.S., Villagra, V.G., Campbell, E.E., Gonzalez, J.J., Irons, T.G., Kenney, R.D., Turner, R.C., Rogers, C.S., Lyles, M.F., White, S.T., Sanchez, C.J., Stritter, F.T., Fletcher, S.W. Can residents be trained to counsel patients about quitting smoking? Results from a randomized trial. *Journal of General Internal Medicine* 6: 9-17, 1991.

Wilson, D.M., Taylor, D.W., Gilbert, J.R., Best, J.A., Lindsay, E.A., Willms, D.G., Singer, J. A randomized trial of a family physician intervention for smoking cessation. *Journal of the American Medical Association* 260(11): 1570-1574, 1988.

APPENDIX A
Smoking Intervention Communication Grid[a]

Physician-Centered ------------------------------ >Patient-Centered

	Information	Reassurance	Closed-Ended Questions	Open-Ended Questions
Provide Advice	Smoking is harmful to your health. As your physician, I advise you to stop smoking.	I believe you can stop smoking.	Do you wonder if smoking is really affecting your health?	How do you think smoking is related to your health?
Assess Motivation	To be a successful ex-smoker, you need to make a serious commitment and make a plan to stop smoking.	You really seem to want to stop smoking.	Have you thought about stopping smoking recently?	How do you feel about trying to stop smoking?
Assess Past Experience	Often there are many things you can learn from your past attempts at stopping.	Being able to stop for a week is a real accomplishment. You made it through the hardest part.	Have you ever stopped smoking in the past?	How did it go the last time you stopped?
Discuss Problems	Certain situations, thoughts, or feelings usually bring on the urge to smoke.	I believe that together we can figure a way for you to deal with the problem situation.	Has your fear about withdrawal kept you from trying to stop again?	What problems do you anticipate coming up if you stop now?
Discuss Resources	Choosing other behaviors to substitute for smoking is easier if you plan ahead.	It sounds like you expect your spouse to be supportive.	What can you do instead of smoking after meals?	What do you believe will enable you to be successful at stopping?
Negotiate Plan	When developing a plan to stop smoking, it is important to choose a "quit" date.	I think that's a very realistic plan.	When will you stop? Could you reduce the amount you smoke to half by the next time we meet?	How do you think you would like to stop?
Arrange Followup	I'd like to set another appointment in 1 or 2 weeks with you to follow your progress.	My staff and I are available to you if the going gets tough.	Is it okay if my nurse calls you in a week or two to see how you are doing?	What kind of followup help from me would be helpful?

[a] *It is suggested that the topics be addressed in the order shown; the order may be changed, however, to meet the needs of the patient and physician.*

APPENDIX B
Outline of the Advice and Counseling Smoking Intervention Approaches

ADVICE-ONLY INTERVENTION

- Advise patient to stop smoking.
- If requested, give patient list of resources.
- Inform patient of periodic telephone contacts.

Sample Statement:

"I notice that you are a cigarette smoker. Smoking is harmful to your health. In many cases, the harmful effects of smoking can be reversed. As your doctor, I must advise you to stop smoking. If you are interested, I have a list of some programs for stopping smoking available in the community. Someone will be contacting you periodically by phone to see how you are doing."

COUNSELING INTERVENTION

- Advise patient to stop smoking.
- Use counseling technique to determine most appropriate method for cessation.
- Set agreement with patient for cessation.
- Provide booklet of stopping smoking tips.
- If requested, give patient list of resources.
- Request return visit in 1 to 2 weeks (or phone contact if unavailable) to check progress and reinforce initial visit.
- Inform patient of periodic telephone contacts.

Sample Intervention:

"I notice that you are a cigarette smoker. Smoking is harmful to your health. In many cases, the harmful effects of smoking can be reversed. As your doctor, I must advise you to stop smoking.

"How do you feel about being a cigarette smoker?

"Have you thought about stopping?

"What reasons would you have for stopping?

"Have you ever stopped smoking?"

YES

- When was the last time?
- How did you stop?
- Any problems?
- How long did the problems last?
- What helped you?
- How did you feel? How did you feel about yourself?

NO

- Have you ever made any other changes? How? When? Any problems?

"Would you like to stop smoking?

"Do you think you could stop now?

"What would be possible problems or barriers to stopping?

"What could help you?

"Would you be willing to develop a plan to stop smoking?"

YES

- Write agreement plan for cessation with patient.
- Give booklet on tips for stopping smoking.
- Request return visit in 1 to 2 weeks (or phone contact if unavailable) to check progress.
- Inform patient that someone will be contacting him/her periodically by phone to see how he/she is doing.

NO

- Give booklet on tips for stopping smoking.
- Request return visit in 1 to 2 weeks (or phone contact if unavailable) to check progress.
- Inform patient that someone will be contacting him/her periodically by phone to see how he/she is doing.

APPENDIX C
Physician Responses to Patients' Concerns

Patient: **I am under a lot of stress, and smoking relaxes me.**

Response: Your body and brain have become accustomed to the drug effects of nicotine, so you naturally feel more relaxed when you get the nicotine you have come to depend on. But nicotine is also a stimulant that temporarily raises heart rate, blood pressure, and adrenaline levels. After a few weeks of not smoking, most ex-smokers feel less nervous.

Patient: **Smoking stimulates me and helps me to be more effective in my work.**

Response: Difficulty in concentrating can be a symptom of nicotine withdrawal, but it is a short-term effect. Over time, the body and brain function more efficiently when you don't smoke, because carbon monoxide from cigarettes is displaced by oxygen in the bloodstream.

Patient: **I have already cut down my smoking to a safe level.**

Response: Cutting down is a good first step toward stopping. But smoking at any level increases the risk of illness. And some smokers who cut back inhale more often and more deeply, thus maintaining nicotine dependence. It is best to stop smoking completely.

Patient: **I only smoke safe, low-tar/low-nicotine cigarettes.**

Response: Low-tar cigarettes still contain harmful substances. Many smokers inhale more often or more deeply and thus maintain their nicotine levels. Carbon monoxide intake often increases with a switch to low-tar cigarettes.

Patient: **I don't have the willpower to give up smoking.**

Response: It can be hard for some people to give up smoking, but for others it is much easier than they expect. More than 3 million Americans stop every year. It may take more than one attempt for you to succeed, and you may need to try different methods of stopping. I will give you all the support I can.

Patient: **I wish everyone would mind their business about my smoking.**

Response: It must be hard to feel like people are nagging you about your smoking. I do not want to add to this. However, I feel as your physician I have a responsibility to help you stay well. I also would like to be able to provide help and support. Is there anything I can do to help?

Chapter 4
Special Practice Settings

CONTENTS

Introduction
Ellen R. Gritz 229

Pediatricians' Role in Smoking Prevention and Cessation
Barbara L. Frankowski and Roger H. Secker-Walker 232
Responsibilities of the Pediatrician 232
Pediatricians' Attitudes and Practices 233
Parents' Attitudes, Needs, and Behavior 236
Objectives of Pediatrician Intervention 238
Conclusion 244
References 244

Smoking Intervention by Providers of Health Care for Women
Mary Sexton, Joan Stine, and Steven Cahill 246
Role of the Provider 246
Effectiveness of Antismoking Intervention 247
Constraints on Office-Based Intervention 249
Training Prenatal Care Nurses 250
Possible Barriers to Effectiveness 254
Components in Obstetrical Offices 256
References 258

A Physician- and Dentist-Delivered Smoking Cessation Intervention for Head and Neck Cancer Patients
Ellen R. Gritz, Clifford R. Carr, David A. Rapkin, Cindy Chang, John Beumer, and Paul H. Ward 259
Purpose of the Project 259
Target Audience 260
Practice or Clinical Setting 260
Recruitment of Patients 260
Protocol for Advice 262
Nature of the Training Program 263
Special Resources and Procedures 263
Products of the Project 264
Barriers and Problems Overcome 265
What Worked and Why 266
What Did Not Work and Why 269
What Would Be Done Differently Now 269
References 270

Medical Advice as a Communication About Risks of Smoking and Benefits of Quitting
Laura C. Leviton, Timothy R. Cline, and Saul Shiffman 272
Introduction 272
Purpose of the Project 272
Target Audience 274
Setting of the Study 275
Recruitment Procedure and Results 276
Nature of Medical Advice Given 278
Nature of Counseling Intervention 280
What Did Not Work and Why 283
What Worked and Why 284
References 284

Appendixes
A. Smoking Materials for Pediatricians 287
B. Algorithms for Delivery of Smoking Cessation Advice 288
C. Protocol Developed by University of North Carolina Faculty Development Program 292
D. Self-Efficacy Intervention 293
E. Transcript From a Self-Efficacy Counseling Session 295

Special Practice Settings

Editor: Ellen R. Gritz

INTRODUCTION One of the major tactics used in physician- and dentist-delivered smoking cessation advice is to tailor the risk and benefit information to the patient's present condition, to maximize the likelihood of capitalizing on a teachable moment or window of opportunity. The four papers in this chapter address specialized practice settings that provide opportunities to reach selected populations and to focus on particular disease risks associated with tobacco use. The four target populations vary substantially. Two of the groups represent essentially healthy populations who might also be seen by primary care and family practitioners—pediatric patients and their parents, and women being treated for gynecologic conditions or pregnancy. The other two populations are persons at high risk of developing potentially fatal malignancies—former chemical workers exposed to a bladder carcinogen—and individuals newly diagnosed with head and neck cancers.

The health care professionals treating these populations also vary markedly in their orientation with regard to the urgency of smoking cessation for their patients. Pediatricians are in the specialty perhaps least empowered with regard to counseling smoking prevention for children and adolescents and smoking cessation for parents. Obstetrician/gynecologists have a clear message to convey to pregnant women, but less specific advice for the gynecologic patient. Physicians and respiratory therapists who perform cancer screening for carcinogen-exposed former chemical workers can provide precisely tailored advice to their high-risk patients. Finally, the head and neck surgeons and maxillofacial prosthodontists who treat patients with cancers of the upper aerodigestive tract are delivering a tertiary prevention message, the avoidance of further disease (cancer or other conditions) caused by continued smoking. Thus, these health professionals also have an urgent mandate to deliver clear and strong cessation messages, and have likely been doing so, albeit in the absence of even the most rudimentary behavioral skills training.

Yet a third dimension useful for scaling the special populations of medical and dental patients addressed in this chapter is their stage of change, or readiness to stop smoking. Intuitively, individuals at very high risk of developing cancer or those already suffering from it should be the most ready to stop and most receptive to advice from the physician or dentist. However, strong tobacco dependence, a sense of fatalism, and external factors (such as management-labor disputes over attribution of disease risk to exposure or to personal behavior) may weight the target population toward precontemplation. About 20 percent of women in the early stage of pregnancy quit smoking (take action) because of nausea, perceived risk to the fetus, and heterogeneous other factors, including low tobacco dependence and support from significant others. Women reached later in pregnancy may be less ready to stop because of a different constellation of reasons, including concern about excessive weight gain, past experience of having a healthy baby—in spite of smoking during pregnancy, greater tobacco dependence, and a smoking spouse/partner. Finally, parents of small children may contemplate stopping smoking to provide a role model and to avoid exposing their offspring to environmental tobacco smoke; but, on the other hand, they may perceive these not to be urgent issues if they and their families are healthy. Thus, patients in each specialty practice will encompass the range of stages of change, which the practitioner must address sensitively, with tailored advice. The goal may not always be action, but movement toward cessation, as in the case of the former chemical workers or women of childbearing age.

The examples provided in these four sections can be generalized to many medical and dental specialties in terms of both educating providers in the delivery of advice and reaching patient populations with certain characteristics and/or health problems.

Pediatricians Pediatricians have a unique opportunity to influence an entire family's smoking behavior, by practicing primary prevention with children who have not yet begun to smoke and by counseling parents to quit before either they or their children suffer any smoking-related health consequences. The surveys of Vermont pediatricians and parents reported here by Frankowski and Secker-Walker reveal the current gap in practice and define the extent of the need. The authors found that pediatricians were very unlikely to have received formal training in delivering smoking cessation advice and, while they did advise smoking parents to quit, the majority of physicians had low levels of confidence about delivering the advice. Parents, on the other hand, responded that it was the pediatrician's job to talk about passive exposure, to counsel children against smoking initiation, and even to advise smoking parents to stop. With these findings in mind, Frankowski and Secker-Walker describe the objectives of an intervention based in the pediatric practice, and they provide useful guidelines for incorporating cessation advice into clinical care.

Providers of Health Care for Women With public health and medical attention focused on the decline in smoking prevalence called for in the Year 2000 objectives, there has been voiced concern over the slower decline in women's smoking rates, compared with men's. Providers of gynecologic and obstetrical services, either in private or public settings, have a special opportunity to deliver a smoking intervention in the context of targeted risks. Surprisingly, there is little information on smoking cessation in the gynecologic setting. However, Dr. Sexton and her colleagues have extensive expertise in developing and implementing pregnancy-based interventions. They discuss interesting issues such as the smoking status of the provider, the role of nurses in the intervention, counseling materials for clients and providers, and the reconciliation of staff time with patients' expectations. The experience gained from these trials will facilitate the development and implementation of further smoking interventions for women in a variety of practices and settings.

Head and Neck Cancer

Individuals with head and neck cancer are the most seriously ill patient population addressed in this monograph. They receive care from highly specialized practitioners, surgeons (otolaryngologists) and reconstructive dentists (maxillofacial prosthodontists). Gritz and her colleagues describe the first systematic smoking intervention trial for head and neck cancer patients, featuring advice delivered by surgeons and dentists and tailored, self-help materials for patients and family members. Faced with cancer diagnosis and treatment, patients are clearly at a teachable moment with respect to smoking cessation. On the other hand, long-term, highly dependent tobacco and alcohol use characterizes many of these patients, imposing obstacles to cessation and potentially reducing the patients' readiness to change. Head and neck surgeons and maxillofacial prosthodontists are highly knowledgeable about the risks of smoking, yet they have had no prior training in behavior skills for delivering cessation advice. The research project described here pioneered the development of materials for patients, the surgeon and dentist cessation training, and the identification and recruitment of eligible patients for the trial. The issues discussed apply to a broad spectrum of seriously ill patients as well as to medical specialties heretofore not involved in smoking cessation counseling.

Chemical Workers At Risk for Bladder Cancer

Counseling an individual who is at high risk for a cancer because of occupational exposure and whose risk is substantially increased by continued smoking might, at first, appear to be easier than counseling a healthy smoker. However, the work of Leviton and colleagues, with a population of former chemical workers exposed to a bladder carcinogen, outlines the complex issues related to perceived responsibility for health status, delivery of information on the risks of smoking and benefits of cessation, readiness to change, and self-efficacy. The target population consists of blue-collar workers who reside in a rural area, are not highly educated, and, in general, have little interest in quitting smoking.

The task of the physicians and respiratory therapists who conduct the periodic bladder cancer screenings is to provide smoking cessation counseling in a manner that facilitates movement toward change and increases the workers' self-efficacy. Challenges involved in recruiting members of the population to the study, training the providers in the counseling protocol, and overcoming the multiple forms of resistance to counseling provide valuable lessons that could be used in multiple settings and by a range of medical and dental providers.

Pediatricians' Role in Smoking Prevention and Cessation

Barbara L. Frankowski and Roger H. Secker-Walker

RESPONSIBILITIES OF THE PEDIATRICIAN

Prevention for Children and Adolescents

Despite public awareness of the long-term morbidity associated with initiation of cigarette smoking during childhood and adolescence, nearly 5 million teenagers (12 to 17 years old) smoke, and there are more than half a million youngsters from 8 to 11 who smoke (DiFranza and Tye, 1990). Each day, more than 3,000 U.S. children begin to use tobacco (Fiore et al., 1989). Pediatricians should take every opportunity to promote nonsmoking among patients. It should be part of routine anticipatory guidance at all visits. Because healthy children see their pediatrician only every 2 years for health supervision, schools may perform this task better, with the pediatrician as a reinforcer or a participant.

Every effort should be made to encourage smoking parents to quit because of the negative role model they offer children. In addition, the pediatrician should support efforts to prevent advertising of all tobacco products. The pediatrician can also play a leading role in the elimination of advertising campaigns that seem likely to influence young people to start smoking.

Smoking Cessation By Children And Adolescents

Pediatricians should play a role in advising patients who are already smoking to quit. However, most pediatricians know no formal way of doing this, and thus merely tell patients, "You should quit." Although other health care professionals also care for children, pediatricians are the least likely to have received training in smoking cessation counseling. Many pediatricians are unaware of community resources to help patients with smoking cessation; however, there are few programs for adolescents at this time.

Protecting Children From Passive Smoking

Pediatricians should be aware of the effects of passive smoke on all stages of a child's growth, including the behavioral implications of having smoking parents, and physicians have an obligation to inform smoking parents of those effects. Surveys have shown that 53 to 76 percent of the homes in the United States contain at least one smoker; between 8.7 million and 12.4 million American children less than 5 years of age are exposed to cigarette smoke in their homes (Landrigan, 1986).

Between 1974 and 1987, four prospective studies and nine case-control studies examined the possible effects of exposure to parental tobacco smoke on the frequency and severity of acute respiratory illness in children (Fielding and Phenow, 1988). Although different research designs were used, the results have consistently demonstrated greater frequency of both upper and lower respiratory problems among the young children of smoking parents than among children of nonsmoking parents. Wheezing and asthma appear to be more common among the children of smoking parents (Weiss et al., 1980). Asthmatic children of smokers reportedly experience improvement when their parents stop smoking, in contrast to children with asthma whose parents continue to smoke (Gortmalker et al., 1982). Smoking by parents has also been identified as a risk factor for persistent middle-ear effusions and otitis media in young children (Kraemer et al., 1983; Stahlberg et al., 1986).

Helping Parents With Cessation

The Surgeon General has suggested that one of the pediatrician's most important educational obligations is to encourage and help parents to give up cigarette smoking (Koop, 1985). Pediatricians are in a unique position to address the issues of smoking prevention and smoking cessation at several levels. Healthy young adults who are starting a family see a pediatrician or family practitioner more often than any other health care professional.

Of the 3.6 to 3.7 million women who have given birth in the United States each year since 1980, approximately 1.0 to 1.2 million smoked while pregnant (Windsor, 1986). According to the Surgeon General, most recent estimates suggest that about 25 percent of U.S. women smoke throughout pregnancy, and the proportion of smokers who stop entirely during pregnancy is approximately 20 percent (US DHHS, 1990). The majority of women who give up smoking during pregnancy start smoking again after the baby is born (Sexton et al., 1985; US DHHS, 1990).

New parents often are motivated to make changes in their lifestyles "for the good of the baby." Each contact with the pediatrician could provide an opportunity for the physician to support a smoking mother in her efforts to quit or a recent ex-smoker in her efforts to refrain from starting again. Women who succeed in staying away from cigarettes will then model nonsmoking behavior for their children. Equal influence should be directed toward fathers as well. However, most pediatricians are not aware of the literature on smoking cessation, nor do they know that there are specific methods of giving brief, effective advice.

PEDIATRICIANS' ATTITUDES AND PRACTICES

Methods

In the current study, the investigators used the questionnaire developed to survey Maine pediatricians (Frankowski and Secker-Walker, 1989) with minor modifications. The questionnaire contained 50 items, including demographic questions, and addressed the pediatrician's estimate of the proportion of parents who smoke, smoke, current activities concerning smoking advice, confidence in his or her ability to offer smoking advice, perceived barriers to offering smoking advice, and opportunities to offer smoking advice. The questionnaire and a stamped, addressed return envelope were mailed to all pediatricians practicing in Vermont; nonrespondents were sent two mailings. Of the 92 pediatricians, 72 responded. After physicians who were no longer practicing pediatrics in Vermont (n=13) were excluded, the response rate was 72 of 79, or 91 percent. Of the 72 pediatricians, 10 are subspecialists and the rest deliver primary care in 19 solo and 16 group practices. The pediatricians in the practices chosen for distribution of parent questionnaires were invited to take part in a more in-depth interview about smoking, administered by the principal investigator. That interview included questions about what the pediatrician actually said about smoking to patients and parents, where the information was recorded, and what type of further training would be of interest to the pediatrician or office staff. Eighteen pediatricians were able to take part in the in-depth interviews (5 of 6 in solo practice and 13 of 19 in group practices), representing 25 percent of the pediatricians who responded to the questionnaire.

Results

Pediatrician Demographics

On average, the pediatricians, 32 percent of whom were women, were 43.5 years old and had been in practice for 13 years. Twenty-seven percent of respondents were in solo practice, 62 percent in a partnership or group, 7 percent in hospital-based practice, 1 percent in a community health center, and 3 percent in other settings. Sixty-one percent were never-smokers, 36 percent were former smokers, and 3 percent gave no response; no one reported being a current smoker.

Effects of Passive Smoke on Children

Fifty-seven percent of the pediatricians estimated that about one-third or fewer of their patients' parents were cigarette smokers. About 40 percent of pediatricians routinely take a smoking history from parents, but only 11 percent record the information in the child's chart. Most pediatricians (64 percent) estimated that they talk to one-half or more of smoking parents about the effects of parental smoking (passive smoke) on their children.

Pediatricians were asked, "What are the major concerns about the effects of parental smoking in children that you discuss with parents?" The percentages of responding pediatricians who checked each concern were as follows: 88 percent, more bronchitis and pneumonia in infancy and childhood; 83 percent, more exacerbation of asthma; 56 percent, parental role modeling for smoking; 53 percent, lower birth weight; 39 percent, more middle-ear infections; 17 percent, fire hazards and burns; and 7 percent, other (allergies, competition in athletics, risk of pulmonary cancer). Figure 1 shows the distribution of parents' beliefs about the effects of parental smoking. Almost all pediatricians (91 percent) felt moderately confident (39 percent) or very confident (52 percent) about addressing passive smoking issues with parents.

Most pediatricians (94 percent) reported they advise smoking parents to quit. The pediatricians estimated advising about two-thirds to quit and spent an average of 4.4 minutes per parent in that activity. The estimated successful quit rate was 12 percent.

Pediatricians were asked, "When you advise parents who smoke about their smoking, what issues do you address?" The percentages of responding pediatricians who checked each issue were as follows: 97 percent, hazards of passive smoking for children; 81 percent, hazards of smoking for smoker; 77 percent, keeping smoke away from infants and young children; 54 percent,

Figure 1
Parents' beliefs about the effects of parental smoking

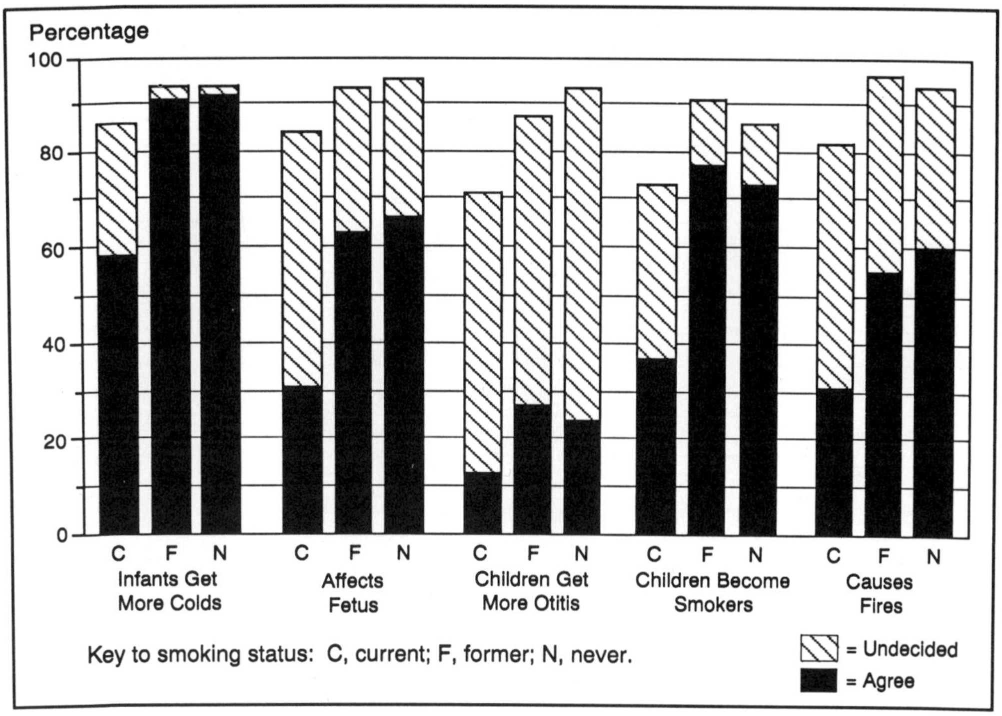

Source: Frankowski et al., in press; used with permission.

benefits of stopping smoking; 40 percent, cutting down the consumption of cigarettes; 29 percent, quitting "cold turkey"; 25 percent, prescribing nicotine chewing gum; 22 percent, setting a quit date; and 10 percent, other issues.

The pediatricians were also asked about the best opportunities to give smoking cessation advice to parents (see Figure 2). The percentages that rated various opportunities as "good or excellent" were as follows: 89 percent, visits for acute respiratory infections; 75 percent, prenatal visits; 72 percent, well-child visits; 65 percent, visits after delivery; 34 percent, visits for other acute problems. Most pediatricians (93 percent) have a no-smoking policy in their offices, 30 percent have printed materials to give smokers to help them quit, and 26 percent had lists of smoking cessation resources available in the community.

Only 45 percent of pediatricians felt moderately confident (25 percent) or very confident (20 percent) about advising parents to quit. Respondents identified several barriers to giving smoking cessation advice to parents: 42 percent cited lack of time; 25 percent said the smoking parent does not expect such advice; 25 percent feel "ill at ease" when giving advice; 7 percent noted lack of reimbursement; and 1 percent said, "none of my business."

Figure 2
Opportunities to give parents quit-smoking advice

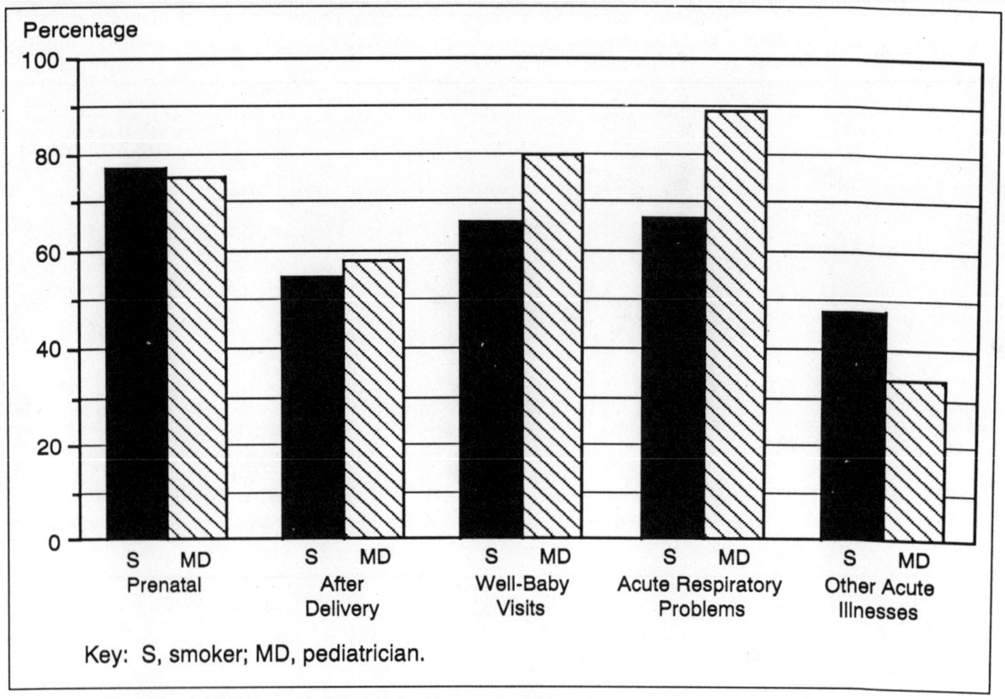

Source: Frankowski et al., in press; used with permission.

Learning How To Give Quit-Smoking Advice

Only 8.5 percent of pediatricians had received formal training in giving smoking advice, but 87 percent would be willing to learn brief methods. Pediatricians were asked to rate opportunities to learn about brief methods for giving smoking cessation advice. The percentages rating different methods "good or excellent" were as follows: 73 percent, 1-hour videotape; 55 percent, journal article; 52 percent, 2-hour training in office; and 41 percent, one half-day continuing medical education workshop or seminar.

PARENTS' ATTITUDES, NEEDS, AND BEHAVIOR

Methods

A second questionnaire was developed to assess parents' attitudes about smoking. The questionnaire contained 34 items and addressed demographics, the parents' beliefs about the effects of parental smoking on children, attitudes about pediatrician-delivered advice about smoking, reactions to pediatrician-delivered advice, smoking history, smokers' intentions to quit, and dietary habits. The questionnaire was first pretested among parents in the investigator's practice, and then it was administered by one research assistant who distributed the questionnaire and a consent form to all parents in the waiting rooms of participating pediatricians' offices. The pediatric practices were chosen randomly to include two solo and two group practices from each of three arbitrarily defined regions: Chittenden County, northern Vermont, and southern Vermont. Approximately 25 parents were surveyed for each pediatrician in each practice.

Results

Parents' Demographics

A total of 676 parents completed questionnaires at 6 solo and 6 group pediatric practices. Several parents who received questionnaires declined participation because of time constraints. The parents, 84 percent of whom were women, had a mean age of 32 years. Six percent had not completed high school, 33 percent were high school graduates, 33 percent had some college education, and 27 percent had 4 or more years of college. The mean number of children per family was 2.0 (SD=0.9), with a mean age of 5.3 years (SD=4.2).

Almost half the responding parents were never-smokers, 30 percent were former smokers, and 21 percent were current smokers. The average number of adult smokers per household was 0.53. Parents started smoking at a mean age of 16.6 (SD=3.1) and smoked about one pack of cigarettes per day (SD=one-half pack). Smoking parents had made an average of 6.6 quit attempts (SD=18.9). The vast majority (82 percent) had tried to quit "cold turkey"; 32 percent had tried gradual reduction; 15 percent had used self-help materials; 10 percent had tried nicotine chewing gum; 9 percent had tried hypnosis; and 3 percent had tried individual or group counseling. Current smokers were significantly younger ($p < 0.0001$) and had significantly less education ($p < 0.0001$) than former smokers or nonsmokers (see Table 1).

Attitudes About Passive Smoke

All parents were asked whether they agreed, disagreed, or were undecided about several statements pertaining to the effects of parental smoking. Most (85 percent) agreed that smoking affected the fetus, 58 percent agreed that infants of parents who smoke got more colds and lung infections, 23 percent agreed that children of parents who smoke got more ear infections, 67 percent agreed that children of smoking parents were more likely to become smokers, and 52 percent agreed that cigarettes cause one-fourth of home fires. As Figure 1 shows, current smokers were less knowledgeable in all areas ($p < 0.0001$); former smokers and never-smokers were very similar in their beliefs.

Table 1
Demographic characteristics of parents, by smoking status

	Total Parents n=668		Current Smokers n=142		Former Smokers n=199		Never-Smokers n=327	
Mean Age (years)	32.0		29.5		33.5		32.1	
	Percentage (Number)							
Education								
Less than high school	6%	(40)	15%	(21)	3%	(6)	4%	(13)
High school	33	(223)	47	(67)	28	(55)	4	(13)
Some college	33	(223)	27	(38)	45	(90)	29	(95)
4-year college	27	(182)	11	(16)	24	(48)	36	(118)

The parents were asked whether they felt it was their pediatrician's job to talk about smoking. Almost all parents felt that the pediatrician should talk about the effects of passive smoke on children (87 percent) and should talk to children and teens about smoking (85 percent). About one-half the parents felt it was the pediatrician's job to advise smoking parents to quit (56 percent). Current smokers were less likely to think that the pediatrician should talk about passive smoke ($p < 0.005$) or talk to parents about quitting ($p=0.01$) (see Figure 3). Forty percent of current smokers and 21 percent of former smokers reported that their pediatricians had talked to them about the effects of their smoking (passive smoke) on their child's health.

Attitudes About Advice From Pediatricians

Surprisingly, 48 percent of current smokers feel it is the pediatrician's job to advise smoking parents to quit. Twenty-eight percent of current smokers said their pediatrician has talked about the effects of smoking on their own health, and 27 percent of current smokers said their pediatrician advised them to quit. Current smokers were asked how they would feel if their pediatrician advised them to quit smoking. About one-half (52 percent) said they would welcome the advice, 30 percent said it would bother them somewhat, and 15 percent said it would not matter to them. Fewer parents had more negative reactions: 11 percent claimed it was none of the pediatrician's business, 4 percent said it would make them angry, and one parent claimed she would change to another pediatric practice (some respondents checked more than one answer). Smoking parents were also asked about the best opportunities to receive quit-smoking advice from their pediatricians. The percentages that rated opportunities as "good or excellent" were as follows: 77 percent, prenatal visit; 67 percent, acute visits for respiratory infections; 66 percent, well-baby visits; 55 percent, after delivery; and 48 percent, acute visits for other problems. As Figure 2 illustrates, smokers and doctors agree closely on opportunities to talk about quitting smoking.

Smokers' Intentions To Quit

Current smokers were asked, "If you decided to give up smoking completely in the next month, do you think you could do it?" Twenty-two percent responded definitely or probably, 35 percent responded maybe, and 42 percent responded definitely or probably not. When asked, "Do you intend to give up smoking in the next month?", 7 percent responded yes, 34 percent maybe, and 59 percent no. However, when asked whether they had any intentions of ever giving up smoking, 68 percent of smoking parents replied yes, 23 percent maybe, and 9 percent no.

OBJECTIVES OF PEDIATRICIAN INTERVENTION

Education of Pediatricians

Pediatricians need to become aware of office-based smoking cessation trials that have examined the efficacy of brief methods of delivering advice to stop smoking. Pediatricians are not familiar with the smoking cessation literature, and they often refrain from giving smoking cessation advice because they think it is not worthwhile—that a 10- to 15-percent quit rate is unacceptably low. In fact, for a minimal intervention of brief advice and limited followup, a quit rate of 10 percent is actually what is to be expected.

Figure 3
Parents' attitudes about advice

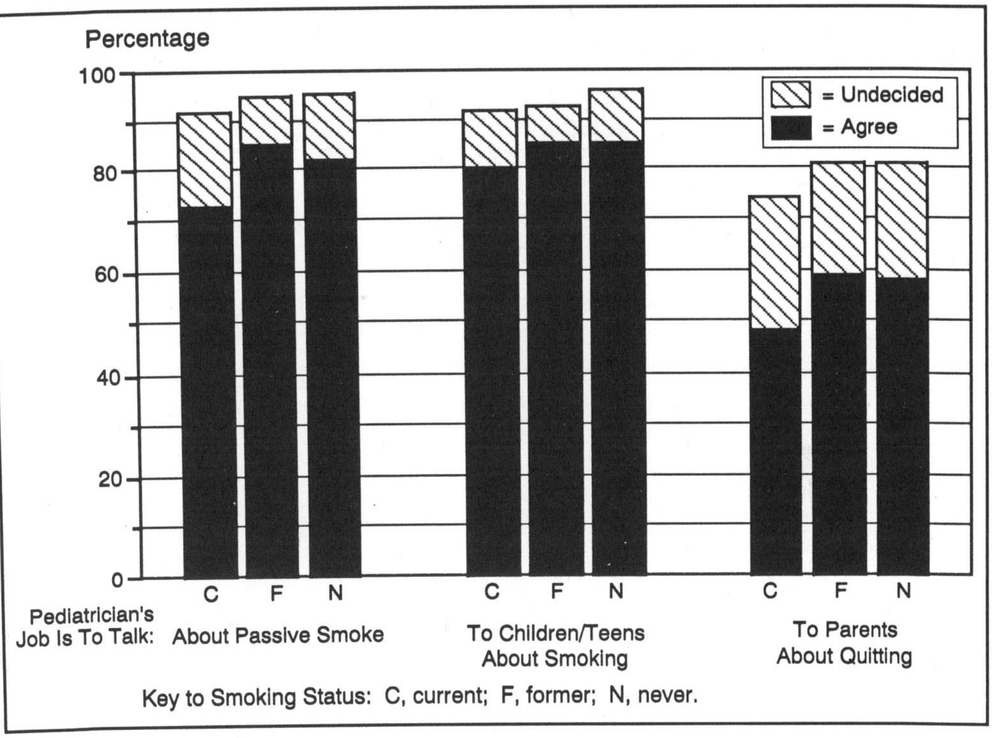

Source: Frankowski et al., in press; used with permission.

A systematic method of training pediatric residents and practicing pediatricians should be established, using the NCI manual for physicians, *How To Help Your Patients Stop Smoking* (Glynn and Manley, 1990), and the supplement, *Clinical Interventions To Prevent Tobacco Use by Children and Adolescents* (Epps and Manley, 1991). Only 8.5 percent of Vermont pediatricians have had formal training in delivering smoking cessation advice, and only 20 percent feel very confident in advising parents to quit.

A recent study showed that residents in primary care specialties (family practice, internal medicine, and pediatrics) had positive attitudes but inadequate practice and training in smoking cessation counseling (Kenney et al., 1988). The survey of 309 residents (66 in pediatrics) showed that the pediatric residents scored significantly lower in most areas of smoking cessation counseling practices, and only 32 percent reported having any training in this area (compared with 76 percent of family practice and 53 percent of internal medicine residents, significantly different at $p < 0.001$). The pediatric residents were also more likely to cite insufficient time as a barrier. However, when pediatric residents were taught smoking cessation counseling methods, they performed as well as the other residents (Strecher et al., 1991). Thus, the need to teach both pediatric residents and practicing pediatricians brief methods of delivering smoking cessation advice is clear. The majority of pediatricians (87 percent in Vermont and 84 percent in Maine) would be moderately or very willing to learn such techniques (Frankowski and Secker-Walker, 1989).

The above-mentioned supplement, *Clinical Interventions To Prevent Tobacco Use by Children and Adolescents,* is currently available. In addition to the four A's (*ask, advise, assist, arrange*), a fifth "A" heads up the list for pediatricians: *Anticipate* the risk for tobacco use at each developmental stage. The guide is divided into three sections: infancy and early childhood, late childhood, and adolescence and young adulthood.

An effort should be made in each pediatric office to identify additional personnel (for instance, a nurse or nurse practitioner) to receive training. Although a brief message from the physician is a key element, other personnel can be used to answer the patient's questions, help with followup, and even counsel smokers on ways to quit (Solberg et al., 1990). Kottke and colleagues (1988) have shown that advice from both a physician and a nonphysician is more effective than from either alone. The dual approach may not be practical for pediatricians practicing solo or in small groups, but it should be considered in other settings. It could alleviate some of the time constraints that concern many pediatricians.

Dealing With Barriers

"Not Enough Time"

Pediatricians should be aware that the anticipatory guidance for prevention of smoking onset and the advice for smoking cessation are brief and meant to be delivered in a few minutes once the methods are learned. There is a growing body of literature indicating that brief advice (less than 10 minutes) can be successful (Pederson, 1982). A 1985 survey of 441 Iowa physicians indicated that almost all (95 percent) said they advise patients to stop; most said they spend less than 10 minutes giving such advice (median, 5 minutes; range, 1 minute to 30 minutes) (Ferguson, 1985). The median success rate for this advice was 10 percent, with a range of 0 to 100 percent. Success rates of this order after physician-delivered smoking cessation advice have been reported from a number of studies. In a meta-analysis of 39 trials of cessation advice or counseling carried out in physicians' offices, the average reported quit rate in the intervention groups was 8.4 percent higher than in the control groups (Kottke et al., 1988). Although some may consider such rates unacceptably low, it should be remembered that facilitating even a quit attempt is significant, because the actual success rate among individuals is related to the number of quit attempts. Even a quit rate as low as 5 percent, as reported by Russell and colleagues for brief (2-minute) smoking cessation advice, would produce a large number of quitters if all primary care practitioners provided such advice (Russell et al., 1979).

"Parents Don't Expect This Advice"

Pediatricians should be aware that one-half of a sample of smoking parents said they would welcome the advice to quit and fewer than 10 percent would react negatively. In fact, 68 percent of smoking parents claim they intend to quit sometime. It has been estimated that up to 80 percent of smokers want to quit (Mason and Lindsay, 1983), and only about 7 percent of current smokers in 1986 predicted they would "definitely" be smoking in 5 years (US DHHS, 1990). However, in a 1987 survey of patients seen in various university-based, outpatient clinic settings, only 58 percent of healthy smokers and 50 percent of smokers with smoking-related symptoms noted that they had been advised by their physicians to stop smoking (Ockene et al., 1987). A survey of 5,875 Michigan adults showed that, of smokers who had seen a physician in the previous year, only 44 percent reported they had ever been told by a physician to quit smoking (Anda et al., 1987). Physicians should not underestimate their influence: The single most important reason people have for quitting smoking is concern for their health. Those who quit for health reasons or in response to physician advice are more likely to make repeated attempts and to maintain abstinence from cigarettes (Orleans, 1985).

"Feel Ill at Ease Giving Advice"

Pediatricians will feel more confident about giving the advice when they have had formal training and when they are made aware that parents feel it is part of the pediatrician's job to offer advice.

Incorporating Smoking Advice Into Office Visits

Smokers in the Household

In the authors' survey of Vermont pediatricians, about 40 percent reported they routinely take a smoking history from parents of each patient, but only 11 percent record the information in the child's chart. In a national mail survey of 779 pediatricians in 1987, about 65 percent reported asking about smoking at the 0- to 5-year well-child visits, and as many as 80 percent reported asking about smoking if the child is 13 or older (Nader et al., 1987). The same survey showed that only 50 percent of pediatricians felt that cigarette smoking was a "very important" topic to discuss at well-child visits from 0 to 5 years. In family practice and internal medicine, flagging a smoker's chart in some way increases the chances that the physician will remember to provide followup smoking cessation advice at subsequent visits (Cohen et al., 1989; Solberg et al., 1990).

New Baby, Smoking Parents

Because pediatricians come in contact with a great number of young adults who may not be routinely seeking health care for themselves and because parental smoking directly affects their children, the argument is strong for pediatricians to deliver brief smoking cessation advice to parents. Perry and Silvis (1987) have outlined methods pediatricians can use to promote nonsmoking or encourage attempts to quit for parents, children, and adolescents; they stress that pediatricians need to learn the skills involved and need to motivate themselves to use these skills. Perry and Silvis suggest encouraging parents to quit smoking and/or refrain from smoking near the child. The pediatricians should (1) ask about parents' smoking habits; (2) motivate themselves to promote cessation and a consistent no-smoking message; (3) motivate parents to quit smoking through discussion of immediate risks to the child; and (4) reinforce ex-smokers to stay away from cigarettes.

The methods that these authors suggest are very similar to the "four A's" method recommended in the NCI manual. The pediatrician should:

- *Ask* parents about smoking in the household, the car, or in day care settings. At sick visits, ask about tobacco exposure. Remember that silence by the physician may be interpreted by parents to mean that smoke exposure is not a significant health risk.
- *Advise* all parents who smoke to stop. Talk about the effects of passive smoke.
- *Assist* interested smoking parents in developing an effective smoking cessation strategy. Set a quit date and provide self-help materials or referrals.
- *Arrange* followup for parents, which can take place at the child's next regularly scheduled well visit. Mark the child's chart with the parents' smoking status as a reminder to ask at all visits.

Respiratory Problems And Smoking Parents

Although it may be more difficult because visits are sporadic, the pediatrician is obligated to inform parents that cigarette smoke is usually one of the causative factors in a child's respiratory illness. It is especially appropriate to emphasize passive smoke issues for infants and children who have problems with recurrent upper or lower respiratory infections, recurrent ear infections, or reactive airway disease. In many cases, the parent who does not accompany the child to the office is the smoker, and a simple phone call from the pediatrician to give information and make a direct plea to the parent to quit smoking may be a powerful motivator. If the parent can be coaxed into setting a quit date, the pediatrician can schedule a followup visit for the child at about the same time to check on child and parent simultaneously. If available, other office personnel can spend more time with the parents.

Child or Adolescent Who Smokes

There is a unique opportunity for the pediatrician because frequently children and adolescents who smoke do not receive proper health care. An extra effort should be made to *ask, advise, assist,* and *arrange*:

- *Ask* about tobacco use at every visit. It may be easier to use a previsit questionnaire.
- *Advise* all tobacco users to stop. Inform smokers that it is easier to stop now than later. Personalize the message and mention reduced athletic capability, cost, odor, and fire hazard.

- *Assist* tobacco users in stopping. Help set a quit date and provide self-help materials. Plan a way to enlist friends to help. Consider having the child or adolescent sign a contract to quit. Rehearse how to say no. Encourage participation in programs that promote the development of skills to solve problems, set goals, make decisions, and counter negative peer pressure. Encourage exercise and social activities incompatible with tobacco use.

- *Arrange* a followup visit within 1 to 2 weeks after the patient's planned quit date; discuss progress and problems. Arrange a second followup visit within 1 to 2 months.

Anticipatory Guidance

Perry and Silvis (1987) suggest that physicians promote nonsmoking by emphasizing (1) harmful physical consequences, (2) the habit-addictive nature of cigarette smoking, (3) advertising techniques that mask the real effects of smoking, and (4) smoke-free environments at home and at the doctor's office. For adolescents, Perry and Silvis suggest promoting non-smoking by emphasizing (1) immediate physiological and social consequences, (2) ways to deal with pressures to smoke, (3) commitment to nonsmoking, and (4) the use of alternatives.

The NCI pediatricians' supplement suggests that the following ideas may be appropriate for well-child visits of patients aged 5 through 12:

- *Anticipate.* Include the children in discussions about smoking and tobacco use. Remind parents that tobacco use often begins in grade school.

- *Ask* the child whether smoking is being discussed in school or among friends. Ask whether the child smokes or whether friends, parents, or other important adults in the child's environment smoke.

- *Advise* the child about immediate negative effects of tobacco use. Remind the child that most adolescents do not smoke. Advise smoking adults about passive smoke and their image as role models. Discourage use of candy cigarettes.

- *Assist* the child in assuming increasing responsibility for his or her health and behavior. Compliment the child on nonsmoking behavior and discuss refusal skills.

- *Arrange* more frequent followup visits for children experimenting with tobacco products.

For adolescents, the NCI manual suggests the following:

- *Anticipate.* Adolescents who are deviance-prone, who show a relative lack of interest in conventional goals, and who overestimate smoking prevalence among adults and teens are at greater risk for tobacco use.

Adolescent females are particularly vulnerable. Peer modeling is one of the most important factors in choosing to use tobacco.

- *Ask* adolescents at every visit whether they smoke and whether their friends use tobacco.
- *Advise.* Congratulate non-users and advise them to resist using tobacco. Discuss the benefits of not smoking.
- *Assist.* When appropriate, encourage participation in programs that promote the development of skills to solve problems, set goals, make decisions, and counter negative peer pressure. Give adolescents information about smoking cessation that they can share with smoking friends.
- *Arrange* followup at appropriate intervals for health care maintenance; make yourself available at other times if necessary.

CONCLUSION Pediatricians should come to view smoking cessation advice as part of the routine anticipatory guidance delivered at all health supervision visits. For this to happen, pediatricians first need to learn the techniques that have been shown to be helpful. Second, they need to overcome their personal barriers to offering the advice. Pediatricians need to know that most smoking parents consider it the pediatrician's job to offer such advice and would actually welcome this help from their children's physicians. The barrier of time becomes less of an issue when the pediatrician learns the brief yet effective method of *ask, advise, assist, arrange.* When possible, other office personnel can be trained to offer further advice on stopping smoking. When other office personnel are not available, the pediatrician can provide appropriate written materials for smoking parents and patients.

REFERENCES

Anda, R.F., Remington, P.L., Sienko, D.G., Davis, R.M. Are physicians advising smokers to quit? The patient's perspective. *Journal of the American Medical Association* 257: 1916-1919, 1987.

Cohen, S.J., Stookey, G.K., Katz, B.P., Drook, C.A., Smith, D.M. Encouraging primary care physicians to help smokers quit: A randomized controlled trial. *Annals of Internal Medicine* 110(8): 648-652, 1989.

DiFranza, J.R., Tye, J.B. Who profits from tobacco sales to children? *Journal of the American Medical Association* 263(20): 2784-2787, 1990.

Epps, R.P., Manley, M.W. A physician's guide to preventing tobacco use during childhood and adolescence. *Pediatrics* 88(1): 140-144, 1991.

Ferguson, K.J., Pomrehn, P.R., Caplan, R.M. Help your patients kick the cigarette habit. *Iowa Medicine* 75(11): 495-497, 1985.

Fielding, J.E., Phenow, K.J. Health effects of involuntary smoking. *New England Journal of Medicine* 319: 1452-1460, 1988.

Fiore, M.C., Novotny, T.E., Pierce, J.P., Hatziandreau, E.J., Patel, K.M., Davis, R.M. Trends in cigarette smoking in the United States: The changing influence of gender and race. *Journal of the American Medical Association* 261(1): 49-55, 1989.

Frankowski, B.L., Secker-Walker, R.H. Advising parents to stop smoking: Opportunities and barriers in pediatric practice. *American Journal of Diseases of Children* 143: 1091-1094, 1989.

Frankowski, B.L., Weaver, S.O., Secker-Walker, R.H. Advising parents to stop smoking: Pediatricians' and parents' attitudes. *Pediatrics,* in press.

Glynn, T.J., Manley, M.W. *How To Help Your Patients Stop Smoking: A National Cancer Institute Manual for Physicians.* U.S. Department of Health and Human Services, Public Health Service, National Institutes of Health, National Cancer Institute. NIH Publication No. 90-3064, 1990.

Gortmalker, S.L., Walker, D.K., Jacobs, F.H., Ruch-Ross, H. Parental smoking and the risk of childhood asthma. *American Journal of Public Health* 72: 574-579, 1982.

Kenney, R.D., Lyles, M.F., Turner, R.C., White, T.S., Gonzalez, J.J., Irons, T.G., Sanchez, C.J., Rogers, C.S., Campbell, E.E., Villagra, V.G., Strecher, V.J., O'Malley, M.S., Stritter, F.T., Fletcher, S.W. Smoking cessation counseling by resident physicians in internal medicine, family practice, and pediatrics. *Archives of Internal Medicine* 148: 2469-2473, 1988.

Koop, C.E. The pediatrician's obligation in smoking education (editorial). *American Journal of Diseases of Children* 139(10): 973, 1985.

Kottke, T.E., Battista, R.N., DeFriese, G.H., Brekke, M.L. Attributes of successful smoking cessation interventions in medical practice: A meta-analysis of 39 controlled trials. *Journal of the American Medical Association* 259: 2882-2889, 1988.

Kraemer, M.J., Richardson, M.A., Weiss, N.S., Furakawa, C.T., Shapiro, G.G., Pierson, W.E., Bierman, C.W. Risk factors for persistent middle-ear effusions: Otitis media, catarrh, cigarette smoke exposure, and atopy. *Journal of the American Medical Association* 249: 1022-1025, 1983.

Landrigan, P.J. Involuntary smoking: A hazard to children. *Pediatrics* 77: 755-757, 1986.

Mason, J.O., Lindsay, G.B. A positive approach to smoking prevention and cessation. *Western Journal of Medicine* 139(5): 721-722, 1983.

Nader, P.R., Taras, H.L., Sallis, J.F., Patterson, T.L. Adult heart disease prevention in childhood: A national survey of pediatricians' practices and attitudes. *Pediatrics* 79: 843-850, 1987.

Ockene, J.K., Hosmer, D.W., Williams, J.W., Goldberg, R.J., Ockene, I.S., Biliouris, T., Dalen, J.E. The relationship of patient characteristics to physician delivery of advice to stop smoking. *Journal of General Internal Medicine* 2: 337-340, 1987.

Orleans, C.T. Understanding and promoting smoking cessation: Overview and guidelines for physician intervention. *Annual Review of Medicine* 36: 51-61, 1985.

Pederson, L.L. Compliance with physician advice to quit smoking: A review of the literature. *Preventive Medicine* 11: 71-84, 1982.

Perry, C.L., Silvis, G.L. Smoking prevention: Behavioral prescriptions for the pediatrician. *Pediatrics* 79: 790, 1987.

Russell, M.A.H., Wilson, C., Taylor, C., Baker, C.D. The effect of general practitioners' advice against smoking. *British Medical Journal* 2: 231-235, 1979.

Sexton, M., Hebel, J.R., Fox, N.L. Postpartum smoking. Paper presented at the International Conference on Smoking and Reproductive Health, San Francisco, October 15-17, 1985.

Solberg, L.I., Maxwell, P.L., Kottke, T.E., Gepner, G.J., Brekke, M.L. A systematic primary care office-based smoking cessation program. *Journal of Family Practice* 30: 647-654, 1990.

Stahlberg, M., Ruuskanen, O., Virolainen, E. Risk factors for recurrent otitis media. *Pediatric and Infant Diseases* 5: 30, 1986.

Strecher, V.J., O'Malley, M.S., Villagra, V.G., Campbell, E.E., Gonzalez, J.J., Irons, T.G., Kenney, R.D., Turner, R.C., Rogers, C.S., Lyles, M.F., White, S.T., Sanchez, C.J., Stritter, F.T., Fletcher, S.W. Can residents be trained to counsel patients about quitting smoking? Results from a randomized trial. *Journal of General Internal Medicine* 6: 9-17, 1991.

U.S. Department of Health and Human Services. *The Health Benefits of Smoking Cessation: A Report of the Surgeon General.* U.S. Department of Health and Human Services, Public Health Service, Centers for Disease Control, Center for Chronic Disease Prevention and Health Promotion, Office on Smoking and Health. DHHS Publication No. (CDC) 90-8416, 1990.

Weiss, S.T., Tager, I.B., Speizer, F.E., Rosner, B. Persistent wheeze: Its relation to respiratory illness, cigarette smoking, and level of pulmonary function in a population sample of children. *American Review of Respiratory Diseases* 122: 697-707, 1980.

Windsor, R.A. An application of the PRECEDE model for planning and evaluating health education methods for pregnant mothers. *Hygie* 5(3): 38-44, 1986.

Smoking Intervention by Providers of Health Care for Women[1]

Mary Sexton, Joan Stine, and Steven Cahill

ROLE OF THE PROVIDER Health care practitioners can significantly reduce cigarette smoking among women. In addition to initiating health care contacts related to medical problems, healthy women are urged to seek even more preventive health care and on a more regular basis than are men; so the number of health care contacts during which it is possible for providers to address smoking is quite high.

During the course of a year, women seek obstetrical and gynecological services that include prenatal care, family planning, and screening for cervical and breast cancers, from family physicians, gynecologists, and other providers. For example, there are 56 million contacts a year by obstetricians and gynecologists (Nelson and McLemore, 1988). Clearly, obstetrical and gynecological practices represent a special opportunity for impact on smoking among women, particularly pregnant women. Yet, obstetricians and gynecologists have not availed themselves of the smoking intervention training provided by the National Cancer Institute. Only 3 percent of 1,568 physicians who have been trained by NCI are obstetricians or gynecologists (Marc Manley, personal communication). The physician's participation in formal training is a step that can lead to the development of office-based smoking intervention.

Not only do health care practices represent an opportunity to reach smokers, but the increasing health risks of women dictate an obligation to do so. Most providers already give a brief message with one or more specific health risks of smoking. The message usually centers on the health of the baby if the woman is pregnant. What is often missing, though, is a standardized protocol that goes beyond giving a health message and that systematically follows the patient's progress at each visit.

The provider can and should adopt the same view and attention toward smoking as toward other medical risks. This focus would convey to the woman a deep and continuing concern over the increased risk that the provider recognizes and would set the framework for development of a treatment plan. In treating acute or chronic disease problems, the provider clearly sees an obligation to give the best medical advice and treatment possible,

[1] The preparation of this manuscript benefited from work partially supported through a cooperative agreement with the Centers for Disease Control.

regardless of how the patient might respond, and the same clarity of professional obligation can be extended easily to treatment consisting of antismoking counseling for smokers.

Patients believe that providers should actively address and discuss the issue of smoking. This was borne out by the authors' recent experience in the Smoking Cessation and Reduction in Public Prenatal Clinics project. As part of the development of the antismoking intervention approach for the project, focus groups of clients seen in prenatal public health clinics were assembled early in the project to delineate key issues about smoking and quitting. The women emphasized the importance to them of the clinic staff's actively giving support to decisions and efforts to quit. After intervention was completed, a survey of the project participants was conducted (regardless of whether they had quit or continued to smoke). Again, the importance of the staff's involvement emerged from the responses. When asked what would help smokers, the women most often suggested that the staff talk with and support clients in their efforts to quit.

With trained physicians implementing a standardized protocol for smoking intervention for their patients, it should be possible to achieve a greater impact on female smokers. The effectiveness may be even greater than reported thus far because of the greater pervasiveness and continuity of the intervention when conducted in health care settings as part of patient care rather than as part of research and demonstration activities.

EFFECTIVENESS OF ANTISMOKING INTERVENTION

Although there is an absence of published information on antismoking intervention for nonpregnant smokers in the gynecological care setting, the effectiveness of antismoking intervention for pregnant smokers has been assessed in diverse health care settings. Table 2 shows that antismoking interventions can produce a significant increase in the percentage of pregnant smokers who quit.

Not all the intervention studies shown, however, nor others reported in the literature, have achieved a statistically significant difference in quit rates. Furthermore, not all studies have included biochemical validation (the cotinine values for the public prenatal clinics project mentioned above are not yet available), and validation results could diminish the reported quit rates and reduce the differences achieved. Nevertheless, the studies, taken as a whole, clearly indicate that quitting by female smokers can be increased. Among studies reporting significant increases, the differences achieved vary by as much as twofold. In the study by Windsor and colleagues (1985), in which a 12-percent difference in quit rates was observed, for example, the intervention consisted of one brief message from a health educator and instruction on the use of a self-help booklet.

In the Sexton and Hebel study (1984), in which a 23-percent difference was observed, the intervention consisted of personal contacts and followup by phone and mail over the entire course of the pregnancy (Nowicki et al., 1984).

Table 2
Quit rates from randomized clinical trials for pregnant smokers

	Quit Rates	
	Experimental Group	Control Group
Public Clinic		
Alabama (Windsor et al., 1985)	14%	2%
Maryland[a]	24	18
Private Setting		
Maryland (Sexton and Hebel, 1984)	43	20
Health Maintenance Organization		
California (Ershoff et al., 1989)	26	17
National Health Care Setting		
England (MacArthur et al., 1987)	9	6

[a] *SCIP (three-state research and demonstration project). Preliminary data without biochemical validation.*

Smokers from both the private sector and the public clinic sector were included. Smokers from the public clinic had quit rates as high as those receiving services from private providers, which suggests that when smokers are given assistance, they will respond, in spite of substantially disadvantaged life circumstances. It is worth noting that by the time they register for prenatal care, about one-fourth of the smokers have already stopped, leaving the heavier and more addicted smokers continuing the behavior. Even so, the provision of assistance after the woman registers for prenatal care results in higher rates of cessation. The importance of reaching female smokers through their health care contacts increases when the considerable postpartum relapse of smokers who quit during pregnancy is taken into account. A continuing focus on the problem of smoking by all providers might assist women in sustaining the quitting they achieve on their own or with assistance during pregnancy.

A broad range of smoking intervention approaches and resources have been used, as illustrated in Table 3. Published information on the specifics of each intervention has been used as a basis for the description, which should be viewed with some caution since it may have been incompletely described. All studies have included some type of materials, and almost all have provided for one-to-one counseling. Most have reported having more than one intervention contact.

A clear picture of the amount of time spent on smoking intervention does not emerge from the information. Somewhat surprisingly, only one study has reported explicit involvement of the physician to assist with the intervention,

Table 3
Description of interventions, by published study

	Provider Message[a]	Materials[b]	Type of Counseling[c]	Number of Contacts	Time (hr)[d]	Quit Rate Difference[e]	Number in Study
Ershoff et al., 1989	HE	P,S,O	I	1	< 1	14%	242
Windsor et al., 1985	HE	S,O	I	1	< 1	12	309
Nowicki et al., 1984	HE	P,O	I	> 1	> 1	23	935
MacArthur et al., 1987	MD, N	P	I	1	NR	3	982
Loeb et al., 1983	HE	P,O	I,G	> 1	> 1	1	963
Aaronson et al., 1985	HE	S,O	I	1	NR	–	58
Langford et al., 1983	N	P	I	1	< 1	0	116
Danaher et al., 1978	HE	P	G	> 1	> 1	–	11

[a] *MD, physician; N, nurse; HE, health educator.*
[b] *P, pamphlet; S, self-help guide; O, other.*
[c] *I, individual; G, group.*
[d] *NR, not reported.*
[e] *Percentage difference between intervention and control groups; no control group reported in Aaronson et al. and Danaher et al.*

beyond what he or she "usually" does. The information suggests that, in the future, the intervention for pregnant smokers could be strengthened by medical personnel's assuming a more prominent role in its implementation.

CONSTRAINTS ON OFFICE-BASED INTERVENTION

The routine of a medical office usually has little free time or flexibility. The procedures for patient care fall into a well-defined set of interlocking activities. The introduction of a new or expanded activity, such as a standardized antismoking protocol, must take into account the constraints that the office routine and staff impose. The ones that are most likely to be faced are described below.

Office Time

The experience with the project in public prenatal clinics showed that several factors impinged on the intervention's being implemented. A balance had to be forged between maintaining a predictable office routine and spending time in counseling patients. As part of the project planning process, the project staff met with prenatal care nurses in public clinics. The nurses were quick to point out that the intervention should be developed with the realization that only a small amount of staff time would be given, since other activities were already extremely demanding. Emerging from the focus groups of patients, on the one hand, was a message that the staff relationship was an important one to patients in quitting. On the other hand, the reality was that staff time was limited. Thus, the project intervention had to focus on the patient's taking a lot of responsibility for her own plan of cessation activities.

Interval Between Visits The infrequency of clinic visits, even for prenatal patients, meant that the staff could not be available on an as-needed basis or even weekly during the time that smokers would be quitting. During the time when the smoker prepares to quit and during the early process of withdrawal from smoking, the individual can benefit most from very frequent contact—daily or even more often—with a support person. It was thus important for the clinic staff to get the patient to find support beyond that which the staff could give.

Skills The public prenatal clinic nurses consistently expressed that training would be needed to enhance their overall counseling skills; in particular, they wanted guidance on how to deal with resistant clients. Most of the staff felt the need for reassurance that they could successfully fulfill the responsibilities given. The authors have met few staff members who felt sufficiently trained and experienced in antismoking intervention.

The public prenatal clinic project intervention was developed within the constraints outlined above. In recognition of limited staff time, the time required by the clinic staff was about 5 to 10 minutes for the initial contact and about 3 minutes for the followup contacts. The intervention itself had a substantial self-help component, in which the patient assumed responsibility for the development and implementation of a specific and personal plan for quitting smoking and avoiding relapse. The patients were told that the self-help materials should be used at home, and they were given guidance by the nurses in how to do that. To address the issue of sustained support, the self-help booklet included a section on how the smoker could develop the skills to achieve ongoing support from family and friends. To reinforce the self-help material, an audiotape and posters for the refrigerator were developed. To address the need for upgrading counseling skills, formal training was provided to the clinic staff.

TRAINING PRENATAL CARE NURSES

Essential steps in the successful implementation of an office-based intervention for the Smoking Cessation and Reduction in Public Prenatal Clinics project included not only the development of an intervention that could actually be implemented in a busy prenatal clinic, but also gaining the staff's cooperation in implementing it. The project staff believed that time spent in training would build confidence in and familiarity with the intervention protocol as well as enhance the cooperation of the staff. While in the majority of sites the antismoking intervention was conducted by the prenatal care nurses, some clinics had very dedicated health educators who did most of the counseling. For simplicity, though, the following discussion refers to nurses as the recipients of the training. The project training may have been more of a challenge than would usually be expected because of the large number of nurses involved, and even more so because the decision to implement the intervention had come from the top down, and in a few instances the clinic nurse had little input to that decision.

Since the nurses had expressed uncertainties about their interactions with the smoker or recent quitter, the intervention encounters were designed to be highly structured and predictable. The training itself focused on a standardized, minimal intervention protocol with the understanding that there was opportunity for expansion. All materials needed for implementation were provided and included those for the exclusive use of the staff. A *Nurses Guide* (State of Maryland, 1989), described below, was developed, as was a form, part of which was used to record smoking status and part of which was a checklist to record specific intervention activities.

Training Structure

There were five participating intervention counties in the project, with the larger ones having multiple prenatal care sites. Since the end of the project, public prenatal care nurses in all the Maryland counties have been trained with essentially the same intervention protocol, but with fewer followup contacts after the initial training session. Training for the Smoking Cessation and Reduction project was arranged for each county separately, to minimize travel time for the staff, and took place as regularly scheduled in-service meetings to prevent disruption of clinic schedules. Because the public prenatal clinics study was a research and demonstration project conducted with some support from the Centers for Disease Control, it was possible to provide several training contacts. The initial training was for one-half day with a followup session scheduled after the staff had time to gain experience with the intervention. Clinics were phoned each month and visited quarterly during the 2-year project. At those times, any problems the staff experienced with intervention could be discussed.

At the initial training session for the project, some background information was provided. An overview of the scientific evidence of the risks of smoking for the fetus during pregnancy, the newborn, and the child was presented, and examples of possible clinical problems seen in smokers were discussed. A summary of reported quit rates achieved in intervention studies was presented. After the introductory material, the rest of the training session was focused on the study intervention.

The smoker's self-help booklet had discrete modules that explicitly considered the patient's stage of readiness to quit, using a Prochaska and DiClemente (1983) approach with different modules on precontemplation, contemplation, and relapse. The training of the nurses emphasized how the booklet could be used with *all* smokers, regardless of their interest or readiness to quit. A separate self-help booklet with almost identical content was developed for recent quitters; it emphasized maintenance of the nonsmoking behavior.

The training of the nurses centered on interaction with the smokers (and recent quitters), using the self-help booklet as the focal material. This focus was to provide consistency of messages and approaches between the nurse's interactions and those in the self-help booklet used at home. Moreover, the nurse's use of the self-help booklet to organize the interaction provided a transition to its use by the client.

To further provide guidance to the counseling exchange, nurses were given a *Nurses Guide*, the content of which was the same self-help booklet provided the patient but expanded to include a brief supplemental section. The added section contained general counseling techniques, a step-by-step standardized counseling protocol for the nurses to follow if they wished, and responses to reasons commonly given for not quitting smoking.

The first two pages of the *Nurses Guide* contained material on how to build a positive relationship with the client, most of which was given as examples of listening and supportive techniques for maximizing the provider/client relationship, such as the one on how to increase confidence and expectations for success:

Technique	Purpose	To Achieve Purpose	Examples
Expressing confidence	To increase confidence and expectations	Express confidence. Be sincere and understanding; avoid "if, maybe, might," or "I think you can quit."	"With your husband's support, I believe you will quit smoking."

Just as the self-help guide provided modules to be used by the smoker, depending on her stage in the cessation process, so the *Nurses Guide* included examples of three standardized protocols (for women who do not want to quit, for women who want to quit, and for recent quitters). Each protocol had the same five counseling steps:

- *Assess* the level of current smoking and interest in quitting.
- Give strong *advice* to quit, along with one or more benefits of cessation.
- *Problem-solve* by identifying potential problems and seeking feasible solutions.
- *Contract* by summarizing the stage the smoker is in with regard to quitting and getting the patient to agree to one or two concrete behaviors (goal), regardless of how simple.
- *Follow up* by assuring the patient that there will be followup at the next appointment.

Specific information was given under each counseling step. For women who do not want to quit, under step 3, "Problem-Solve," the nurse following the steps would (a) identify potential problems and (b) seek "do-able" solutions. A list of possible solutions was given as examples: "Read the self-help manual, listen to the audiotape, put up the posters, think about quitting." The nurse could suggest these or substitute others, as appropriate.

The third short section of the supplement included specific reasons the smoker might give for not quitting, along with specific responses that the nurse could use. If the smoker said, "I get pleasure from smoking," the nurse could respond, "You will get pleasure from quitting, too—improved taste and smell, and better smelling breath, clothes, and hair. But you get more than pleasure; you are freed of any concern over how smoking could harm you and your baby."

The *Nurses Guide* included references to specific pages of the booklets as illustrations or further examples of the messages that the nurse could give for each step of the counseling protocol. The client could follow along in her own self-help booklet as the nurse pointed out the specific content. The nurse could embellish the content of the intervention booklet as much or as little as desired, while maintaining the core protocol, and could always turn to the *Nurses Guide* for further multiple and specific messages and directions. Thus, the materials and approach developed for use by the nurse could be used throughout all the prenatal care sites, regardless of the different levels of skills and motivations found in the staffs from clinic to clinic.

In addition to the *Nurses Guide*, a one-page form was developed and given to the nurses so that a simple but consistent record of the patient's smoking status and intervention could be maintained. At each visit the nurse was expected to record the number of cigarettes the patient had smoked in the preceding 24 hours, the patient's status with respect to willingness to quit (if still smoking), the intervention topics discussed at the visit, the problems or barriers to achieving the goal, and the goal for the next visit. This form provided a continuous record that could be used at successive visits even if a different nurse saw the patient.

As a part of the nurses' training, role-playing was demonstrated by two trainers. Volunteers were then asked to participate to further illustrate how the counseling protocol could be implemented. The role-playing showed how resistance could be addressed. It was emphasized that the provider should always leave the door open for future counseling by avoiding an argumentative approach and acknowledging that people change their minds, and that if the client became interested, there would be a chance to discuss quitting techniques in the future.

The training concluded with a discussion of the smoking status of the nurses and how that might affect their effectiveness in counseling smokers. No one was asked individually about smoking status, but often the nurses would volunteer whether they were current smokers, quitters, or never-smokers. The discussion not only led to suggestions, such as using another behavior—for instance, weight control—around which to identify personal involvement in making changes, it also engaged the nurses in envisioning how they would interact with smokers. It proved to be a very lively and fruitful part of the training session.

POSSIBLE BARRIERS TO EFFECTIVENESS There are a number of issues that may present barriers to the development and implementation of an effective office-based intervention. These barriers are not necessarily overcome through developing or choosing a strong intervention protocol and training staff to use it.

Reimbursement All medical office staffs, but especially those in the private sector, have to be mindful of the cost of patient services. The amount of time and effort that providers spend on antismoking counseling will depend, to some extent, on whether reimbursement is available and specifically linked to that counseling.

Provider Attitudes And Characteristics The authors' experience suggests that reimbursement is not the primary barrier to office-based intervention. The attitude of providers sometimes produces a stumbling block to assisting the smoker, even when reimbursement is not an issue. It has been observed that, for a number of reasons, some providers do not enthusiastically embrace the idea of counseling, even when the intervention is minimal. Some of their own characteristics get in the way of assisting the smoker, as described below:

- *Futility of effort.* Patient compliance is a general problem for the health care practitioner, regardless of what the provider recommends. In reality, some smokers will not change within any given timeframe, and it cannot be predicted with much certainty which individual smokers will change. Most experienced interventionists view smoking cessation as a process and assume that any assistance is one more input to move the smoker along in a progression of changing behavior that has the ultimate goal of an achievement of quitting. Nevertheless, a significantly higher proportion of smokers will stop smoking when assistance is given; according to current information, a 10- to 20-percent increase in quit rates can be achieved from intervention. As techniques improve, the effect may be even larger. Even very modest increases in quit rates are enough to make a significant impact on smoking-related morbidity and mortality. To avoid disappointment and feelings of futility, the provider should accept the reality that antismoking counseling will not be effective with every smoker but will be effective enough overall to improve health. It is helpful to set realistic expectations of success and avoid the feeling that the effort is meaningless.

- *Burnout.* A few prenatal care providers have expressed that an effort to change the smoker's behavior is wasted time because the smokers "are not going to change." Some nurses in training sessions were burned out with their jobs. Just as some patients will not respond to assistance, some few providers will not be responsive to opportunities to increase their counseling effectiveness. For those unusual individuals, the mind set prevents even a reasonable consideration of what is proposed. Where it is possible, staff members who believe they cannot make an impact and who resent having to provide counseling should not have direct counseling contact and responsibility, but should be asked to contribute to antismoking intervention only in indirect ways.

- *Ambivalence.* Some health care providers are ambivalent about smoking cessation counseling because smoking falls outside traditional medical problems, and it is, in the end, the patient who controls the success of the outcome. The provider is unable to apply to smoking the familiar technical skills and knowledge that define medical expertise. Since the highly skilled training from which the provider's prestige and professional standing stem is of little applicability, the health task itself is given less worth, despite evidence to the contrary. Such ambivalence can be addressed with training and a consistently applied antismoking protocol that is viewed as an integral and essential component of good patient care.

- *Smoking status.* The provider who smokes is especially likely to be in conflict and be defensive about the importance and effectiveness of antismoking intervention. Included in the prenatal clinics training described above was an explicit discussion of how a provider's smoking status, regardless of what it is, might influence his or her attitude and effectiveness as a smoking cessation counselor. This broader approach was a good way to take the spotlight off staff members who smoke. For example, current smokers themselves said that patients might perceive that providers who smoke are not credible. These providers were encouraged to consider the appropriateness of their being actively involved in the intervention and to exercise the option of no direct responsibility if they could not overcome their barriers.

  Most providers of prenatal care, however, even smokers, felt they could seriously and sincerely work with pregnant smokers, quite possibly because of the open discussion in training and because their peers supported their involvement. The providers who had never smoked found that they should be prepared to address the client's challenge to the provider's lack of empathy. These providers were encouraged to think of other behaviors that required them to make significant lifestyle changes. The provider who had successfully quit could draw on the experience but, at the same time, needed to avoid becoming overzealous and personalizing the change process too much.

The trainers found it helpful to identify and discuss barriers during the planning and training phases of the intervention and felt that more time should have been given to the discussion. Often the staff expressed helpful suggestions, and the group interaction helped build staff commitment to the intervention and overcome some of the attitudes. Overcoming barriers can be a real challenge, but if the barriers remain, they weaken or completely undermine the intervention efforts.

COMPONENTS IN OBSTETRICAL OFFICES

From the experience in Maryland with three large antismoking programs for (a) about 1,000 prenatal patients in private practice, (b) about 2,000 smokers in State-funded maternity clinics, and (c) about 1,000 smokers in a high-risk university clinic, giving attention to several components appears to be important in the development of an effective antismoking intervention in an obstetrical/gynecological setting. The points highlighted below relate more to structuring the setting and the intervention than to the content of the intervention. The reason is not that the content is unimportant, but that examples of content can be more readily found than can guidelines for how to structure the intervention. While some points are overlapping, the components identified are those relating to structuring the office and those that concern structure of the intervention.

Office Structure

Components of the medical office structure for smoking intervention are as follows:

- *Have a smoke-free office.* The message that health and smoking are incompatible should be conveyed by behavior as well as word. When members of the office staff smoke or condone patients' smoking in the office, it undermines the strength of the health message.
- *Include the physician.* A message from the physician is seen as a credible one and sets the stage for a systematic and serious approach to antismoking intervention from all of the office staff.
- *Include as many other staff members as possible.* All of the office staff can contribute to intervention efforts, and it is important that they do so. Even indirect support, such as adhering to a no-smoking office policy, gives a consistent message in words and behavior from one staff member to the next.
- *Prepare the staff.* Professional consulting skills should be sought and utilized maximally. Nutritionists, social workers, and health educators, while seldom available in other ambulatory settings, are often resources in HMO and public clinic settings. Staff members from human service disciplines, such as these, usually have formal training in the knowledge, skills, and techniques of behavioral change, which enables them to provide more intensive antismoking intervention to patients. They are also a valuable resource for training other staff members; they are often eager to accept the primary responsibility for developing antismoking intervention in the office setting. If no trained staff is available, smoking intervention training can be obtained from outside agencies such as NCI, health voluntary organizations, and State agencies.
- *Use chart notes.* Chart notes about the assessment of smoking and recommendations to the patient should be routine and should become part of the patient's medical record.

Intervention Structure

Components of the intervention structure are as follows:

- *Use a standardized protocol.* In some settings, services are organized so that the patient may see not only different physicians but also different nurses over the course of several visits. Many guidelines for use by the provider have been developed. As part of implementing the smoking intervention, choosing a specific guide, such as NCI's *How To Help Your Patients Stop Smoking* (Glynn and Manley, 1990), will assure that a uniform core approach is taken with every smoker and recent quitter. After gaining experience, the office staff will be able to tailor the approach to individual smokers. The chart notes on the assessment and treatment progress of the smoker provide a history of activities and may be the only means of tracing the course of the medical risk factor of smoking, and of the patient's progress in quitting.

- *Address smoking at every visit.* Smoking should be systematically addressed by the provider at every visit. Encourage any progress on the part of the patient. Expressing optimism that she will one day be ready to quit precludes a completely negative message.

- *Assess smoking status.* Smoking status of the patient is almost always included at least once in the chart notes. The provider should determine and record the amount of smoking at the initial visit and at *every subsequent visit,* just as for any other risk factor. It is the continuity of assessment that most providers can improve. If the smoking status of the patient is routinely assessed and recorded, the patient will be aware of this effort, and the importance that the physician attaches to this risk factor will be elevated. At the same time, the patient's awareness level regarding her behavior is increased. Assessment of the risk factor can itself be an intervention activity (Mahoney et al., 1979) and is certainly necessary for a systematic approach to intervention.

- *Reinforce the message to quit.* The provider message can be reinforced in ways that take only a small amount of personnel time: by self-guided booklets, by audiotapes, videos, posters, and a no-smoking office policy. The more systematic, pervasive, and varied the antismoking intervention is, the more likely that quit rates will increase.

A minimal approach, consisting of (1) assessment and recording of smoking status and intervention activities at every visit, (2) a brief smoking message from the provider at every visit, (3) provision of self-help materials, and (4) referrals to already existing community programs, takes few resources. Voluntary agencies (e.g., American Lung Association, American Cancer Society, American Heart Association) or even hospitals can be found that will provide additional services if needed, and to which smokers or recent quitters can be referred. Training of staff members can usually be obtained from some of these same agencies. If it is not feasible to arrange training by outside agencies, self-training can be developed because of the vast array of materials now available. Beginning with a minimal approach and expanding it as resources warrant would seem to be possible for any office providing health services to women and would greatly increase the number of female smokers who are reached.

REFERENCES

Aaronson, N.K., Ershoff, D.H., Danaher, B.G. Smoking cessation in pregnancy: A self-help approach. *Addictive Behaviors* 10(1): 103-108, 1985.

Danaher, B.G., Shisslak, C.M., Thompson, C.B., Ford, J.D. A smoking cessation program for pregnant women: An exploratory study. *American Journal of Public Health* 68(9): 896-898, 1978.

Ershoff, D.H., Muller, P.D., Quinn, V.P. A randomized trial of a serialized self-help smoking cessation program for pregnant women in an HMO. *American Journal of Public Health* 79(2): 182-187, 1989.

Glynn, T.J., Manley, M.W. *How To Help Your Patients Stop Smoking: A National Cancer Institute Manual for Physicians*. U.S. Department of Health and Human Services, Public Health Service, National Institutes of Health, National Cancer Institute. NIH Publication No. 90-3064, 1990.

Langford, E.R., Thompson, E.G., Tripp, S.C. Smoking and health education during pregnancy: Evaluation of a program for women in prenatal classes. *Canadian Journal of Public Health* 74(4): 285-289, 1983.

Loeb, B.K., Waage, G., Bailey, J. Smoking intervention in pregnancy. In: *Proceedings of the Fifth World Conference on Smoking and Health* (volume 1), W.F. Forbes, R.C. Frecker, and D. Nostbakken (Editors). Ottawa, Ontario: Canadian Council on Smoking and Health, 1983, p. 389.

MacArthur, C., Newton, J.R., Knox, E.G. Effect of antismoking health education on infant size at birth: A randomized controlled trial. *British Journal of Obstetrics and Gynecology* 94(4): 295-300, 1987.

Mahoney, M.J., Arnkoff, D.B. Self-management. In: *Behavioral Medicine: Theory and Practice*, O.F. Pomerleau and J.P. Brady (Editors). Baltimore: Williams and Wilkins, 1979, pp. 75-96.

Nelson, C., McLemore, T. *National Medical Care Survey*. U.S. Department of Health and Human Services, Public Health Service, Centers for Disease Control, National Center for Health Statistics, 1988.

Nowicki, P., Gintzig, L., Hebel, J.R., Latham, R., Miller, V., Sexton, M. Effective smoking intervention during pregnancy. *Birth* 11(4): 217-224, 1984.

Prochaska, J.O., DiClemente, C.C. Stages and processes of self-change of smoking: Toward an integrative model of change. *Journal of Consulting and Clinical Psychology* 51(3): 390-395, 1983.

Sexton, M., Hebel, J.R. A clinical trial of change in maternal smoking and its effect on birth weight. *Journal of the American Medical Association* 251(7): 911-915, 1984.

State of Maryland, Department of Health and Mental Hygiene. *Nurses Guide To Quit and Be Free*. 1989.

Windsor, R.A., Cutter, G., Morris, J., Reese, Y., Manzella, B., Bartlett, E.E., Samuelson, C., Spanos, D. The effectiveness of smoking cessation methods for smokers in public health maternity clinics: A randomized trial. *American Journal of Public Health* 75(12): 1389-1392, 1985.

A Physician- and Dentist-Delivered Smoking Cessation Intervention for Head and Neck Cancer Patients[2]

Ellen R. Gritz, Clifford R. Carr, David A. Rapkin,
Cindy Chang, John Beumer, and Paul H. Ward

PURPOSE OF THE PROJECT

The research described in this paper differs from the other studies reported in this monograph with respect to both the patient population and the health care providers. Although the great majority of smoking cessation interventions for physicians and dentists have been designed for primary care practitioners, who see generally healthy patients, there have been no systematic trials with specialized surgeons and dentists treating cancer patients. In general, quit-smoking rates of medical patient populations have increased with severity of disease (US DHHS, 1984). Thus, one would predict a high cessation rate in a cancer patient population with smoking-related tumors. Indeed, a 2-year continuous abstinence rate of 47 percent was recently reported for patients with stage I non-small-cell carcinoma of the lung (Gritz et al., 1991b).

Patients with squamous cell carcinomas of the head and neck present a natural group for intervention. In many cases, surgery and/or radiation therapy can provide definitive treatment, and the 5-year relative survival rate is approximately 51 percent for malignancies of the oral cavity and pharynx and 67 percent for larynx cancers (US DHHS, 1990). The period of diagnosis and treatment of smoking-related tumors is an optimal time for smoking intervention, presenting a teachable moment when motivation for cure and prevention of further disease is heightened. Head and neck surgeons and maxillofacial prosthodontists who treat this cancer patient population have not previously been involved in smoking cessation research, so there is an opportunity to extend training into new areas of specialty.

The study described here is part of the UCLA Cancer Control Science Program, a program project grant with the theme of enhancing adherence to cancer control regimens. Recently completed, the prospective, randomized trial developed, implemented, and evaluated a provider-delivered smoking cessation intervention for patients with head and neck cancers (Gritz et al., 1990 and 1991a). The main goal of the study was to compare the smoking cessation rates of treatment and control groups at 1 year after the intervention.

---

[2] This research was conducted with support from National Cancer Institute grant number CA-43461.

The study intervention was designed to maximize the likelihood of behavioral change as a result of the cancer diagnosis and treatment and to capitalize on doctor-patient bonding to reinforce and sustain the smoking cessation effort (Becker, 1974; Burling et al., 1984; Burt et al., 1974). The structure and components of the study intervention were modeled after methods established as effective in NCI-sponsored physician smoking cessation trials (Glynn and Manley, 1990). Delivering personalized, face-to-face advice in multiple interactions and using multiple intervention modalities (e.g., a target quit-date contract signed by both provider and patient, in addition to repeated advice) comprised the most successful components of smoking cessation interventions in medical practice (Kottke et al., 1988). In addition to patient behavior, the provider's own beliefs and attitudes, smoking status, motivation and efforts in patient counseling, and adherence to the cessation protocol were important influences on outcome (American Cancer Society, 1981; Ewart et al., 1983). The current study assessed these provider beliefs and behaviors and, through a standardized training module, attempted to develop, enhance, and sustain effective provider counseling skills.

TARGET AUDIENCE

Providers in this study consisted of 103 head and neck surgeons and 7 maxillofacial prosthodontists (26 attending physicians and 84 residents). Subjects were accrued from 10 clinics at participating southern California sites: 3 university hospitals (including both the head and neck and the maxillofacial clinics at UCLA, the main site); 3 Veterans Administration Medical Centers; 2 Los Angeles County hospitals; 1 health maintenance organization; and 1 armed services hospital.

PRACTICE OR CLINICAL SETTING

A total of 389 eligibility checklists were completed on patients with newly diagnosed squamous cell carcinomas of the head and neck. The study sites represented a broad spectrum of facilities providing surgical and followup care to this patient population in the southern California region.

Study subjects had varying treatment regimens that entailed medical care by multiple providers—head and neck surgeons, maxillofacial prosthodontists, and radiation oncologists—in as many different clinics. The three most typical paradigms for treatment were surgery only, surgery followed by radiation therapy, and radiation therapy only. Subjects were also seen by different providers within the same clinic, particularly at university and VA hospitals. Much of the subjects' care was provided by residents under the supervision and guidance of attending physicians.

RECRUITMENT OF PATIENTS

Patients older than 18 with newly diagnosed squamous cell carcinomas of the head and neck were eligible for the study. Participating providers completed an eligibility checklist on each patient to determine whether a second tier of enrollment criteria was met: (1) life expectancy of more than 1 year; (2) tobacco use within the past year; (3) absence of gross psychopathology; (4) medical followup by local providers; (5) ability to speak and read English; and (6) agreement to undergo treatment.

Study interviewers reviewed medical records and operating room schedules and attended morning rounds and tumor conferences to ensure that all eligible patients were identified. After confirming a diagnosis of squamous cell carcinoma, providers introduced the study to eligible patients. All patients willing to participate were contacted by a study interviewer, who arranged a baseline interview prior to the start of medical treatment. Patients provided written, informed consent to participate in the project at the start of the baseline interview.

Approximately 57 percent of the 389 patients with newly diagnosed squamous cell carcinomas of the head and neck identified were eligible for enrollment (n=221), and 84.2 percent of those were randomized (n=186). Not using tobacco in the 12 months preceding diagnosis was the predominant basis for exclusion from enrollment, accounting for 57.1 percent (n=96) of the 168 ineligible patients. Sixty-three (65.6 percent) of these 96 ineligible patients had stopped smoking more than 1 year prior to diagnosis, and the remaining 33 (34.4 percent) were classified as nonsmokers. The smoking histories of seven of the latter were unknown, and so they were conservatively assumed to be nonsmokers. Thus, the overall rate of current tobacco use among both eligible and ineligible subjects was 75.3 percent (n=293), and the overall rate of ever-use of tobacco was 91.5 percent (n=356).

The 186 randomized patients were predominantly male (73.7 percent) and in the sixth decade of life or older (average age was 58.5 years). Whites constituted 72.6 percent of the sample; 18.8 percent were black, 6.5 percent Latino, 1.1 percent Asian, and 1.0 percent other. Approximately one-third of subjects (33.9 percent) had not completed high school; 14 percent were college graduates. Although 57.8 percent had an annual family income under $15,000, 17.3 percent fell into the $40,000-and-over category. Finally, 51 percent were married or living with someone.

The primary site of disease was the oral cavity or pharynx for 60.9 percent and the larynx for 39.1 percent of patients. At diagnosis, 31.1 percent had early stage disease (stages I and II). Total laryngectomies were performed on 24.7 percent of patients; 28.5 percent were treated with radiation only; and 46.8 percent had surgery other than total laryngectomy (which was followed by radiation in some cases).

At diagnosis, 12 percent of patients were former smokers (had quit 1 to 11 months earlier) and 88 percent were current smokers (had smoked within the past month). Overall, this was a moderately addicted group of long-term, heavy smokers; they had been smoking an average of 39.7 years and had a mean score on the Fagerstrom tolerance scale of 6.6 (11 maximum).

PROTOCOL FOR ADVICE

The research protocol defined delivery of smoking cessation advice in both usual care and experimental intervention conditions. As Table 4 shows, there was a range of conditions in which advice (initial advice to stop smoking, initial advice to maintain abstinence, or booster session advice) was given. Algorithms were developed for delivery of advice in each condition. Each of these advice algorithms, detailed in Appendix B, could be completed in the course of a provider-patient discussion lasting approximately 7 minutes. Providers learned and practiced delivering advice (see "Nature of the Training Program," below).

Initial advice was delivered to surgical patients 2 to 3 days prior to hospital discharge and to radiation patients prior to the start of treatment by attending (faculty) and chief resident physicians and dentists.

The *usual care* condition consisted solely of the delivery of the standardized usual care initial advice—risks of smoking behavior and benefits of cessation during continuing medical care. Providers were told to follow their usual practices.

The *experimental intervention* was designed to be integrated into regular medical care, as well. The initial advice session, as in usual care, consisted of standardized, strong advice to quit smoking. This advice was enhanced by greater interaction in determining the patient's receptivity to attempting cessation; expressing confidence in the patient's ability to stop; discussing craving and the withdrawal syndrome; negotiating the target quit date and joining the patient in signing the written contract; and assuring the patient of ongoing support for smoking cessation during treatment and followup care (Appendix B). The initial advice was further reinforced with targeted, written, self-help and social support materials for the patient and spouse or caregiver, and the formal smoking cessation contract (see "Products of the Project," below). For the first year after treatment, head and neck cancer patients return monthly for followup visits. Six monthly booster sessions for smoking cessation were administered during these followup medical appointments. In addition, six postcards with smoking cessation maintenance tips were mailed monthly to intervention subjects from the office of their provider.

Table 4
Classification of smoking cessation advice sessions

Initial Advice (All Patients)	Booster Sessions (Intervention Patients Only)
Current and former smokers—usual care group	Abstainers and slippers
Current smokers—intervention group	New relapsers (since last visit)
Former smokers—intervention group	Reduced- and full-consumption smokers

NATURE OF THE TRAINING PROGRAM

Training was conducted at the provider's site, often as part of a tumor conference. Providers included faculty and house staff. Training was conducted in a single 2-hour session and included a baseline questionnaire, a didactic presentation about the study, a videotape of advice, and role-playing. Training began with administration of a baseline questionnaire eliciting providers' knowledge, attitudes, and beliefs about smoking behavior (their own and patients') and about smoking cessation in head and neck cancer patients. Behavioral and pharmacological aspects of tobacco dependence, study aims, and the methodology of the randomized trial were then explained. Providers were encouraged to ask questions about their individual roles and theoretical and methodological aspects of the study, or to express concerns about implementation of the research protocol at their facility.

To become familiar with the contents of the smoking cessation advice that was to be delivered in usual care and experimental intervention conditions, providers were shown videotaped vignettes in which a surgeon delivers smoking cessation advice across the range of conditions. The videotapes were constructed to be direct models for providers to replicate, exemplifying application of an algorithm to each advice condition. Algorithm outlines preceded and followed each vignette on the videotape.

After the videotaped vignettes were shown, printed advice algorithms were distributed, and providers were asked to break into dyads for role-play of delivery of advice to "patients" (see Appendix B for usual care and experimental, advice-giving algorithms). Each dyad member was asked to enact the role of both provider and patient, in turn, giving and receiving advice in as many conditions as possible. Although a few providers were initially hesitant to engage in the unfamiliar task of role-play, nearly all became engaged in the process quite rapidly. Project staff members observed the dyads and provided feedback. Training concluded with a discussion of the role-play, involving all providers and offering an opportunity to raise final questions.

Additional training sessions were conducted for new residents, typically at 1-year intervals. Continual monitoring of audiotaped provider-patient interactions allowed the research staff to identify providers who needed brushup training. Such supplemental training was also provided on rare occasions when providers themselves requested it.

SPECIAL RESOURCES AND PROCEDURES

Videotapes

Creation of training videotapes required special resources. Preproduction work consisted of scripting, casting and recruitment, and rehearsal. For the sake of simplicity, economy, and the intended feeling of the video vignettes (realistic yet light), it was desirable to have a considerable amount of improvisation. To this end, no formal scripts were created. Instead, advice algorithms were used as the basis for improvising vignettes spanning the range of advice conditions. This approach simplified rehearsals and ensured that video vignettes were faithful to what providers themselves would do when delivering advice to real patients: express themselves as naturally as possible while following a particular advice algorithm.

Casting required one provider and a small number of persons willing to role-play patients. Real patients were not used because of logistical complications—contacting them, screening for suitability, obtaining consent—and because of the ready availability of research staff and other volunteers. The director of the university video laboratory was enthusiastic about playing a patient and was extremely supportive and helpful in producing the tape. Other "patients" were recruited from the project staff. The provider delivering advice on the videotape is a UCLA faculty member and a colleague of many providers at other study sites. He was selected because of his demeanor and his interest in the project.

All six vignettes were taped in one 3-hour session. Editing was done by university video lab staff in consultation with the research team. Videographics displaying algorithm outlines were inserted before and after each vignette.

Guidelines And Reminders For Advice

Special procedures were aimed primarily at making it easy for providers to implement their tasks with patients and/or to assure that they did so in accordance with requirements of the study. Provider training has already been described. Providers were encouraged to keep copies of advice algorithms. Self-help booklets (described below) relieved providers of any need for detailed knowledge of quitting or abstinence strategies. Special stickers were designed and printed, and these were placed on the covers of hospital charts of participating patients. Project staff members reminded providers immediately before and during clinics about which patients required advice. Providers were also reminded when telephone boosters were required. Provider-patient interviews were audiotaped for several reasons: (1) to provide documentation that providers were actually giving advice according to protocol (e.g., to document that intervention advice was not contaminating usual care); (2) to ensure that providers experienced a degree of motivation-accountability in their advice-giving (especially useful with residents); and (3) as noted above, to allow the research staff to identify providers who were in need of brushup training.

Patient Tracking

Special procedures were also required to follow some research subjects. Some patients, especially those living out of state, and those in low socioeconomic groups, had addresses that were difficult to obtain (or that frequently changed) or had no phones and were otherwise difficult to track, contact, and interview. Project interviewers developed impressive persistence and ingenuity in obtaining data from these patients.

PRODUCTS OF THE PROJECT

The components of the smoking cessation intervention are designed to be individually and collectively exportable. The components include standardized, strong advice to stop smoking; targeted, written, self-help and social support materials; a contracted quit date; booster advice sessions; and postcards with maintenance tips. Written materials include three booklets: the first for stopping smoking (*Team Up To Stop Smoking*); the second for maintaining abstinence (*Team Up To Stay Off*); and the third a social support booklet for the patient's spouse, family member, or other caretaker (*Team Up To Help a Friend*).

The booklets are written specifically for head and neck cancer patients and contain smoking cessation information that takes into account patients' medical, physical, and psychological condition. The two smoking cessation booklets feature illustrated descriptions of the connection between patients' smoking and their cancers; the value of quitting and special opportunity to quit now; simple, direct instructions on how to stop smoking; information about coping with high-risk situations for relapse; a discussion of alcohol use and the relapse risk associated with drinking; and a supportive discussion of the stress that smoking cessation creates for the patient. The social support booklet, directed to patients' significant others, describes effective strategies to aid the patients in their effort to stop smoking and stay off cigarettes.

These materials are grounded in the premise that, during this critical period of cancer treatment and recuperation, positive social support must be delivered to the patient in a variety of interpersonal contexts in which smoking is likely to occur. Psychological issues relating to head and neck cancer and disturbances of affect and physical functioning are empathically addressed.

The stop-smoking and stay-quit contract is printed on an official-looking document. It consists of a pledge to quit or stay off cigarettes as of an agreed-on date and spaces for both the patient's and the provider's signatures, and it is embossed with two hands clasped in a symbolic gesture of support between the provider and patient. The contract is a three-part, no-carbon-required form, with one copy each for the patient, the provider, and the study staff.

The six monthly postcards, which give tips for stopping smoking and maintaining abstinence, are signed by a member of the provider's staff. The postcards are mailed in conjunction with monthly booster sessions.

The training videotape described above is completely self-explanatory and could be used in any medical or dental setting where patients with head and neck cancers are treated. It is 30 minutes long but can be shown in segments consisting of the initial advice session and the three types of followup sessions (abstinence, relapse, and continuing smoker).

BARRIERS AND PROBLEMS OVERCOME

A number of unanticipated administrative, provider, and subject barriers prevented easy implementation of the protocol. Administrative barriers included the lack of participation by radiation oncologists and difficulty in maintaining continuity of care. The protocol originally was designed to include radiation oncologists among the providers. Resistance to participation was encountered at two sites, principally because of infrequent contact between radiation oncologist and patient and the lack of regular followup once radiation therapy is completed. Therefore, the protocol was adapted to have smoking cessation advice delivered to radiation-only patients by the referring surgeon or, when appropriate, by a participating dentist.

Continuity of care is frequently a problem in tertiary care facilities. Patients are often treated or followed concurrently by multiple providers, including head and neck surgeons, radiation oncologists, and maxillofacial prosthodontists. As a consequence of resident rotations, VA patients and clinic patients at university hospitals frequently have multiple providers within the same clinic as well. Thus, the provider-patient bond becomes more tenuous than in a private-practice setting. In our study, this was disadvantageous because provider-patient bonding was hypothesized to be important for maximizing the impact of the smoking cessation intervention.

Although study providers as a group were very helpful, a few were not willing to follow the research protocol closely. Contrary to protocol, some attending physicians wanted to routinely delegate advice-giving to residents and necessary paperwork to project interviewers. Persistent explanations of the rationale for these aspects of the protocol were helpful with those providers. Surgical residents are oriented primarily toward learning complex operating techniques and amassing experience with disease diagnosis and treatment. Because of the psychosocial nature of this study, it was often perceived as their lowest priority. Thus, constant supportive urging by attending physicians and study staff was necessary.

Patient adherence to trial procedures exceeded our expectations. In addition to participating in advice-delivery sessions, patients were interviewed at baseline and at 1, 6, and 12 months after the initial advice session. Surviving patients then participated in annual interviews thereafter. However, there was a small segment of subjects who were very difficult to follow. The reasons included mobility, mostly among the Veterans Administration patients; homelessness, applying not only to VA but also to county hospital subjects; and family interference. Occasionally, relatives on whom the subjects were dependent, either for communication (because they were speech impaired) or for transportation, thwarted access to the subjects such that further participation was precluded. It was difficult to discern, in these situations, how closely the protectiveness of relatives reflected a subject's lack of interest in study participation.

WHAT WORKED AND WHY

Understanding The Milieu

The study staff made every effort to understand thoroughly the timing, implications, and impact of medical treatment delivered to head and neck cancer patients. Project staff members attended rounds and tumor conferences to become immersed in the providers' milieu; tracked patient movement from clinic entry (and from previous physician referral, when appropriate) through treatment and followup; and interviewed patients, providers, and staff at participating clinics. These activities facilitated the design of an intervention that was easily integrated into standard medical care, as well as tailoring the smoking cessation materials to the needs and concerns of head and neck cancer patients.

Two important adjustments to the intervention were made because of this groundwork. First, the timing of the smoking cessation advice was moved from the second clinic appointment, usually when patients were informed of their cancer diagnosis, to 2 or 3 days prior to hospital discharge for surgical patients. After being informed of their cancer diagnosis, most patients were so absorbed in their cognitive and emotional efforts to begin to cope with their situation that they were unable to assimilate smoking cessation advice. As a part of standard care, surgeons warned all of their patients of complications that can result from continuing to smoke prior to anesthesia. Most patients stopped smoking, at least briefly, for that reason, or because of hospital policy. When they had recovered sufficiently from their surgery and were ready to leave the nonsmoking hospitals, patients were able to attend to long-term concerns, including smoking cessation and its health implications.

Second, patients receiving radiation therapy as the initial treatment modality were often not seen by their primary surgical provider for at least 6 weeks. This could have allowed those patients to return to their routines, including smoking, without the benefit of smoking cessation advice. Thus, the advice was delivered to these patients prior to the first radiation therapy appointment.

Quality Control

Study interviewers took many precautions to ensure that all head and neck cancer patients with newly diagnosed squamous cell carcinomas were identified as potential subjects. They attended tumor conferences and hospital rounds; reviewed operating room schedules for types of surgery that are specific to head and neck cancer; checked medical records of clinic patients; and maintained as much of a presence as possible in the participating clinics. Although the protocol called for providers to identify eligible patients through eligibility checklists, the research staff often assumed the responsibility for screening clinic records of new patients and completing the checklists in consultation with physicians. Additional paperwork was deemed burdensome to the providers.

Delivery of control and intervention advice by participating providers was persistently monitored to ensure protocol adherence and to prevent subject contamination. First, a subject's file was marked with a sticker once he or she was randomized. Second, intervention materials (including advice guidelines, three smoking cessation booklets, and a quit-smoking/stay-off contract) were presented by a staff interviewer to each provider just prior to delivery of intervention advice. Third, providers were asked to audiotape the delivery of initial advice in both conditions and the delivery of the intervention booster sessions. The study staff reviewed the tapes for adherence to the advice guidelines and gave feedback to providers. Finally, all subjects were asked to complete exit checklists after the initial advice was delivered.

Provider Training And Involvement

Perhaps the single most important factor predisposing to success in provider involvement was the leadership role taken by the Chief of Head and Neck Surgery and the Chief of Maxillofacial Prosthodontics at UCLA. Although participation in this research was technically not required of all faculty and residents, the enthusiastic support and continuous encouragement of those two prominent clinicians clearly facilitated acceptance and support of the study. Without the sponsorship and collegial stance taken by those two individuals, the project probably would not have sustained the involvement and interest of the other providers. It is noteworthy in this regard that not a single surgeon or dentist (faculty or resident) refused to participate in the trial.

Success with respect to provider involvement included several additional dimensions: suitability of intervention and supplementary materials to the clinical environment; education of providers with respect to behavioral research strategies and designs (which may differ significantly from biomedical research strategies); receptivity of providers to training in delivery of smoking cessation interventions; and motivation of providers to follow research guidelines in implementing the experimental smoking cessation intervention and the usual care condition.

As described earlier, providers were trained to deliver a cogent smoking cessation message (Appendix B) in a timeframe quite compatible with a typical provider-patient interaction, usually 7 minutes or less. Dispensing supplementary materials (contract, booklets, and postcards) proved to be easy and required little time.

Education of providers included orientation to the overall research strategy and to providers' roles and tasks. Providers responded well to training sessions, often participating energetically in the dyadic role-plays. Responses to questionnaires administered during training sessions indicated that providers were well aware of the morbidity associated with patients' continued use of tobacco. Providers saw themselves as important and practical sources of advice to quit smoking.

Provider behavior after training was generally consistent with the impression that they were motivated to assist patients' smoking cessation efforts and to conform to the requirements of the research protocol. The house staff and attending surgeons and dentists worked cooperatively with research staff, integrating aspects of the protocol with their clinical routines. Tape recordings of control and experimental interventions indicated that providers succeeded in avoiding contamination across conditions. This was particularly important because the design of the study required all providers to administer both types of intervention (only patients were randomized). Overall it seems clear that, in the context of a sharply and economically presented rationale and training, and when equipped with appropriately designed materials, even very busy providers will function effectively as sources of a behavioral intervention in smoking cessation research.

Patient Participation Experience gained in this trial suggests that intervention with head and neck carcinoma patients, a potentially difficult patient population (with long-term histories of tobacco and alcohol use), is quite feasible. Nearly 85 percent of eligible patients were successfully enrolled. The patients proved to be cooperative participants, even during periods of illness and hospitalization, in this long-term research effort. As an example of the altruism expressed by many patients, about 10 participation checks were returned with explicit directions to donate the funds to the research study.

WHAT DID NOT WORK AND WHY Provider training required more time than the physicians and dentists wanted to devote to that activity. Multiple training sessions were necessary at some sites because large numbers of providers were unable to attend preplanned sessions, even though these coincided with tumor conferences. Future training sessions should be shorter and more compatible with provider schedules.

Booster sessions and followup interviews were timed to coincide with medical followups to minimize subject burden. Frequently, the standardized scheduling was not maintained, and study interviewers had to adjust followup schedules accordingly. It was desired that all patients receive smoking cessation advice at designated times, that is, a fully standardized intervention. However, diversity of treatment regimens and nonstandardized medical followup required that flexible scheduling and telephone boosters be introduced into the protocol. Thus, it proved difficult to maintain the planned schedule for booster sessions. Telephone boosters were instituted to ameliorate the problem, especially for radiation patients who were also being treated by the dentists. Providers were asked to limit the number of telephone boosters to two of the six prescribed sessions.

WHAT WOULD BE DONE DIFFERENTLY NOW This section discusses how the current research paradigm would be adapted to a nonresearch, clinical environment. Modifications fall into two categories: (1) the physician and dentist training and counseling role, and (2) the patient intervention.

The importance of support from the most senior and powerful clinicians ("top down") has been discussed, but it was important also to engage co-operation from the interns and residents on the medical-dental teams ("bottom up"). The latter, young physicians and dentists, were responsible for delivering much of the counseling. They had to be convinced of the intervention's importance (both biomedically and behaviorally), of their own effectiveness (self-efficacy), and of the value of acquiring such skills in their surgical or dental residency (rather than detracting from their development of operating technique or basic scientific research).

In the present study, providers' cooperation was won with time and the repeated exhortation and example of the senior clinicians. Counseling skills should be framed as valuable contributions to well-rounded dental and surgical training during the training session. As one of the division chiefs often states, "We want to be physicians as well as surgeons."

Head and neck surgeons and maxillofacial prosthodontists are extremely busy clinicians who, in hospital settings, see many patients in the course of half-day clinics. Thus, the fact that the counseling interventions were time-limited (7 minutes or less, on the average) was very appealing. However, paperwork, such as determining patient eligibility for the intervention, tracking smoking status, remembering to schedule return appointments, and sending reminder postcards, was perceived as too burdensome. Nurses or medical clerks could easily assume these tasks. Second, compressing training sessions into a single hour, as was done eventually out of necessity, fits the tumor conference paradigm better than the original 2-hour structure. Repeated and individual review of counseling algorithms, as appropriate patient interviews arose, led to better provider retention and performance. Finally, the number and spacing of booster advice sessions can easily be accommodated to the actual scheduling of medical or dental followup appointments and need not occur on a set monthly basis for 6 months.

The patient intervention would benefit from several modifications. The first involves emphasizing the usefulness and importance of the targeted self-help booklets. Patients tended to dissociate the receipt of these materials during their time as inpatients from their home recovery activities, which was certainly not the intent of the intervention. For example, it is unclear how many significant others ever received the third item, the social support booklet. It would be better for clinicians to be certain to hand the booklet directly to a family member or caretaker and to deliver the advice and the two patient booklets in the presence of that support person.

Consequent to initial advice, booklets should be actively used in booster sessions. Mailed followup support material, such as postcards, should be tailored to the patient's current smoking status so as to be maximally relevant and personalized. The intervention developed in this study was designed with the direct collaboration of clinicians, specifically with these providers and their patients in mind. Because of this close working relationship, relatively few modifications would be required for a generalized dissemination of the intervention.

REFERENCES

American Cancer Society. The impact of providing physicians with quit smoking materials for smoking patients. *CA—A Cancer Journal for Clinicians* 31: 75-78, 1981.

Becker, M.H. The health belief model and sick role behavior. In: *The Health Belief Model and Personal Health Behavior*, M.H. Becker (Editor). Thoroughfare, NJ: C.B. Slack, 1974, pp. 82-92.

Burling, T.A., Singleton, E.G., Bigelow, G.E., Baile, W.F., Gottlieb, S.H. Smoking following myocardial infarction: A critical review of the literature. *Health Psychology* 3(1): 83-96, 1984.

Burt, A., Thornley, P., Illingworth, D., White, P., Shaw, T.R.D., Turner, R. Stopping smoking after myocardial infarction. *Lancet* 1(7852): 304-306, 1974.

Ewart, C.K., Li, V.C., Coates, T.J. Increasing physicians' antismoking influence by applying an inexpensive feedback technique. *Journal of Medical Education* 58(6):468-473, 1983.

Glynn, T.J., Manley, M.W. *How To Help Your Patients Stop Smoking: A National Cancer Institute Manual for Physicians.* U.S. Department of Health and Human Services, Public Health Service, National Institutes of Health, National Cancer Institute. NIH Publication No. 90-3064, 1990.

Gritz, E.R., Carr, C.R., Rapkin, D.A., Chang, C., Beumer, J., Ward, P.H. A smoking cessation intervention for head and neck cancer patients: Trial design, patient accrual and characteristics. *Epidemiology, Biomarkers and Prevention* 1(1): 67-73, 1991a.

Gritz, E.R., Nisenbaum, R., Elashoff, R., Holmes, E.C. Smoking behavior following diagnosis in patients with stage I non-small-cell lung cancer. *Cancer Causes and Control* 2(2): 105-112, 1991b.

Gritz, E.R., Ward, P.H., Beumer, J., Carr, C.R., Rapkin, D.A. Increasing adherence to a provider-implemented smoking cessation intervention for head and neck cancer patients. In: *Advances in Cancer Control: Screening and Prevention Research (Progress in Clinical Biology Series, Volume 339)*, P.F. Engstrom, B. Rimer, and L. Mortenson (Editors). New York: Wiley-Liss, 1990, pp. 83-93.

Kottke, T.E., Battista, R.N., DeFriese, G.H., Brekke, M.L. Attributes of successful smoking cessation interventions in medical practice: A meta-analysis of 39 controlled trials. *Journal of the American Medical Association* 259(19): 2882-2889, 1988.

U.S. Department of Health and Human Services. *The Health Benefits of Smoking Cessation: A Report of the Surgeon General.* U.S. Department of Health and Human Services, Public Health Service, Centers for Disease Control, Center for Chronic Disease Prevention and Health Promotion, Office on Smoking and Health. DHHS Publication No. (CDC) 90-8416, 1990.

U.S. Department of Health and Human Services. *The Health Consequences of Smoking: Chronic Obstructive Lung Disease. A Report of the Surgeon General.* U.S. Department of Health and Human Services, Public Health Service, Office on Smoking and Health. DHHS Publication No. (PHS) 84-50205, 1984.

Medical Advice as a Communication About Risks of Smoking and Benefits of Quitting

Laura C. Leviton, Timothy R. Cline, and Saul Shiffman

INTRODUCTION To gain maximum effect from medical advice to quit smoking, it is important to understand the process by which medical advice causes smokers to consider cessation and to take actions to quit (Evans, 1986). A medical or dental professional's advice to quit can provide motivation, whereas an intervention (on-site counseling, referrals to other resources) can provide the patient with tools and skills to quit. A study sponsored by the National Cancer Institute is focusing on three elements of this process: making the health risks personal, emphasizing the benefits of quitting, and increasing patients' perceptions that they are capable of quitting. Although other aspects of medical advice may also facilitate smoking cessation, these seem to be key aspects.

PURPOSE OF THE PROJECT The project was implemented in a rural area of Pennsylvania and originated as an effort to provide a service to a cohort of former chemical workers who have been exposed to a bladder carcinogen (Leviton et al., 1991; Marsh et al., 1991). Because of the chemical workers' increased risk of bladder cancer, both the risks of smoking and benefits of quitting are greater for these smokers than they are for smokers in the general population. However, the workers were not uniformly aware of this fact before the study started.

Access to the cohort members presented an important opportunity to study the combined effects of several forces. Medical or dental advice in this context should have greater importance for patients because the professional is giving essential information about patients' personal risk for smoking-related disease, in combination with information about patients' self-efficacy, or their ability to quit smoking and thus avoid disease. Although the cohort's situation is unique, the same kinds of intervention could be given by medical and dental professionals to different kinds of smokers who run increased risk of disease because of the combination of smoking and other factors.

The major outcome measure in this study is not smoking cessation but *progress toward* smoking cessation (Horn, 1976; Leventhal and Cleary, 1980; Pechacek and Danaher, 1979). Even when medical advice does not lead to immediate smoking cessation, it may well lead to progress along the road to quitting and may help to tip the balance in favor of quitting. In fact, the guidelines provided by NCI explicitly tailor medical advice about smoking cessation to the smoker's stage of self-change. Smokers proceed through at least five such stages: (1) precontemplation, in which they do not seriously consider quitting and or even give it much thought; (2) contemplation, in which they begin to consider quitting; (3) short-term quitting, in which smokers have recently quit but may yet relapse; (4) relapse, in which quitters have returned to smoking but may try cessation again; and (5) long-term maintenance of cessation (DiClemente, 1986; DiClemente and Prochaska, 1985; DiClemente et al., 1985; Prochaska et al., 1988). In recent research, a preparation stage is added, in which smokers are getting ready to take action (Prochaska et al., 1992).

The project differs from the larger studies in this volume, in that it was mounted to test several hypotheses about health professionals' advice. The authors predict that advice to quit has different effects on progress toward quitting, depending on the participants' level of health risk attributable to smoking and the way in which each smoker interprets risks and benefits. The level of risk is varied through comparison of smokers at high risk of bladder cancer because of occupational exposure with other smokers residing in the same area who are at relatively low risk. The interpretation of the risks and benefits is varied through different types of counseling for smokers, one of which is aimed at increasing self-efficacy, that is, improving the smokers' perceptions that they are capable of quitting.

Hypothesis 1 The investigators predict that a medical professional's advice will, on average, lead to greater progress toward cessation among high-risk smokers than among smokers at lower risk. Health messages that imply greater danger are generally more effective in changing behavior and attitudes than messages that do not (Leventhal, 1970; Sutton, 1982). However, when people know they are vulnerable to a health threat, various negative reactions can result (Leventhal and Watts, 1966). The health message may induce feelings of helplessness, anger, and other reactions that impede the adoption of healthful behavior (Leventhal et al., 1980). Such reactions are likely to impede progress through the stages of smoking cessation. Smokers may be less likely to seek out new information on quitting or to take actions to quit. People perceive themselves to be vulnerable to cancer and other smoking-related diseases for many reasons. A secondary goal of this project is to discover whether any negative effects of medical advice emerge, especially for smokers at higher risk, and how those might be avoided.

High-risk smokers are more likely than others to feel vulnerable to disease. Although high-risk smokers are more likely than others to quit after receiving medical advice, most of them do not do so (Burt et al., 1974; Pechacek, 1979; Pederson, 1982; Rose and Hamilton, 1978). Some of them may be defeated by barriers such as nicotine addiction, but others may not even try to quit or think about quitting. The more sensitive measures of progress toward smoking cessation can give us this information.

Hypothesis 2 Second, the investigators predict that, although smokers may not progress all the way to long-term quitting, medical or dental advice to quit will move them along in the process. Medical advice can move smokers from precontemplation to contemplation of quitting by encouraging a reevaluation of personal health risks and benefits of quitting. If high-risk smokers start to contemplate quitting, the perceived benefits of quitting will be greater than those for smokers at lower risk, and therefore high-risk smokers are more likely to decide to quit.

Medical advice can also assist in moving the smoker from contemplation to action by providing a rationale or motivation to act (Rogers, 1975). If high-risk smokers have reached the stage of action, they have greater motivation and a stronger rationale for quitting (Leventhal et al., 1980; Rogers, 1975; Sutton, 1982).

Setting a quit date and providing nicotine gum give the smoker cues to action (Eraker et al., 1985). Whether the smoker quits for the long term or relapses depends less on medical advice, as such, and more on factors such as the development of coping skills (Shiffman, 1985) and overcoming nicotine addiction (Fagerstrom, 1982). In the medical and dental practice settings, advice to quit can be followed by counseling on these factors.

Hypothesis 3 Third, the investigators predict that smokers who receive self-efficacy counseling will make greater progress toward cessation than those who do not receive such counseling. The latest generation of medical advice protocols often includes efforts to increase self-efficacy (e.g., Janz et al., 1987). Self-efficacy has been found to be an important predictor of lifestyle changes in general (Bandura, 1990b) and of smoking cessation in particular (DiClemente, 1986; Prochaska et al., 1985). Most important, research has revealed that it is possible to instill greater perceived self-efficacy through counseling in a variety of settings (Bandura, 1990a and 1990b; Gilchrist and Schinke, 1983; Maddux and Stanley, 1986).

TARGET AUDIENCE

The study is being conducted in a 50-mile radius around Lock Haven, Pennsylvania, a community of approximately 12,000 people in the Allegheny Mountains of rural north central Pennsylvania. Two groups participated: former chemical workers at high risk of bladder cancer and similar smokers, resident in the same area, who are at lower risk of bladder cancer. The former chemical workers participate in a program sponsored jointly by the National Institute on Occupational Safety and Health, the Agency for Toxic Substances and Disease Registry, and the Pennsylvania Department of Health. The plant at which these workers were exposed began operation in 1944 and went bankrupt in 1981. The workers come to the Lock Haven Hospital for screening at least once per year, more often if screening reveals a suspicious or positive result. As of this writing, 82 percent of the living cohort members have enrolled in screening and more than 90 percent have returned for repeat screening (Marsh et al., 1991).

The workers were exposed to beta-naphthylamine (BNA), one of the most powerful chemical carcinogens. The resulting increased risk of bladder cancer, which persists for many years after exposure, ranges up to 87 times the risk in the general population (Case et al., 1954; Schulte et al., 1985). Preliminary evidence suggests that smoking and BNA exposure have a multiplicative effect on risk (Schulte et al., 1985). Quitting smoking would presumably lower future risk for developing bladder cancer, regardless of the relation to BNA.

More than 80 percent of the former workers still reside within a 50-mile radius of Lock Haven. Of these, 48 percent are current smokers, and 68 percent have a high school education or less. The majority are blue-collar workers and have lived in rural communities most of their lives. As with the rest of the community, they generally have little interest in quitting smoking.

The project recruited smokers at lower risk who were similar in background to the worker cohort members through visits to 14 blue-collar worksites. The coordinator of the screening program approached the worksites and convinced management to offer the intervention on site. Workers signed up for appointments on specific days.

SETTING OF THE STUDY

Medical advice and counseling components were provided in two settings: at a small hospital in Lock Haven and at 14 worksites in the same general area. The hospital is the setting for the bladder cancer screening program for the former chemical workers. Worksites at which lower risk smokers were recruited included roadwork and home construction sites and a variety of factories and mills. The entire team, including the medical professional, clinic coordinator, interviewer, and counselor, visited the sites on given days. Intervention took place in areas set aside for that purpose, and workers signed up for prearranged times to receive advice and counseling.

Medical advice was provided by three physicians and one respiratory therapist. Their participation was based on their availability at the time of the participants' appointments. A respiratory therapist was included to increase the investigators' flexibility in implementing the study, and because her expertise in smoking-related disease carried some professional authority that was somewhat similar to that of the physicians. An important element for the analysis of outcomes will be to compare participants who received advice from physicians with those who received advice from the respiratory therapist, to examine whether professional identification made a difference.

Counselors included an elementary school teacher trained in the American Lung Association's smoking cessation program, a social worker, and four psychology students from the nearby college. In this rural area, professional cessation counselors were not available; however, all counselors participating in the study were carefully trained and supervised by an experienced smoking cessation counselor. We believe that the diversity of counselors is a strength of the counseling intervention. If individuals with minimal experience can be trained to administer self-efficacy intervention, the method is more easily transportable to medical settings in the community.

Training of the counselors was done in several stages. The supervisor conducted all training from his base in Pittsburgh during the course of five visits to Lock Haven. The initial orientation to the counseling sessions was geared to changing the counselors' mindset about counseling. All of the counselors had been taught that counseling meant giving an individual whatever he or she needed to assist the process. However, it was necessary to make the distinction between such counseling and adherence to a research protocol based on certain prescribed methods—in this case, a focus on enhancing self-efficacy, or an attention placebo. The trainer pointed out to counselors that departures from the self-efficacy material would actually dilute the expected effects of intervention.

The concept of self-efficacy was presented to the counselors and discussed at length. They were introduced to the sequence of steps in the counseling session (see below). Finally, the trainer and counselors role-played the various counseling protocols. They role-played both the counselor and the smoker being counseled.

Counselors then practiced the self-efficacy intervention on friends who smoked, and they tape-recorded the sessions. The tapes were then mailed to the trainer and were brought into the next training session for group supervision and feedback. When the trainer and the counselors were confident that they had mastered the counseling method, each trainee counseled a pilot participant, and the sessions were videotaped. The group of counselors then critiqued the videotapes, together with the supervisor.

When they were judged to be proficient in the counseling protocols, the trainees began counseling the study participants. Each session was tape-recorded and mailed to Pittsburgh. The supervisor monitored the recordings to guard against departures from the protocol. When necessary, the supervisor telephoned the counselors to point out departures from the protocol or to point to missed opportunities to reinforce participants' feelings of self-efficacy.

RECRUITMENT PROCEDURE AND RESULTS

From the start, the project team was aware of the difficulty of generating interest in smoking cessation among little-educated, rural, blue-collar workers. Recruitment yielded 255 current smokers, short of the project's goal of 300. Participants were 75.1 percent men and 24.9 percent women. The mean age of participants was 42 years, and mean of education was 12.7 years. Married participants constituted 74.5 percent of the sample.

For the former chemical workers (higher risk smokers), medical advice and counseling were to be given at the time of their screening for bladder cancer. However, many were not interested in hearing what a medical professional had to say about smoking. Although the coordinator of the bladder cancer screening program had developed good relationships with the workers and had successfully recruited them into bladder cancer screening, her efforts to recruit them into a smoking cessation intervention were less successful. We projected that 108 of the workers residing in the area would take part; of these, 43 men participated in the smoking intervention. At various worksites we recruited 5 additional men who had been exposed to BNA at another nearby plant, accruing a total of 48 smokers at higher risk of bladder cancer. The remaining 207 participants, or 81.6 percent, were smokers at lower risk of bladder cancer than the chemical workers.

There may be several explanations for the meager participation among the worker cohort. To be in the study, workers had to sign a separate consent form, which provided them with an opportunity to say no to the project. Although the screening program gets good participation, it still requires effort from the screening coordinator to cajole the workers into getting their repeat screenings. In many cases, the screening coordinator was fairly sure she would lose a worker from the screening program if she pushed too hard for the smoking program.

This project was less successful in recruiting precontemplators than in recruiting smokers at the stages of contemplation or action. Because precontemplators do not choose to expose themselves to information about the dangers of smoking and benefits of quitting—for example, to listen to what a medical professional has to say—it is likely that they would refuse to participate. A higher percentage of precontemplators might be encountered in usual medical and dental practice settings because all smokers visiting the setting can be exposed to such advice, whether or not they choose to participate in a study. The dentist or physician has a foot in the door already.

In surveys of the general population, a fairly large percentage of smokers are at the stage of precontemplation. Prochaska and colleagues found that, across studies and populations, 50 to 60 percent of smokers are precontemplators, 30 to 40 percent are contemplators, and only 10 to 15 percent are ready to quit (Prochaska et al., 1992). There is no reason to believe that Lock Haven smokers differ much from the national trend, and some reason to believe that a higher percentage are precontemplators, because of local norms and a high smoking prevalence. Nevertheless, only 43 of the participants, or 16 percent, were precontemplators; that is, they reported that they had not given any serious thought to quitting smoking (17.3 percent of the high-risk smokers and 15.7 percent of low-risk smokers). Contemplators were defined as those who reported that they seriously thought about quitting before the intervention but had not quit for longer than 24 hours during the previous year. They constituted 105, or 39 percent, of the participants (42.0 percent of the high-risk smokers and 38.4 percent of low-risk smokers). The remaining 120 smokers, or 45 percent, had quit for more than 24 hours at some time during the previous year (40.7 percent of high-risk smokers and 45.9 percent of low-risk smokers); that is, they had been short-term quitters and had relapsed recently. Clearly this intervention has attracted primarily the smokers who were thinking about quitting and were seeking help.

A third explanation for the workers' lack of participation relates to the history of their common health problem. Strong political pressure from the workers was necessary to create the bladder cancer screening program (Leviton et al., 1991). In the course of that struggle, some opponents told the chemical workers that they did not deserve a screening program because they contributed to their own problems by smoking. Many former workers still recall this altercation with anger and would resist participating for that reason.

NATURE OF MEDICAL ADVICE GIVEN

The three physicians and the respiratory therapist had received brief training in the use of medical advice to quit smoking. All had seen a training videotape developed by investigators at Stanford University (Cummings et al., 1989a and 1989b). The tape presented examples of physician advice interventions, tailored to the needs of smokers who were at the precontemplation, contemplation, and action stages of quitting. All had access to a flowchart developed by the University of North Carolina's Faculty Development Program, which indicates how to tailor advice to the smoker's stage of change. (See Figure 1 in Chapter 3.) The nature of physician advice was kept deliberately simple. Each element and its role in the study are outlined here.

Personalizing Risks and Benefits

The physician or respiratory therapist was informed in advance of each participant's risk status and readiness to quit smoking. The professional first gave a brief description of the effects of smoking on health and the benefits of quitting. If a participant was identified

Protocol

as a high-risk smoker, the professional added that smoking increased the risk for bladder cancer and that quitting smoking increased the chances of staying healthy.

Comment

One goal of the study was to examine whether advice by a medical professional causes smokers to reassess their own personal risk for health problems. For many years, it has been clear that knowledge alone is not sufficient to induce people to change their behavior (McGuire, 1985). Although smokers may understand in general the risks of smoking and benefits of quitting, they may not yet have come to believe that they run a personal health risk. In contrast to nonsmokers, smokers tend to underestimate the health risks of smoking and to discount their personal risk (Shiffman, 1987).

A medical professional's advice is likely to affect smokers by personalizing the health risks and benefits (Weinstein, 1988). When smokers quit, they often cite health concerns, and these are often precipitated by a specific circumstance, such as having an acute illness or knowing someone who has cancer (Shiffman, 1987). In a similar fashion, advice from a medical professional may constitute a precipitating event for the smoker.

Averting Dysfunctional Reactions

Protocol

The medical professionals were urged not to use scare tactics, to avoid any form of fear imagery, and to speak with participants in the same way that they would with their other patients. For higher risk smokers, all members of the project team checked for anxious or fearful reactions that could affect participants' ability to use the counseling that followed. The study coordinator was careful to ask about anxiety in a followup phone call within 48 hours. If individuals expressed anxiety, the study coordinator was to spend time with them to discuss the meaning of the information that the physician and counselor had given.

Comment

The high-risk smokers in the study are not similar to the kind of patient that may walk into any office practice. They are vulnerable to disease because of exposure to a potent chemical carcinogen. They may be especially likely to experience dysfunctional reactions as a result of receiving information about their risk. Each of the dysfunctional reactions could impede progress toward smoking cessation. A helpless reaction is especially likely if smokers perceive quitting as too difficult or if they take a fatalistic attitude toward their risk for disease (Peterson and Seligman, 1984). Also, smokers could avoid thinking about the risk information, as they have done when faced with other bad news about health (Folkman and Lazarus, 1980). Smokers do avoid information on the dangers of smoking (Brock and Balloun, 1967), and those who quit and then relapse into smoking discount their personal risk of health problems (Gibbons et al., 1991). Finally, some smokers may respond by coping with emotions rather than problem-solving or planning to eliminate the feared consequence (Leventhal, 1970). Such reactions may explain smokers' resistance to medical advice. To minimize such reactions, improvements in risk communication are needed.

Making Progress Toward Cessation

Protocol

If smokers were ready to quit, the medical professional set a quit date and indicated that the study coordinator would telephone the participant within 48 hours. If participants were not ready to set a quit date, the medical professionals nevertheless urged them to set a quit date when the study coordinator called in 48 hours.

Finally, the medical professional checked for contraindications for nicotine gum and, if none were found, offered a prescription for the gum (under supervision of a physician), regardless of the participant's readiness to quit. Participants were told that they would see a counselor in a few minutes who would show them how to use the gum.

Comment

As mentioned above, setting a quit date can move the smoker to the stage of action; other smokers are at the preceding stages. Research on the stages of change indicates that there may be a brief window of time in which a person is ready to make a change. If circumstances interfere, the opportunity passes. Moreover, we have no reason to expect that the opportunity will be available for all smokers at the time they receive medical or dental advice to quit. However, providing nicotine gum and other resources to help the smokers quit will help them to follow through, if and when the opportunity occurs.

Recommendations For Advice

Medical and dental professionals should stress the benefits of quitting as well as the risks of smoking; it always helps to emphasize the positive. People interpret health risks in a positive or a negative way, depending on how the issue is framed (Fischoff, 1988; Nisbett and Ross, 1980). The smoker's cup may be described as half full (you can prevent illness by quitting) or half empty (you run a risk of disease by smoking). The medical or dental professional can influence the way the patient interprets risk.

Professionals who provide advice to quit smoking need to distinguish between communication about risks and benefits and communication that arouses fear. The former is positive, because it provides information about a danger that can be avoided through smoking cessation. However, information about a danger may or may not induce the emotional reaction of fear.

The best means of avoiding negative reactions to medical advice is to provide concrete means to overcome or avoid the danger (Leventhal et al., 1980; Rogers and Mewborn, 1976). Giving the smoker increased skills to quit, and confidence to use those skills, will help greatly. Simply providing a prescription for nicotine gum, without a demonstration of its use, is less likely to impart needed skills. Simply referring a patient to counseling resources is even less likely to ensure that the patient will come to possess skills to quit smoking.

Personal contact and continued communication are often found to be essential when communicating with people about increased health risks (Leviton et al., 1991). Misconceptions can be corrected, and anxiety alleviated, through such contact. In the same way, a physician's or dentist's communication about the risks of smoking and benefits of quitting would ideally be followed by contact between the smoker and other staff, who could assess anxiety and alleviate it if needed.

NATURE OF COUNSELING INTERVENTION

The counseling intervention consisted of three components: (1) instruction on the use of nicotine gum (if the participant was interested in the gum); (2) use of a self-efficacy intervention, an attention placebo, or no special counseling; and (3) directing participants' attention to self-help materials. After intervention, counselors left the room, permitting participants to independently select self-help materials; choice of these materials (as a behavioral measure of information-seeking) constitutes one of the dependent variables of the study.

Nicotine Gum Demonstration

Protocol

The counselor explained the use of nicotine gum and used ordinary chewing gum to demonstrate, because experience suggests that patients do not generally receive appropriate training in how to use the gum. Participants received a sheet of simple instructions and practiced, again with a piece of regular gum. The counselor rein forced each participant's mastery of using the gum and emphasized that, should the participants decide to quit, they now possessed an important resource to help the process.

Comment

The nicotine gum constitutes a central feature of the intervention, in that it is a tool provided to smokers to assist them in avoiding the dangers of smoking and achieving the benefits of quitting outlined in the medical advice component. A prescription is provided even to those who may not be ready to quit, on the assumption that providing a tool for quitting will hasten the day when they may take action.

Self-Efficacy Counseling

Protocol

The second phase constituted the comparison of self-efficacy intervention, attention placebo, or no special counseling. Participants were randomly assigned to these three conditions, and counselors were blind to the condition to which participants were randomized, up to this point. The self-efficacy intervention and attention placebo occurred in the context of assessing participants' past experience in attempting to quit. These two conditions were identical in terms of counselor questions for the participant and differed only in that the self-efficacy counseling gave participants feedback about their ability to quit smoking.

An outline of the self-efficacy counseling is given in Appendix D. Overall, the counselors asked questions about the participants' past experience in quitting and in other behavior changes. They reinforced coping strategies that participants had applied successfully. They reinforced other skills and abilities that could be transferred to the smoking cessation task. They pointed to barriers the participants mentioned, suggested other strategies the participants might use to overcome those barriers, and emphasized that participants had the ability to use those skills.

Participants were first asked about their most recent attempt to quit and then about their most successful attempt to quit. If the participants had never attempted to quit, they were asked about the last time they had simply coped with not smoking (when it was prohibited or a cigarette was not available). If they had not coped well, they were asked about attempts to change other behaviors related to health.

For each of these experiences, the counselors strongly emphasized the participants' success in refraining from smoking (or otherwise changing behavior). The counselors noted the strategies the participants had used at the time. They then asked participants to identify, in each experience, the barriers that prevented them from quitting for good.

Throughout, the counselors strongly reinforced the fact that participants possessed the coping skills and abilities they needed to quit smoking. These abilities were evidenced by their prior attempts to quit, previous health behavior changes, or experience in refraining from smoking.

Counselors summarized these experiences and reframed them as success experiences, indicating that the participants had the abilities required to quit. The counselors then summarized the barriers to quitting that smokers had identified as situations that would make it difficult to resist smoking. The counselor then turned to pamphlets that addressed those barriers (see below).

Comment

Smokers may have reason to doubt their ability to quit when they are offered medical advice. The quitting situation may not be familiar, and self-efficacy is relatively low under these conditions (Bandura, 1977 and 1986). In addition, smokers may have tried to quit smoking in the past and perceive their relapse as a failure caused by lack of ability. Finally, a medical profes-sional's information about the dangers of smoking may cause some fear or alarm. Emotional arousal contributes to doubts about self-efficacy (Maddux and Stanley, 1986).

Fortunately, self-efficacy perceptions can be changed. People can be persuaded that they have the ability to change health-related behaviors, and this does encourage them to change (Maddux and Rogers, 1983). People who provide models of effective behavior (all those smokers who needed several attempts to quit) can also instill greater self-efficacy and enhance behavior change (Bandura, 1990b; Gilchrist and Schinke, 1983). Personal experience of success also enhances self-efficacy, and skills training to maintain cessation increases the likelihood that personal efforts will meet with success (Maddux and Stanley, 1986). Reframing the prior attempts to quit as successes, rather than failures, will work as long as the smokers are directed to overcoming the barriers that caused them to relapse.

Self-Help Materials

Protocol

In the third phase, counselors directed participants' attention to self-help materials. Some of the self-help materials were of a general nature, including both American Lung Association and American Cancer Society self-help books. In addition, however, there were eight pamphlets that focused directly on the barriers participants were likely to identify: urges and temptations; withdrawal symptoms; stress; crisis situations; family members, friends, and coworkers who smoke; weight gain; social situations; and boredom.

Comment

The pamphlets on barriers related directly to the situations that had prevented participants from quitting in the past. Participants' self-efficacy in quitting smoking should be directly enhanced by knowledge that skills are available to help them succeed (Maddux and Stanley, 1986). Taking and reading the relevant pamphlets can set the stage for further contemplation or for action to quit smoking.

Self-Efficacy Counsel

Appendix E is a transcript from a self-efficacy counseling session, which is used to give practitioners a feeling for the types of information that smokers provide and the kinds of feedback that counselors give to reinforce self-efficacy. In practice, it is preceded by training in the use of nicotine gum and followed by access to self-help materials specifically focused on barriers to quitting that the patients identify. The transcript also affords a glimpse of the kinds of participants seen in this study.

Recommendations For Counseling

In the context of medical advice, counseling by other staff can follow on the actual communication about health risks and benefits of quitting. When smokers doubt their ability to quit smoking, they may not try. Yet their own experience provides the raw material for changing perceptions. Smokers tend to view relapses as failures, reflecting their inability to quit. Counseling can help them to view relapses as learning experiences, which can help them to refrain from smoking on their next try.

Letting smokers know that other people require more than one try at quitting helps to reinforce this message. Identifying the barriers to quitting helps smokers to take a problem-solving approach and points the way to skills they will require to succeed in quitting for good.

WHAT DID NOT WORK AND WHY

A major disappointment in this study was the failure to recruit a larger proportion of the smokers who were at increased risk of bladder cancer because of their smoking. It is notable that the screening coordinator, so trusted and liked by cohort members, simply could not get them to take part. A very large proportion of the cohort was likely to be smokers at the precontemplation stage of quitting. It is unlikely that they would be more favorable to advice to quit, even if they received the advice from their own physicians. Low education and the local norms in favor of smoking may offer explanations for their resistance to hearing medical advice.

We have observed this problem at an anecdotal level in two other worker cohorts: another group at risk of bladder cancer and a cohort exposed to asbestos. Both groups were blue-collar or low-income groups; both had been subject to accusations that they contributed to their health problems more by smoking than by their occupational exposure.

However, participation in smoking cessation among work-exposed groups does not have to be low. Li and colleagues screened 1,231 smokers who worked at a Navy shipyard and who had been exposed to asbestos (Li et al., 1984). Eighty-seven percent of the smokers agreed to participate in a minimal smoking intervention, and 84 percent of eligible candidates did take part. However, the investigators had secured a consent to participate at the time of the first medical screening, and the intervention took place 1 month later, at the time the smokers received their test results. It may be that the combination of events was sufficient to motivate a large percentage of smokers in this context. Clearly, the workers had an incentive both to find out all they could at the time of initial screening and to return for their test results and the smoking intervention. By contrast, in the examples studied by these authors, smoking cessation is provided as a later service, after a health surveillance program has been in place for some time and the workers have a fairly good idea of their state of health. The authors also conclude that recruitment of such workers into smoking cessation must be a major intermediate outcome and that careful planning and design are imperative to carry it out.

Generally, the training and supervision of the counselors was successful. The continued feedback on tape-recorded sessions was an important feature, however. The recruitment of participants occurred in fits and starts, and therefore counselors did not have routine, consistent experience in delivering the self-efficacy intervention. The most common problem was that they occasionally missed key things that the participants said that provided opportunities to reinforce a feeling of self-efficacy. The authors suggest that supervision be continual, that monitoring of samples of counseling sessions be continued, and that feedback to counselors be given promptly.

WHAT WORKED AND WHY

This study is at the preliminary stage of analysis. While some hypotheses may not be supported, a key finding is the quit rate of 22.7 percent at 1 year. However, experience in implementing the study leads the authors to suggest improvements for smoking interventions in medical and dental settings. First, health risks and benefits were communicated effectively, even for those patients who are at increased risk of bladder cancer because of conditions other than smoking. Enhancing self-efficacy is apparently a useful way to guard against misinterpretation of the advice and dysfunctional reactions to it. Only one high-risk smoker in this study displayed a negative emotional reaction to the information. The study coordinator worked with the subject in person and by telephone until she was satisfied that he correctly understood the risk and benefit information and was no longer acutely anxious about the role of smoking in his risk for contracting bladder cancer.

It might be argued that the precontemplators, who did not take part in great numbers, may well be anxious about the role of smoking in their risk for bladder cancer. For this reason, they avoided exposure to the information that the physician had to provide. It will be interesting to examine the interview responses of the precontemplators who did participate in the study, to find whether they were more anxious or fearful about the risk information than were other participants.

This study is pertinent to the issue of whether more extended counseling to quit smoking can feasibly be delegated to other staff members in the physician's office. The authors' experience indicates that it is feasible to train people to administer a self-efficacy intervention, even if they possess little prior counseling experience. Continuing supervision and training for this purpose is needed, however, as the quality of counseling was found to be uneven. The counseling protocol was adaptable to 14 work settings as well as the hospital setting. These are important conclusions, because availability of experienced counselors is likely to vary greatly among medical and dental practice settings.

REFERENCES

Bandura, A. Perceived self-efficacy in controlling AIDS. *Evaluation and Program Planning* 13: 9-17, 1990a.

Bandura, A. Self-efficacy mechanism in human agency. *American Psychologist* 40: 359-373, 1986.

Bandura, A. Self-efficacy mechanism in physiological activation and health-promoting behavior. In: *Adaptation, Learning and Affect*, J. Madden IV, S. Matthysse, and J. Barchas (Editors). New York: Raven Press, 1990b.

Bandura, A. Self-efficacy: Toward a unifying theory of behavioral change. *Psychological Review* 84: 191-215, 1977.

Brock, T.C., Balloun, J.L. Behavioral receptivity to dissonant information. *Journal of Personality and Social Psychology* 6: 413-428, 1967.

Burt, A., Thornley, P., Illingworth, D., White, P., Shaw, T.R.D., Turner, R. Stopping smoking after myocardial infarction. *Lancet* 1(7852): 304-306, 1974.

Case, R.A.M., Hosher, M.E., MacDonald, D.B., Pearson, J.T. Tumors of the urinary bladder in workmen engaged in the manufacture and use of certain dyestuff intermediaries in the British chemical industry: Part 1. *British Journal of Industrial Medicine* 11: 75-104, 1954.

Cummings, S.R., Coates, T.J., Richard, R.J., Hansen, B., Zahnd, E.G., Vander Martin, R., Duncan, C., Gerbert, B., Martin, A., Stein, M.J. Training physicians in counseling about smoking cessation: A randomized trial of the "Quit for Life" program. *Annals of Internal Medicine* 110(8): 640-647, 1989a.

Cummings, S.R., Richard, R.J., Duncan, C.L., Hansen, B., Vander Martin, R., Gerbert, B., Coates, T.J. Training physicians about smoking cessation: A controlled trial in private practice. *Journal of General Internal Medicine* 4(6): 482-489, 1989b.

DiClemente, C.C. Self-efficacy and the addictive behaviors. *Journal of Social and Clinical Psychology* 4: 302-315, 1986.

DiClemente, C.C., Prochaska, J.O. Processes and stages of self-change: Coping and competence in smoking behavior change. In: *Coping and Substance Abuse*, S. Shiffman and T.A. Wills (Editors). San Diego, CA: Academic Press, 1985.

DiClemente, C.C., Prochaska, J.O., Gibertini, M. Self-efficacy and the stages of self-change of smoking. *Cognitive Therapy and Research* 9: 181-200, 1985.

Eraker, S.A., Becker, M.H., Strecher, V.J., Kirscht, J.P. Smoking behavior cessation techniques and the Health Decision Model. *American Journal of Medicine* 78: 817-825, 1985.

Evans, R.I. What can social psychology contribute to increase the probability of adherence of behavior change through patient-physician communication? In: *Education of the Patient With Cardiac Disease in the Twenty-First Century*, N. Wenger (Editor). New York: LeJacq, 1986.

Fagerstrom, K.O. A comparison of psychological and pharmacological treatment in smoking cessation. *Journal of Behavioral Medicine* 5: 343-351, 1982.

Fischoff, B. Decisionmaking on AIDS. Invited paper presented at the Vermont Conference on Primary Prevention, Burlington, Vermont, September 1988.

Folkman, S., Lazarus, R.S. An analysis of coping in a middle-aged community sample. *Journal of Health and Social Behavior* 21: 219-239, 1980.

Gibbons, F.X., McGovern, P.G., Lando, H.A. Relapse and risk perception among members of a smoking cessation clinic. *Health Psychology* 10: 42-45, 1991.

Gilchrist, L.D., Schinke, S.P. Coping with contraception: Cognitive and behavioral methods with adolescents. *Cognitive Therapy and Research* 7: 379-388, 1983.

Horn, D. A model for the study of personal choice health behavior. *International Journal of Health Education* 19: 89-98, 1976.

Janz, N.K., Becker, M.H., Kirscht, J.P., Eraker, S.A., Billi, J.E., Wolliscroft, J.O. Evaluation of a minimal-contact smoking cessation intervention in an outpatient setting. *American Journal of Public Health* 77(7): 805-809, 1987.

Leventhal, H. Findings and theory in the study of fear communications. In: *Advances in Experimental Social Psychology* (volume 5), L. Berkowitz (Editor). New York: Academic Press, 1970.

Leventhal, H., Cleary, P.D. The smoking problem: A review of research and theory in behavioral risk modification. *Psychological Bulletin* 88: 370-405, 1980.

Leventhal, H., Meyer, D., Gutmann, M. The role of theory in the study of compliance to high blood pressure regimens. In: *Patient Compliance to Prescribed Antihypertensive Medication Regimens: A Report to the National Heart, Lung, and Blood Institute*, R.B. Haynes, M.E. Mattson, and O.E. Tillmer (Editors). U.S. Department of Health and Human Services, Public Health Service, National Institutes of Health. NIH Publication No. 81-2102, 1980.

Leventhal, H., Watts, J. Sources of resistance to fear-arousing communications on smoking and lung cancer. *Journal of Personality* 34: 155-175, 1966.

Leviton, L.C., Marsh, G.M., Talbott, E.O., Pavlock, D., Callahan, C. Drake Chemical Workers' Health Registry: Coping with community tension over toxic exposures. *American Journal of Public Health* 81: 689-693, 1991.

Li, V.C., Kim, Y.J., Ewart, C.K., Terry, P.B., Cuthie, J.C., Wood, J., Emmet, E.A., Permutt, S. Effects of physician counseling on the smoking behavior of asbestos-exposed workers. *Preventive Medicine* 13: 462-476, 1984.

Maddux, J.E., Rogers, R.W. Protection motivation and self-efficacy: A revised theory of fear appeals and attitude change. *Journal of Experimental Social Psychology* 19: 469-479, 1983.

Maddux, J.E., Stanley, M.A. Self-efficacy theory in contemporary psychology: An overview. *Journal of Social and Clinical Psychology* 4: 249-255, 1986.

Marsh, G.M., Leviton, L.C., Talbott, E.O., Callahan, C., Pavlock, D., Hemstreet, G., Logue, J.N., Fox, J., Schulte, P., Drake Chemical Workers' Health Registry Study: I. Notification and medical surveillance of a group of workers at high risk of developing bladder cancer. *American Journal of Industrial Medicine* 19: 291-301, 1991.

McGuire, W.J. Attitudes and attitude change. In: *Handbook of Social Psychology* (3rd edition), G. Lindzey and E. Aronson (Editors). New York: Random House, 1985.

Nisbett, R., Ross, L. *Human Inference: Strategies and Shortcomings of Social Judgment.* Englewood Cliffs, NJ: Prentice-Hall, 1980.

Pechacek, T.F. Modification of smoking behavior. In: *The Behavioral Aspects of Smoking* (NIDA Research Monograph 26), N.A. Krasnegor (Editor). U.S. Department of Health, Education, and Welfare; Public Health Service; Alcohol, Drug Abuse, and Mental Health Administration; National Institute on Drug Abuse. DHEW Publication No. ADM 79-882, 1979.

Pechacek, T.F., Danaher, B.G. How and why people quit smoking. In: *Cognitive-Behavioral Interventions: Theory, Research and Procedures,* P.C. Kendall and S.D. Hollon (Editors). New York: Academic Press, 1979.

Pederson, L.L. Compliance with physician advice to quit smoking: A review of the literature. *Preventive Medicine* 11: 71-84, 1982.

Peterson, C., Seligman, M.E.P. Causal explanations as a risk factor for depression: Theory and evidence. *Psychological Review* 91: 347-374, 1984.

Prochaska, J.O., DiClemente, C.C., Norcross, J.C. In search of how people change: Applications to addictive behaviors. *American Psychologist* 47: 1102-1114, 1992.

Prochaska, J.O., DiClemente, C.C., Velicer, W.F., Ginpil, S., Norcross, J.C. Predicting change in smoking status for self-changers. *Addictive Behaviors* 10: 395-406, 1985.

Prochaska, J.O., Velicer, W.F., DiClemente, C.C., Fava, J. Measuring processes of change: Applications to the cessation of smoking. *Journal of Consulting and Clinical Psychology* 56: 520-528, 1988.

Rogers, R.W. A protection motivation theory of fear appeals and attitude change. *Journal of Psychology* 191: 93-114, 1975.

Rogers, R.W., Mewborn, C.R. Fear appeals and attitude change: Effects of a threat's noxiousness, probability of occurrence, and the efficacy of coping responses. *Journal of Personality and Social Psychology* 34: 562-566, 1976.

Rose, G., Hamilton, P.J.S. A randomized controlled trial of the effect on middle-aged men of advice to stop smoking. *Journal of Epidemiology and Community Health* 32: 275-281, 1978.

Schulte, P.A., Ringen, K., Hemstreet, G.P. Optimal management of asymptomatic workers at high risk of bladder cancer. *Journal of Occupational Medicine* 28: 13-17, 1985.

Shiffman, S. Coping with temptations to smoke. In: *Coping and Substance Abuse*, S. Shiffman and T.A. Wills (Editors). New York: Academic Press, 1985.

Shiffman, S. Psychosocial factors in smoking and quitting: Health beliefs, self-efficacy, and stress. In: *The Pharmacological Treatment of Nicotine Dependence*, J.K. Ockene (Editor). Cambridge, MA: Harvard University Press, 1987.

Sutton, S.R. Fear-arousing communications: A critical examination of theory and research. In: *Social Psychology and Behavioral Medicine*, J.R. Eiser (Editor). New York: John Wiley, 1982.

Weinstein, N.D. The precaution adoption process. *Health Psychology* 7: 355-386, 1988.

APPENDIX A
Smoking Materials for Pediatricians

American Cancer Society. *Special Delivery Smoke Free: Stop Smoking Book.* American Cancer Society, 1988. 88-1C-No. 2422.01LE.

Strecher, V.J. *A Healthy Beginning: The Smoke-Free Family Guide for New Parents.* American Lung Association and American Academy of Pediatrics, 1988.

Strecher, V.J., Rimer, B. *Freedom From Smoking for You and Your Family.* American Lung Association, 1987.

APPENDIX B
Algorithms for Delivery of Smoking Cessation Advice

Part 1
Contents of initial advice—usual care patient

1. Provide information concerning the *risks* of continuing to smoke and benefits of cessation—smoking increases probability of recurrence, second primary cancers, delayed and compromised healing, more illness of other types.
2. Deliver strong advice to stop smoking or stay off cigarettes.

Part 2
Contents of initial advice—current smoker, experimental patient

1. Review smoking history.
2. Provide information concerning the risks of continuing to smoke and *benefits* of cessation—quitting decreases risk of recurrence, second primary cancers, more illnesses of other types, and promotes healing.
3. Identify patient's receptivity to smoking cessation.
4. Deliver strong advice to stop smoking.
5. State confidence in patient's ability to stop smoking.
6. Provide self-help booklets on stopping smoking and maintaining abstinence.
7. Provide booklet to spouse/other person providing care on social support for the patient stopping smoking.
8. Mention withdrawal symptoms and craving for cigarettes.

9 A. If [patient is] willing to quit, set target quit date and obtain patient's signature on smoking cessation contract.

9 B. If [patient is] unwilling to quit, suggest reduced consumption.

10. State continuing support and reassurance that you are available during followup visits to help patient in effort to stay off cigarettes.

Part 3
Contents of initial advice—former smoker, experimental patient

1. Review smoking history—quit date.
2. Provide information concerning the risks of continuing to smoke and *benefits* of cessation—quitting decreases risk of recurrence, second primary cancers, more illnesses of other types, and promotes healing.

3. State confidence in patient's ability to stay quit.
4. Provide self-help booklets on stopping smoking and maintaining abstinence.
5. Provide booklet to spouse/other person providing care on support for the patient in remaining abstinent.
6. Ask about problems—refer to booklets.
7. Obtain patient's signature on staying-quit contract.
8. State continuing support and reassurance that you are available during followup visits to help patient in effort to stay off cigarettes.

Part 4
Booster session—experimental patients:
Problem-solving guide, abstainers and slippers

1. How long has patient been off cigarettes?
2. Ask about problems—has patient slipped or is patient currently having any problems staying quit?
3. YES — What are their problems (debrief)?
   A. Withdrawal—discuss duration of symptoms and craving.
   B. Mention abstinence violation effect (AVE): accepting slips as normal occurrence triggered by "high-risk" situation; explain that person feels like a failure after slip and gives up entirely (relapses) instead of continuing to cope; person expects cigarette to be a "reward."
   C. Discuss avoiding relapse situations/triggers.

   NO — (Go to #4)
4. State confidence in patient's ability to stay quit.
5. Remind patient to refer to booklets on staying quit and social support for questions regarding effective maintenance of abstinence.
6. State your continuing support and reassurance that you are available during followup visits to help patient in effort to stay off cigarettes.

Part 5
Booster session—experimental patients:
Problem-solving guide, new relapsers (since last visit)

1. How long was patient quit and when did he/she go back to smoking?

2. Review circumstances of relapse situation and acknowledge difficulty.

3. Determine patient's willingness to stop smoking again.

   WILLING (Go to #6) UNWILLING (Go to #4)

4. Ask patient to state reasons for unwillingness. Counter arguments. Is patient willing to quit?

   WILLING (Go to #6) UNWILLING (Go to #5)

5. Discuss reducing consumption. (Go to #9)

6. Mention abstinence violation effect (AVE), accepting slips as normal occurrence triggered by "high-risk" situation; explain that person feels like a failure after slip and gives up entirely (relapses) instead of continuing to cope; person expects cigarette to be "reward."

7. Provide guidelines for effective cessation and long-term abstinence:

   A. Refer to self-help booklets and social support booklet.

   B. Discuss need for more intensive methods/aids such as referral to smoking cessation clinic or prescription for nicotine replacement pharmacotherapy. If requested, provide referral and/or Rx.

8. Obtain patient's commitment to stop smoking. Set new target quit date and sign new contract. Express confidence in patient's ability to stop smoking.

9. State your continuing support and reassurance that you are available during followup visits to help patient in effort to stop smoking cigarettes.

Part 6
Booster session—experimental patients:
Problem-solving guide, reduced-consumption and full-consumption smokers

1. Has patient cut down at all on smoking (number of cigarettes, tar and nicotine content of brand)?

   YES (REDUCED CONSUMPTION) NO (FULL CONSUMPTION) (Go to #3)

2. Review techniques used by patient to reduce smoking.
3. Review benefits of quitting/risks of continuing to smoke.
4. Determine patient's willingness to stop smoking completely.

   WILLING (Go to #7) UNWILLING (Go to #5)

5. Ask patient to state reasons for unwillingness. Counter arguments. Is patient willing to quit?

   WILLING (Go to #7) UNWILLING (Go to #6)

6. Suggest reduced consumption. (Go to #9)
7. Provide guidelines for effective quitting methods.
   A. Refer patient to self-help and social support booklets.
   B. Discuss need for more intense methods/aids such as referral to smoking cessation clinic or prescription for nicotine replacement pharmacotherapy. If requested, provide referral and/or Rx.
8. Obtain patient's commitment to stop smoking. Set new target quit date and sign new contract. Express confidence in patient's ability to quit.
9. State your continuing support and reassurance that you are available during followup visits to help patient in effort to stop smoking cigarettes.

APPENDIX C
Protocol Developed by University of North Carolina Faculty Development Program

1: Prescribing Nicotine Gum

RATIONALE: Nicotine gum supplies nicotine (the possible basis of addiction) without carbon monoxide or carcinogenic tars. Nicotine from gum is released slowly (if gum is chewed slowly) without sharp nicotine boli produced through cigarette smoking.

GUIDELINES FOR USE OF GUM:

- Quit smoking before using gum.
- Chew gum slowly (about one chew for every normal puff interval), keeping taste and tingle at minimal level.
- Use for craving, about 10 to 15 pieces per day.
- Taper from gum and stop using gum after 3 months (withdrawal from gum has been difficult for some patients).

2-4: Obstacles to Quitting

2. FEAR OF WEIGHT GAIN:
   - Two-thirds of quitters gain weight; only one-third gain weight and keep a significant amount of weight.
   - Weight gain can be prevented by a modest diet and exercise.
   - Patient may crave sweets; warn about this.
   - Compulsive eating may suggest nicotine withdrawal; patient may respond to nicotine gum.
3. FAILED IN PRIOR ATTEMPTS TO QUIT:
   - Most successful quitters require several tries.
   - Circumstances of relapse should be studied to prepare for next try.
4. NERVOUSNESS:
   - May be a sign of nicotine withdrawal (see #1).
   - Tranquilizers are not effective in breaking smoking habit.

RELAPSE

Indicate that most successful quitters required several tries; many people need to LEARN HOW TO QUIT.

Analyze relapse experience ("When and where did you smoke your cigarette?"). Have smoker develop strategy for coping with that experience.

Recycle smoker into new quit date and schedule followup.

APPENDIX D
Self-Efficacy Intervention
(preceded by nicotine gum demonstration)

1. Most folks are surprised to learn that it often takes three or more tries before a smoker finally quits for good. Have you tried to quit smoking?

   IF NO, GO TO 1-C IF YES, CONTINUE TO 1-A

1-A. Think about the most recent time you tried to quit smoking. How long were you able to stay off cigarettes this last time?

EMPHASIZE SUCCESS

What did you do when you had the urge to smoke but didn't?

RECORD EFFICACY INDICATORS ON LAST PAGE
AND
REINFORCE SELF-EFFICACY

What happened that got you started again?

RECORD BARRIERS ON LAST PAGE

1-B. Think about your most successful try at quitting smoking. How long were you able to stay off cigarettes that time?

EMPHASIZE SUCCESS

What did you do when you had the urge to smoke but didn't?

RECORD EFFICACY INDICATORS ON LAST PAGE
AND
REINFORCE SELF-EFFICACY

What happened that got you started again?

RECORD BARRIERS ON LAST PAGE

IF GOOD DATA ARE RETRIEVED, GO TO 1-D; IF NOT, CONTINUE

1-C. Think about a time when you really craved a cigarette, but decided not to have one. What happened?

RECORD EFFICACY INDICATORS ON LAST PAGE
AND
REINFORCE SELF-EFFICACY

Point out that they were successful in handling that craving . . . they have what it takes to control all desires to smoke.

1-D. Review and summarize all EFFICACY INDICATORS for the participant. Reiterate how useful/helpful those qualities/abilities will be when participant tries to quit (again).

1-E. Let's consider some of the things that might be holding you back from quitting now. If you were to quit smoking today, which of these situations would make it really hard for you to resist having a smoke?

CHECK OFF BARRIERS IDENTIFIED:

______ urges/temptations

______ withdrawal symptoms

______ stress

______ crisis situations

______ family member/friend/coworker smokes

______ weight gain

______ social situations

______ boredom, pass time

DIRECT PARTICIPANT TO PAMPHLETS.

APPENDIX E
Transcript From a Self-Efficacy Counseling Session

Counselor: Most people are surprised to learn that it often takes three times or more to finally quit smoking. Have you ever tried to quit?

Patient: When you say three times . . .

Counselor: You may have tried twice before, you know, not necessarily in this program—any time in your life. Have you ever tried to stop smoking?

Patient: Yeah, I tried "cold turkey," and I think the very first time right after dinner, and I might have gone a couple of months. Oh, some crisis or something happened, you know, and, whizzzzt.

Counselor: OK. So, in thinking about that first time you tried to quit, about how long did you stay off the cigarettes at that time?

Patient: I think I was off maybe 6 or 7 weeks, something like that.

Counselor: Oh, that's very good.

Patient: But you know, like I told the doctor, the biggest thing I could do is to change my habits, because every time I get a cup of coffee I get a cigarette.

Counselor: So, what did you do when you had the urge to smoke, but didn't at that time, during those 6 or 7 weeks?

Patient: Boy, I tell you, that's 25 years ago.

Counselor: You say that's 25 years? OK. You don't remember what you did.

Patient: No, I didn't smoke.

Counselor: There wasn't anything you did instead?

Patient: No, I didn't have anything like this or . . .

Counselor: OK, but you still were motivated, and you were coping with that craving at that point.

Patient: Yes, because I had smoked from the time I got out of high school, through the service and everything else.

Counselor: But for 6 or 7 weeks—that's quite a while. You were doing something else, ignoring it or just using self-discipline.

Patient: Yeah, just using, probably more self-discipline than anything else.

Counselor: Well, you did it, you know, and habits, you know, that's what it is, a habit. As you said, you want to change that habit. You said there was just some sort of crisis that happened that caused you to start again.

Patient: Yeah, something probably, if I remember right it's when Jenny's mother fell and broke her leg, and we were running back and forth between the hospital, we had the young one, and one thing probably brought on another.

Counselor: All right. Think about your most successful try at quitting smoking. Was it only that one time that you had tried? Was that the most successful time?

Patient: Yeah, I said to myself many times "I'm going to quit now, stop for a day," or something like that . . .

Counselor: But the 6 to 7 weeks was the most successful time?

Patient: That's the most successful time.

Counselor: And again you just—something motivated you at that point—there was obviously something important enough in your mind that you were thinking that you wanted to quit smoking at that point.

Patient: Probably so, but like I say at this point in time I can't—

Counselor: Can't remember what it was? Well, perhaps you will be able to remember. So, you did the same thing, you don't really remember 25 years ago what you did when you had the urge to smoke. Now the last time when you tried to quit smoking—if you can remember—when you really craved a cigarette, but decided not to have one, what happened?

Patient: You mean like when I quit for a day or so?

Counselor: Even for a day, yes.

Patient: Oh . . ., most of the time it would just be getting a cracker or celery or something.

Counselor: So, you replaced it with something else? So, you realized that you needed to replace it with something else in order to make yourself more comfortable at that time when you were having that craving.

Patient: Right.

Counselor: That's good. Again, you have been successful, you tried about 6 or 7 weeks, and you've done it for a couple days—a day here, a day there?

Patient: Yeah, I was able to do that.

Counselor: So, it does prove that you can do it, if you really want.

Patient: I'm going to use the gum no matter what, anyway.

Counselor: OK, Dennis, we had talked before, it sometimes does take someone three or more times to quit smoking. That's because there's a lot of barriers when you want to quit. There's all kinds of situations, crises, things that just get in the way when you want to quit smoking. What are some of the things that you feel hold you back from quitting smoking? I mean, such as withdrawal symptoms; what are some of the things that hold you back the most? The hardest, toughest times for you to handle.

Patient: Well, like I say, in the morning I always, the first thing, I come down, I have coffee. It's just the idea that you just crave it, you want it, you know, and I think—or as you're saying, a crisis. You got to sit down and do something.

Counselor: Do you feel your stress might be related to that?

Patient: Yeah, sometimes stress would do it, you know, you're having an odd day, a bad day, something doesn't go right, you know, and you say, oh, the heck with it and go over here and have a cigarette. You can just as soon say in reality I'm going to go over here and have a glass of water, you know.

Counselor: You just kind of stop caring.

Patient: It's a crutch.

Counselor: Now remember what I said to you before, that a lot of situations and things can happen that lead us, that stop us from being able to give up smoking. Right over here I have all kinds of helpful information and I'd like you to look at them, help yourself, take as many as you like, anything that's especially helpful for you. Go ahead, help yourself, we have plenty more.

Patient: OK, no problem.

Counselor: This is the same booklet right here. But I really think it sounds to me like you've thought, put it together.

Patient: I guess I know what I want to do.

Counselor: I guess it's just going to take you to make up your mind.

Patient: Yes, make up my mind.

Counselor: Like all of us. I want to thank you, and go ahead help yourself to the brochures.

Chapter 5

Dissemination, Facilitation, and Maintenance of Office-Based Cessation Assistance

CONTENTS

Introduction
David M. Burns 301

Smoking Cessation as a Clinic Quality Improvement Project
Leif I. Solberg 303
Introduction 303
External Intermediary Support 304
Lessons Learned for Future Diffusion 308
The Quality Improvement Paradigm 309
Applying Quality Improvement 310
CQI for Smoking Cessation 311
Conclusion 318
References 319

Computerized Reminder System To Aid Physicians In Assessment and Counseling of Patients Who Smoke
Stephen J. McPhee, Joyce Adair Bird, Don Fordham, Jonathan E. Rodnick, and Emilie H. Osborn 321
Introduction 321
Subjects 321
Description of the Intervention 323
Implementation of the CPRS 326
Analytical Methods 327
Results 328
Discussion 329
Conclusions 332
References 333

Physicians' and Dentists' Roles in COMMIT—
The Community Intervention Trial for Smoking Cessation
Elizabeth A. Lindsay, Judith K. Ockene, Larry Berger,
Norman Hymowitz, Paul Pomrehn, and Douglas M. Wilson 334
Introduction 334
Trial Goals 334
Trial Design and Endpoints 335
Trial Organization and Intervention 336
Goals for Health Care Providers 336
Intervention Protocol 336
Discussion and Conclusions 340
References 341

Dissemination of Physician-Based
Smoking Cessation Interventions
Michael G. Goldstein, Nancy A. MacDonald,
Raymond Niaura, and Catherine Dubé 342
Introduction 342
Diffusion Theory and Application 343
Transtheoretical Model 344
Physicians Counseling Smokers 346
Summary 352
References 353

Clinical Interventions in Tobacco Control:
A National Cancer Institute Training Program
For Health Care Providers
Marc Manley, Roselyn P. Epps,
Robert Mecklenburg, and Corinne Husten 356
Disseminating Interventions 356
Oral Health Team Research 362
Project Evaluation 367
Conclusions 367
References 368

Appendix A. Case Studies 369

Dissemination, Facilitation, And Maintenance of Office-Based Cessation Assistance

Editor: David M. Burns

INTRODUCTION The successful approaches used by health care providers to alter the smoking behavior of patients are presented in the preceding chapters of this monograph. Likewise, the enormous impact that could be achieved if the 70 percent of smokers who see a physician each year and the 60 percent of smokers who see a dentist each year were to receive advice and assistance in quitting is well described. However, the majority of smokers who saw a physician in the past year did not receive advice to quit on their last visit, and one-half of all smokers have never heard from their physician that they should quit. To modify the behavior of physicians and dentists will require the application of the recruitment strategies, motivational approaches, and training methods developed by the investigators responsible for the trials described in the early chapters. It will require also the application of effective methods of disseminating and institutionalizing office-based smoking cessation assistance as part of the systems by which we deliver and receive health care. The process of moving from a research or demonstration project to widespread acceptance of a health promotion/disease prevention program is often the most difficult part of technology transfer in cancer control.

Chapter 5 presents what we know about disseminating and facilitating smoking cessation assistance in medical and dental practice settings. Just as the previous chapters delineate the importance of changing office-based patient flow and information systems to sustain physician compliance in regular counseling, this chapter details the kinds of changes that can be made in systems outside the physician's office that will encourage more physicians to provide regular counseling as well as make their advice more effective. The important questions of how to recruit and train practicing physicians, dentists, and their staffs; how to sustain motivation and meet the ongoing training necessitated by staff and practitioner turnover; and how to use office systems and staff to enhance the effectiveness of clinicians' advice are addressed in this chapter. These issues constitute the groundwork for the successful institutionalization of cessation advice into U.S. medical and dental practices.

The first section, by Solberg, deals with smoking cessation as a clinic quality improvement project and addresses the issues of disseminating and, more important, maintaining smoking cessation assistance in physicians' offices. It uses the rapidly growing quality assurance effort in medical practice to both motivate and institutionalize smoking cessation advice in an office practice. Solberg presents a clear process for introducing smoking counseling into a practice as part of the effort to continually improve the quality of delivered care. Tools for monitoring the success of the effort and for modifying it to improve its effectiveness are described. This approach provides the ongoing feedback needed to sustain the cessation effort as well as the documentation that third party payers need to ensure that the preventive services they have contracted for are being delivered.

In the second section, McPhee and colleagues describe a computerized system for reminding physicians to provide advice, track the success or failure of the advice that is given, and provide the summary data on overall physician behavior that would facilitate the continuous quality improvement process. The linkage between the process and technologic solutions described in these first two papers may well be synergistic in promoting the acceptance of office-based smoking assistance.

Regardless of the approach selected, dissemination of office-based interventions will require recruitment and training of physicians, dentists, and their staffs on a large scale. Three approaches to this problem are presented in this chapter, dealing with communities at three different levels: local, state, and national. Strategies for recruitment and training of health care providers as one component of a comprehensive community-based smoking intervention effort are described by Lindsay and colleagues, through the experiences of the COMMIT trial. Their section describes approaches that can be effective in communities with populations of about 100,000, and that can be incorporated into efforts directed at community mobilization for a comprehensive tobacco control effort. A second approach to physicians, on a statewide basis, described by Goldstein and coworkers, uses professional organizations to recruit physicians and incorporate "academic detailing," whereby skilled individuals visit physician offices to motivate and train physicians and their staffs for providing advice and assistance in smoking cessation. This approach deals with physician-based smoking cessation as a separate project, rather than as a part of a comprehensive tobacco control effort, but identifies realistic methods for using outside resources to help develop and sustain smoking cessation advice in an office practice.

The last dissemination approach, described by Manley and colleagues in the final paper of this chapter, is the National Cancer Institute effort to develop and implement a national training program for health care providers to improve their knowledge and skills for helping patients to quit smoking. The authors present approaches used to develop materials that synthesize what was learned from clinical trials and the strategies used to recruit physicians and dentists to participate in the training. The increasing medicalization of smoking as a health care problem and its acceptance by physicians as a problem they must treat with each patient will lead to smoking intervention being more and more a part of systems for health care delivery.

Smoking Cessation as a Clinic Quality Improvement Project[1]

Leif I. Solberg

INTRODUCTION Numerous studies in a wide variety of medical settings have demonstrated that physician advice to stop using tobacco can be very effective. Individual studies (Cohen et al., 1990; Cummings et al., 1986; Glynn and Manley, 1990; Ockene, 1987) and a meta-analysis of the controlled clinical trials (Kottke et al., 1988) have both demonstrated the characteristics of interventions that lead to the greatest probability of successful quitting among tobacco-using patients who are seeing a physician for care of some other problem. In general, these studies show that medical interventions are most effective when they are

- Provided at nearly every encounter over the longest possible time by both physicians and staff;
- Aimed at those interested in changing their behavior;
- Presented in a clear, supportive, and nonconfrontational manner that concentrates on specific plans, assistance, and followup for quit attempts;
- Supported by various easily available forms of assistance, both behavioral and pharmacological; and
- Followed by positive reinforcement after quitting occurs.

Nearly all physicians agree that tobacco use is a very serious health hazard. However, their patients often do not receive advice that meets the above-mentioned criteria. In addition to the need to focus on the problems that patients bring, there are many other barriers, such as lack of time, reliance on the physician's memory, lack of staff support, and an approach that does not emphasize these criteria. Research on physician behavior suggests that, if this situation is to be changed, organizational changes that support office smoking cessation systems will be necessary (Battista and Mickalide, 1990; Belcher et al., 1988; Inui et al., 1981; Pommerenke and Weed, 1991). These systems must include the following:

- Staff involvement and support;
- Reminders to physicians to intervene during office visits;

[1] Supported in part by National Institutes of Health grant no. R01-CA38361 and by Blue Plus.

- Brevity, so that physicians can provide advice at nearly every visit;
- A variety of assistance for patients who need it; and
- Followup without requiring physician time or memory.

It is clear that, for these actions to occur regularly, systems must be in place that screen and label charts of all patients for tobacco use and that all components of the system are maintained and upgraded regularly.

In addition, it may be necessary to train physicians in the importance of conducting and how to conduct brief discussions of smoking cessation as a part of normal office visits. However, there is reason to believe that little more than a brief orientation may be necessary with proper office system support.

Individual physicians, medical care organizations, and public policy-makers must decide how to initiate and maintain these office systems in primary care settings if we are to gain maximum physician impact. Although there have been some examples of external intermediaries successfully implementing these systems in representative practices, this diffusion has required considerable effort, experience, and resources.

EXTERNAL INTERMEDIARY SUPPORT

After demonstrating the feasibility and value of an office system to accomplish the smoking cessation objectives described above in one clinic (Nokomis) (Solberg et al., 1990), the National Cancer Institute-sponsored Doctors Helping Smokers (DHS) project team decided that the next task was to demonstrate that typical private primary care practices would want to (and could) accomplish the same thing. Because the DHS co-principal investigator was also the Medical Director for Quality Assurance for a health maintenance organization (Blue Plus) that contracted with more than 100 private primary care practices throughout the state of Minnesota, a collaborative relationship was developed between the research project and the HMO.

Eleven of the practices contracting with Blue Plus were selected as the target group (on the basis of location, with no awareness of their interest in either smoking cessation or this project). None of these practices had more than 15 percent of their patients covered by Blue Plus.

These practices were "recruited" by the Medical Director through an introductory letter, which was followed by a phone call and a visit. The practices were told that they were under no obligation to cooperate, but if they were willing, we would teach and help them to implement an office smoking cessation system that had already been demonstrated to be feasible and effective.

All 11 practice groups contacted (representing 29 separate clinics) discussed the project with us, and each agreed to try it in at least one of their sites. Over the course of the next 2-1/2 years, 24 of these 29 clinics initiated an office system very similar to that at Nokomis; at the end of that period, 8 clinics were maintaining a full system and 6 were maintaining a partial system. This represented 48 percent of the clinics.

A full smoking cessation office system consists of the following:

- Routine screening of all patients for tobacco use status at every visit;
- Labeling of all charts as either users or non-users;
- Establishing a separate smoke card for each tobacco user;
- Use of the smoke card to remind physicians to discuss tobacco use, to document each tobacco use discussion, and to communicate to the staff any plans made with the patient;
- Delivery of self-help booklets during office visits to any tobacco user interested in quitting;
- Followup by brief telephone calls after quit dates;
- Provision of some type of counseling assistance; and
- Establishing a smoke-free clinic policy.

The intervention with the practices consisted of an introductory full-day workshop and subsequent quarterly half-day refresher meetings attended by no more than three staff members from any one clinic. Only 10 percent of physicians in these clinics ever attended any of these workshops. In addition, 1.5 FTE (full-time equivalent) nurse coordinators from DHS visited or called the clinics regularly, and one of the DHS physicians visited infrequently. Clinics were provided with materials for training and distribution to patients and were encouraged to establish a support structure including

- Establishment of a clinic-wide policy for the system;
- Identification of a staff and a physician coordinator able to provide strong leadership for the program;
- Development of an implementation plan and start date;
- Orientation and training;
- Arrangement for necessary resources;
- Cooperation with performance audits by DHS nurses; and
- Efforts to provide feedback and spirit-building events.

The components of the smoking cessation system that seemed to be most difficult for clinics to establish and operate were those providing followup and any form of assistance or counseling. The component that tended to decay most easily once started was consistency of smoke card use, especially by the physicians. All of this was most dependent on strong and creative leadership by the physician and staff coordinator.

It was difficult to predict which clinics would be successful and which would not, primarily because of the limited knowledge that the DHS team had about each clinic during the first phases of the project. As clinic and individual patterns of behavior became clear, it became possible to identify the problems that interfered with successful adoption of a smoking cessation system. We believe that most of these problems would have the same effects on adoption of any other system (and in fact were doing so for existing operations). The main problems were general clinic stress, the motel syndrome, and ineffective leadership.

General Clinic Stress

Anything that caused great stress and required everybody's attention distracted the staff from the clinic's ability to start a new system. For example, one large clinic that never even got started (despite original expressions of understanding and great interest) was undergoing great financial stress because it was losing affiliation with another HMO that controlled many of the patients. Another large clinic got off to a fair start but then decided to end its affiliation with an HMO and lost 25 percent of its patients. This led to the loss of an equivalent share of physicians and staff and, not surprisingly, to the dissolution of their smoking cessation system. A third clinic did very well for more than 3 years but quit when it became stressed by an increased patient load.

The Motel Syndrome

Although individual practice is nearly nonexistent in Minnesota primary care, some group practices are really solo practices in disguise. The physicians practice in their own individual ways, sharing only billing, lab, and call systems. Because the DHS approach requires policy and procedure agreement if it is to be effective, it was only marginally effective in such clinics. If one or two physicians wanted to use it between themselves and their nurse, that was possible, but such efforts tended to be short-lived. One dedicated physician went on very well for more than a year by himself before quitting, and soon thereafter he left the clinic altogether.

Ineffective Leadership

Each clinic needed to have at least one physician who was respected by the others, believed this approach was important, and understood how to foster organizational change. It was clearly not enough to find a physician advocate who believed strongly in fighting tobacco use. If that physician was primarily a social activist against tobacco or took an individualistic or moralistic approach, he or she was unlikely to understand or support our approach. Beyond that, such attitudes would result in other physicians at the clinic labeling the enthusiast as unrealistic or radical. In any case, a physician who knew how to forge support for a group approach was essential.

It was also necessary to have a staff person with the authority, ability, and desire to implement the system. If any of those elements was missing, the system tended to be less effective and to fade over time. An effective staff coordinator could make up for the absence of an effective physician leader for a while. However, because even such a person has very limited ability to affect physician behavior, the staff would eventually get discouraged by the lack of cooperation from the physicians.

One of the best clinics exemplified this problem when, after 3 years of effective operation, the physician coordinator went on maternity leave and eventually returned on part-time status. Although the staff coordinator continued to be very involved, the physicians stopped using the system as much, leading to discouragement and inactivity on the part of the nurses. When the additional stress of an increased patient load developed, this clinic decided to "take a break" from the system.

A minor factor in some clinics was the personal use of tobacco by physicians or staff. We found that such use of tobacco was much less of a problem than the user's attitude about it. For example, although one of the most dedicated smoking cessation workers was a receptionist who smoked, she organized and used the smoke card system very effectively. However, in another clinic, posters and signs mysteriously disappeared as the staff coordinator put them up, the result, she believed, of sabotage efforts on the part of disgruntled smoking staff members.

Clearly, it would be best to identify these problems ahead of time and make adjustments. One detection device may be to see how other patient care systems are functioning; another may be to require some data-gathering task and then measure the accuracy and timeliness with which the clinic complies.

Given the potential for these problems, one might ask whether it is possible to set up the system that we are recommending. We believe that the fact that 48 percent of these randomly selected typical clinics in a high-stress, high-competition environment like that in Minnesota were still operating reasonably good DHS systems 2-1/2 years after being approached demonstrates both the compatibility and utility of the system and the possibility of stimulating it from the outside.

After completion of the grant, Blue Plus agreed to continue the intervention on its own, hiring a 1.0 FTE nurse coordinator and a 0.2 FTE physician expressly to continue and extend this project to its other clinics. The only major change was to work with clinics that volunteered interest, so as to make more efficient use of Blue Plus resources. In the subsequent 1-1/2 years, another 13 Blue Plus clinics set up DHS systems with our help, and the previous ones continued to receive some support. In addition, six more Blue Plus clinics would like to start, and several clinics from other HMOs have adapted and adopted the system with minimal help from us.

LESSONS LEARNED FOR FUTURE DIFFUSION

What factors motivated these clinics to undertake a project requiring significant time and energy while promising no financial advantage? In part it was undoubtedly the belief that this is an important problem that needs better methods. In the first 30 clinics, there was the additional reinforcement that they were part of a unique nationwide project associated with the National Institutes of Health and with a sense of group camaraderie. This latter was strengthened by fairly intense support from the full DHS team.

That these factors were important is attested by the seemingly greater difficulty that we have had with the subsequent clinics, despite their volunteer participation. Most are still operating, but several have quit and others are struggling.

All clinics have also benefited from a Hawthorne effect—attention from people whom they respected and from a major insurer of their patients (if you include the 25 percent of their business associated with the parent Blue Cross and Blue Shield plan). In addition, Blue Plus has required for years that all of its primary clinics operate quality assurance systems that institute two improvement projects per year. However, only two or three clinics have listed their DHS system in their required annual reports of quality projects, so they may not have made that connection.

Thus, it appears (as in A.J. Dietrich's New England area cancer prevention project) that an outside organization that understands and is flexible about the problems of primary care can stimulate and maintain organizational systems change in typical clinics (Dietrich et al., 1990). However, in both the DHS and the Dietrich examples, this has been accomplished by people who may not be widely replicable. The real problem is how to stimulate internal ownership and leadership to develop and maintain the new systems.

Although we started with the belief that it was important to tailor the DHS system to meet the needs of each clinic and to audit to evaluate the need for system modifications, we have come to realize that these concepts are absolutely essential. Without tailoring, the system remains something that the clinic has borrowed from elsewhere, easy to return or discard when any problems arise. Without adjustments based on actual performance, changes will not be likely to improve function. The problem is similar for both—unless one does the modification and audits oneself, one doesn't care enough about how the system functions, and the result is decay. We now believe that, unless there is within-clinic management of the change, the system is not likely to be successful in the long run.

Thus, outsiders may have an important role to play in encouraging development of systems like DHS for smoking cessation and in teaching some of the techniques necessary to develop and maintain any system, but that role is more limited than what we had originally foreseen. However, both Tornatsky's work with diffusion of a new approach to mental health care (Tornatsky et al., 1980) and Rogers' writings about diffusion of innovations (Rogers, 1983) should have prepared us for that. These problems may seem to leave in limbo the question of how to encourage widespread replication of smoking cessation systems in clinics.

Fortunately, a new paradigm is developing in American medical care that promises to produce major improvements in the way that health care is delivered. What makes this paradigm particularly promising for smoking cessation is that it serves as a map for internal leadership to follow to identify processes requiring change and to make continuous, self-sustaining improvements.

This map includes exactly what we have learned is necessary. The map can be specific about the process of making change without specifying the details of the change. Moreover, because this approach requires that those within a clinic or health care organization conduct this assessment and improvement, it has the potential to become effective, maintained, and widely replicated. We believe that this can be the vehicle with which to accomplish smoking cessation aims.

THE QUALITY IMPROVEMENT PARADIGM

To understand this new paradigm, it is necessary to understand its origins as well as its methods. This paradigm is commonly called continuous quality improvement (CQI) or total quality management. Although at least 40 years old in most other types of business, it is only a few years old in health care. In fact, although it began with American quality experts (W. Edwards Deming and Joseph Juran, in particular), their concepts found greatest initial acceptance in Japan and are credited with being the main stimulus to the enormous gains in quality and productivity exemplified by Japanese business (Deming, 1986; Juran, 1988; Walton, 1986). In the past 5 to 10 years, these same ideas have gained acceptance in American business (both manufacturing and service) and appear to be capable of the same benefits in health care.

Health care concerns in the United States have forced an increasing number of health care leaders to look to this CQI approach as a partial answer to their problems, a redirection that was sparked most prominently by the appearance of a journal article in 1989 (Berwick, 1989). Berwick's subsequent book, *Curing Health Care,* is the best single exposition of this approach in health care to date (Berwick et al., 1990).

Although CQI has grown out of quality assurance, it differs from it in many very important ways. Quality assurance in medicine has developed a very bad reputation among physicians. It has come to represent a search for "outliers" (bad apples) who have poor practices resulting in low quality. Quality assurance theory holds that, if these bad apples can be identified and removed or corrected, we shall see quality improve; thus, it emphasizes regulatory approaches and inspection methods.

Other businesses have learned that inspection has only a minimal effect on quality while adding substantially to costs, creating fear and other barriers to cooperation, and reducing productivity. The new quality approach instead assumes that the great majority of workers in any industry wish to do a good job, but this desire is regularly interfered with by the systems within which they work as well as by a serious lack of training and management leadership. Thus, the focus in CQI is on continuous improvement in the processes of work by involving the workers who best know those processes in cross-functional teams that study and improve the processes. The emphasis is on quantitative methods and pragmatism, which are concepts that should be very comfortable to practicing physicians. However, it also requires close multidisciplinary teamwork; emphasis on prevention; and especially, attention to the wishes of the customer, which are approaches that have not been nearly as traditional for physicians.

APPLYING QUALITY IMPROVEMENT

In its simplest form, CQI can be best viewed as a cyclical process in which systematic improvements are introduced into a process after studying the nature and frequency of problems. The effects of these improvements are closely monitored in quantitative ways, so it can be determined whether the improvements are helpful. The improvements are modified as necessary and proliferated when proven but continue to be subject to the same monitoring for future assessment and change until an adequate level of performance has been reached. This is known as the Shewhart or plan-do-check-act (PDCA) cycle (Walton, 1986).

In health care, the Hospital Corporation of America (HCA) has been particularly active and a leader in this new CQI movement. It has added to the Shewhart cycle in a way that makes it easier to understand by calling it the FOCUS-PDCA cycle (McEachern and Neuhauser, 1990). The acronym comes from the following steps:

- F, find a process to improve;
- O, organize a team of people who know the process well;
- C, clarify knowledge of the process as it exists;
- U, understand the causes of variation and problems in the process;
- S, select a systematic improvement based on that understanding;
- P, plan the introduction of that improvement and how to monitor its impact;
- D, do both the improvement (on a small scale if possible) and the monitoring;
- C, check on whether improvement has actually occurred; and
- A, act to modify, expand, and maintain any real improvements.

The cycle is repeated as needed.

It is easy to see how such an approach might be used in improving a manufacturing process. However, if one understands that all work (mental as well as physical) involves processes in which an input is converted to an output in a series of linked steps, then it is easier to see how this might become applicable in a service business. If it can work in the airline or hotel business, it might be useful to at least some aspects of medical care. In fact, some physicians are starting to feel that it might also apply to the clinical aspects of medical diagnosis and treatment as well.

All other types of business where this has been tried have found that applying this approach to existing processes produces large savings from reduction in waste and rework (25 to 35 percent) as well as great improvements in customer and employee satisfaction (Berwick et al., 1990). Early applications in health care through the National Demonstration Project, HCA, and others suggest the same will be true (Berwick et al., 1990).

Berwick has conceptualized the CQI steps in a way that is more generic and familiar to health professionals by suggesting four phases for them (Berwick et al., 1990): (1) project definition and organization (F and O); (2) diagnostic journey (C and U); (3) remedial journey (S, P, and D); and (4) holding the gains (C and A).

Thinking of it in this way makes it clear that this CQI process is very analogous to the way that physicians approach the medical problems of their patients. After organizing their practice to support their work, the physicians gather data in relation to hypothesized causes of a problem, make a first guess at a root cause, try an intervention (treatment), monitor and measure progress, and then modify both the tentative diagnosis and the treatment if they don't hold up under the scrutiny of followup observation.

CQI FOR SMOKING CESSATION

Let us see how an individual primary care medical practice of any size can apply this CQI to improve its smoking cessation effectiveness with its patients.

F—Find a Process To Improve

Although studies show that most physicians feel ineffective in getting their patients to quit smoking, that does not mean that they understand the problems interfering with their effectiveness (e.g., lack of awareness of which patients smoke and lack of reliable quit-reinforcement systems) or that they agree with approaches proven to be more effective. Therefore, it may be necessary to first verify quantitatively that the desirable activities are not occurring.

This can be demonstrated in a way that will also be useful for monitoring the effects of any change by conducting a simple chart review and a survey of patients as they leave the office (see Figures 1 and 2). Having a questionnaire filled out by each adult patient until 30 to 40 tobacco users have responded should indicate to what extent those users report that they experienced the five criteria listed in the first paragraph of this article:

Figure 1
Baseline audit of tobacco cessation activities at a clinic

A. Chart Review

1. Obtain about 50 random charts of adults (age 18 and over) from patients with a recent office visit, just before they are to be refiled.
2. Total charts reviewed: _______
3. Total charts labeled for tobacco use (problem list or any identification on chart cover):

   Labeled as user: _______

   Labeled as non-user: _______
4. Review of the *last* progress note:
   a. Total with any indication of tobacco discussion: _______
   b. Total identified as current tobacco user: _______
   c. Total with advice to quit: _______

B. Patient Survey

Without letting physicians and nurses know the days to be studied, pick five days out during one month, including one of each day of the week. On these days, the receptionist gives each departing adult patient a survey form and asks them to complete it and deposit it in a box near the door. It is important to know how many surveys were given out and how many were collected on each day.

Source: Solberg and Kottke, 1989; used with permission of the authors.

- Supportive assistance to quit is given at nearly every encounter over the longest possible time by both physicians and staff;
- Attention is directed primarily to those interested in quitting;
- Assistance is clear, supportive, and nonconfrontational and concentrates on specific plans, followup, and counseling;
- Multiple forms of assistance are available, both behavioral and pharmacological; and
- Quit dates or spontaneous quits are positively reinforced soon after they occur.

If a more elaborate study is desired, the respondents can be followed up by phone or mail survey 6 to 12 months later to determine their actual quit rates. It will be the unusual clinic that finds much compliance with the criteria, even if the physicians and staff are aware of the period during which the study is being conducted.

Figure 2
Tobacco survey

1. Were you asked about tobacco use during your visit today?

   ______ Yes ______ No

   If yes, who asked? ______ Nurse ______ Doctor ______ Other

2. Do you use tobacco every day?

   ______ Yes ______ No (Go to #4)

3. Were you advised to quit during today's visit?

   ______ Yes ______ No (Go to #4)

   If yes:

   a. Was the advice friendly and supportive?

      ______ Yes ______ No

   b. Did you agree to quit?

      ______ Yes ______ No (Go to #4)

      If yes:

      Were you offered help to quit?

      ______ Yes ______ No

      Were you offered any followup? (such as an appointment, phone call, etc.)

      ______ Yes ______ No

4. Age: ______

5. Sex: ______ Female ______ Male

Thank you very much for helping us!

Source: Solberg and Kottke, 1989; used with permission of the authors.

If a practice (clinic) already has accepted the need to change to a more systematic approach, then it can postpone these studies to the U phase (below). However, our experience suggests that unless some simple quantitative review measures are used, it is very difficult to understand the problems and to make appropriate system modifications.

O—Organize A Team To Improve the Process Logical members of the team in most practices would be a physician, nurse, receptionist, medical records person, and office manager. The goal is to include a representative from each functional area that is involved with the process. Knowledge of the actual work of these areas is critical to useful contributions to the team effort. Furthermore, it is clear that a team consisting only of physicians is not likely to produce either a feasible solution or one that will be maintained.

C—Clarify The Existing Process The first step in clarification is to construct a flowchart or algorithm of the *existing* process (not what is supposed to occur). The flowchart in Figure 3 can be used as a starting point for whether patients receive smoking cessation advice in their clinic's existing, unsystematic approach to this problem. As they clarify the existing process, the team will be able to appreciate the degree to which the existing system depends on chance, whim, and memory and results in variation that virtually guarantees ineffectiveness.

U—Understand The Problems And Causes of Variation Reviewing the flowchart (Figure 3) may allow team members to see why smoking cessation advice is ineffective. However, it will facilitate monitoring the effect of any future changes if this judgment is based on specific data as well. If they were not used during the F phase (above), the patient survey (Figure 2) and additional measurements of the frequency of nurse and physician smoking comments in the chart (Figure 1) can easily document the variability (both within and between individuals) that is occurring in these activities.

Here it is important for the team members to understand the role that reducing variability holds for improving results and efficiency. Although some may be reluctant to standardize the care process, it will be difficult for them not to see that systematic approaches involving many of the clinic staff will be necessary. Variation beyond that which is necessary to accommodate important differences between patients or providers should be seen as affecting both efficiency (i.e., costs) and effectiveness.

S—Select an Approach for Improvement The DHS model was designed specifically to address these criteria and to solve the problems of variable ineffective advice. However, there are other approaches or variations in these DHS approaches to accomplish the same goals. For example, a smoking record card can be kept with the patient's chart (instead of separately) or smoking patients can be referred out of the practice for any necessary assistance with quitting. It is important that the practice develops a sense of ownership of the approach chosen and that it adopts some way to measure the degree to which the approach is working. Figures 4 and 5 can be used to chart a clinic's own system.

P—Plan To Initiate and Monitor the Improvement Once the team members have decided on an approach, they must develop a plan for introducing that approach in the practice. They may wish to start with only part of the approach or to apply the full approach in only one site or section of the practice to more easily control and assess it. However, it will be necessary to obtain support for the

Figure 3
Flowchart for actual office smoking cessation

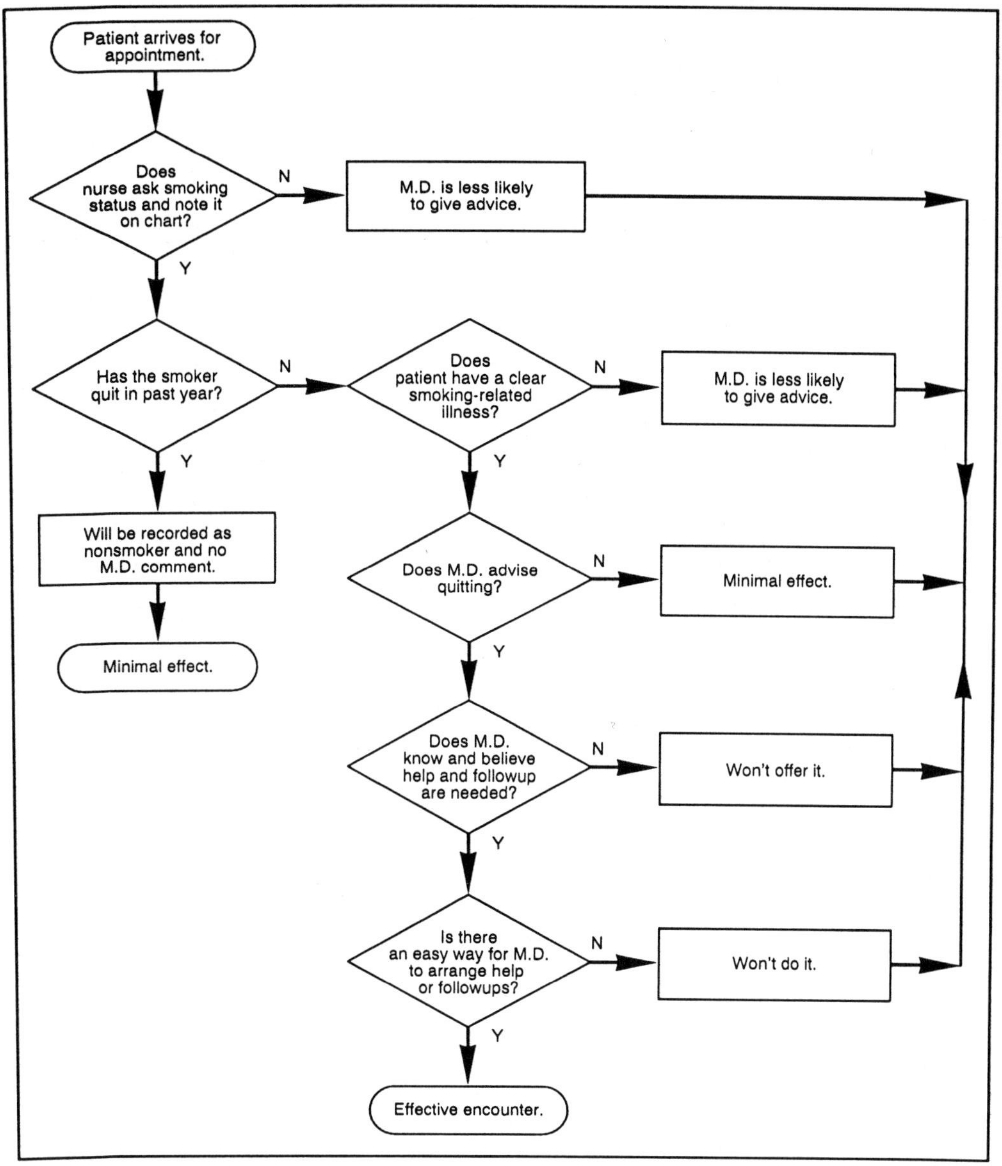

change, both from management and from each person who will play a role in it. It also will be necessary to identify a coordinator; to conduct orientation and training; and to make the necessary scheduling, resources, and time available to support it.

If the approach chosen involves a standard record form and/or labeling system like that in the DHS system, it will be relatively easy and quick to

Figure 4
Office tobacco-use cessation process flowchart

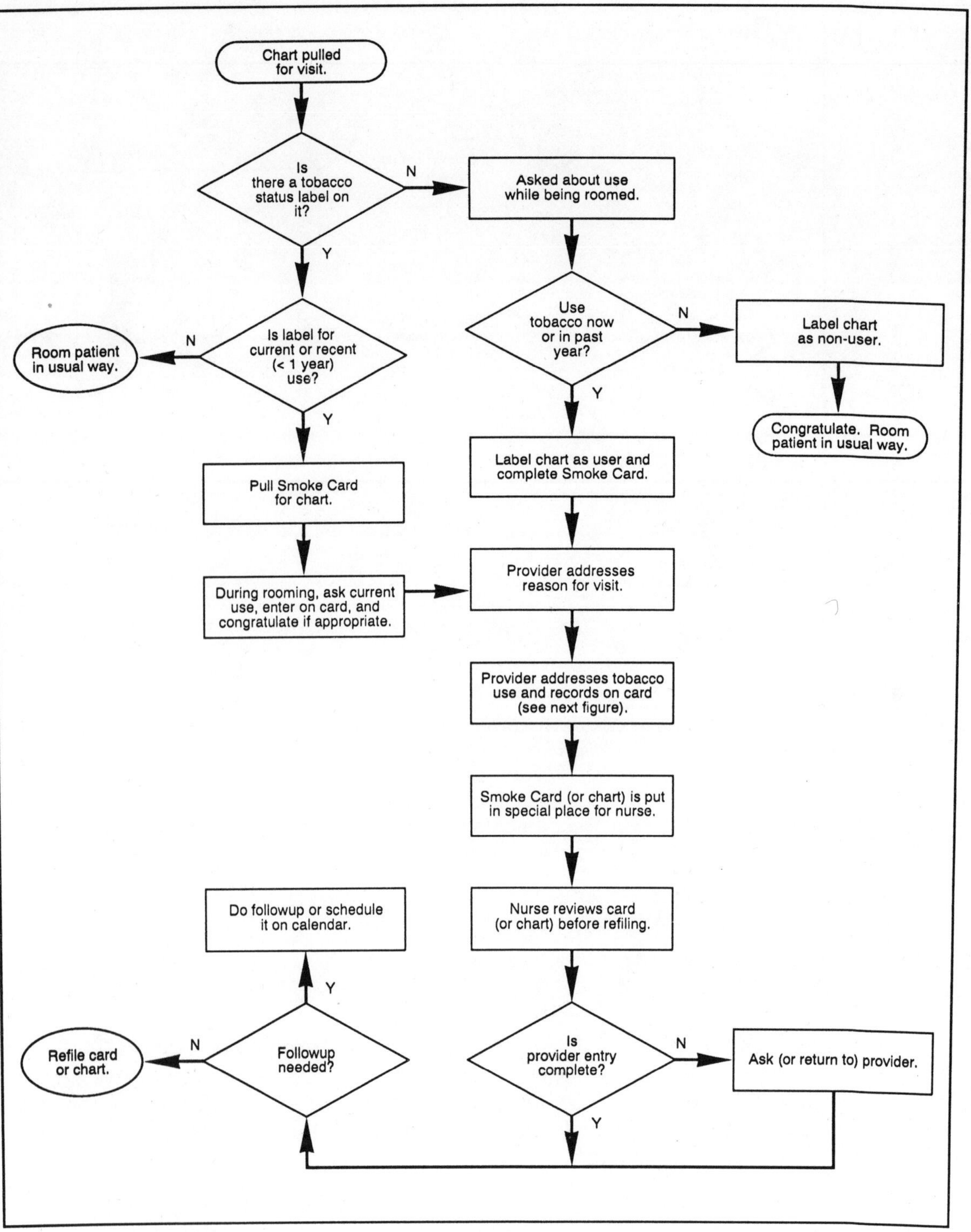

Figure 5
Provider-patient tobacco interaction flowchart

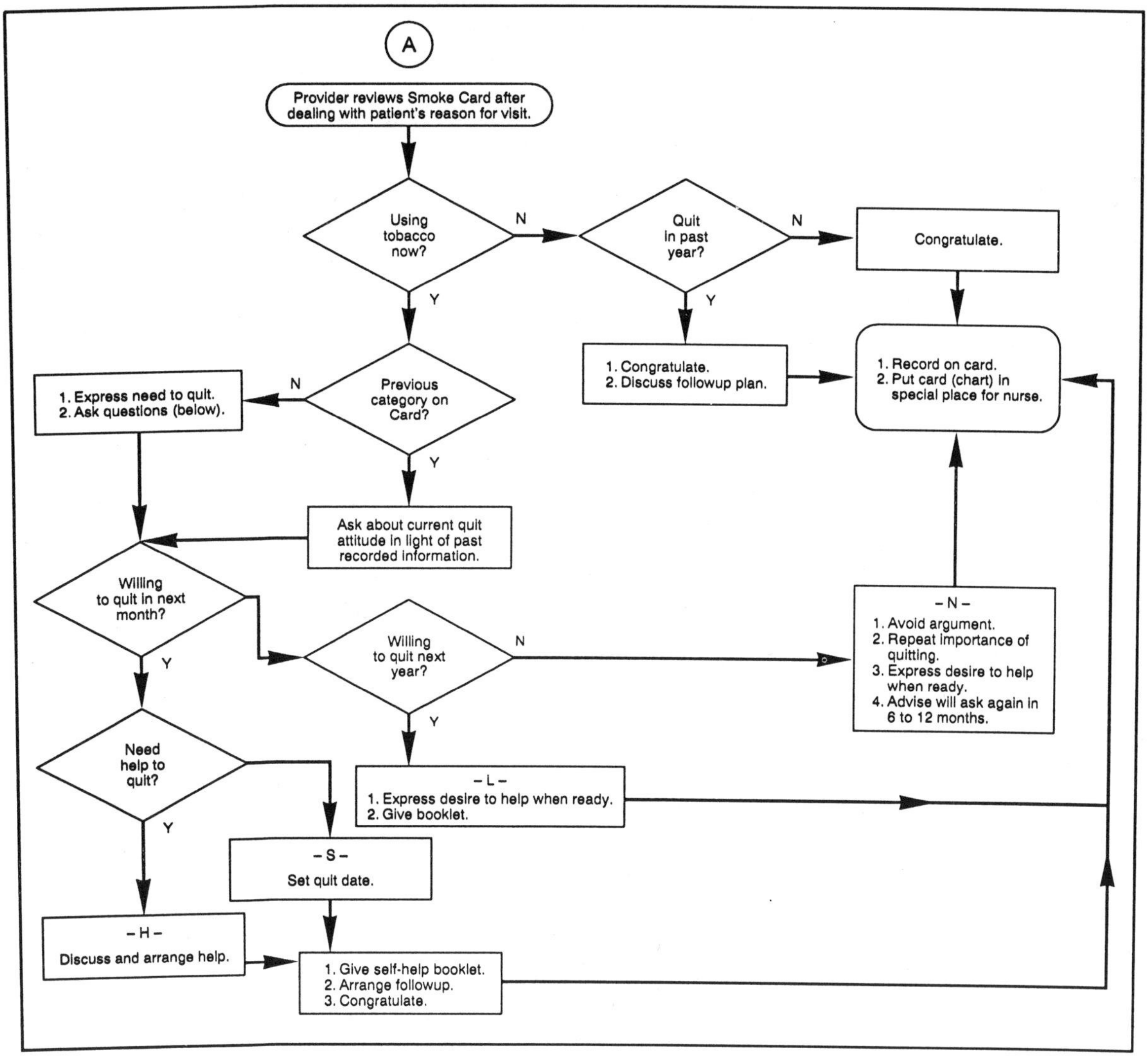

set up a periodic review that will determine whether these aspects of the improvement process are being used as desired. It is also desirable to determine the reactions of physicians, staff, and patients to the change.

D—Do the Improvement And Monitoring

Establish a "start day" (just like a quit day for a smoker) and initiate the carefully planned changes. Also, plan to repeat the audits at regular intervals, for example, at 1, 3, 6, and 12 months.

C—Check on How the Change Is Working After the change has been in effect long enough to gather data about how the new process is working and how it is being perceived, it is time to evaluate and plan any necessary modifications. If no data have been collected, it will be necessary to base this entirely on anecdotes and subjective reactions. However, the CQI approach assumes quantitative assessments are more likely to be useful.

A—Act To Expand or Improve The Change If the assessment suggests that the process is functioning well, it may be time to expand to other areas of the practice. However, if substantial changes are necessary, it may be better to defer that until one or more additional rounds of the PDCA cycle have occurred.

When periodic audits suggest that the new system is working well (usually at 6 to 12 months), it also may be time to assess the extent to which it is producing the desired outcome of tobacco cessation. This can be done by reviewing the smoking records or by a simple followup of a sample of tobacco users (as was described in the F phase). If the team is satisfied with the monitoring data, it is then ready to set up permanent responsibilities for maintenance. The team then may be dissolved or may continue to build additional preventive services into the same system. We have expanded the DHS system to one for all cardiovascular risks, and it can clearly be adapted to include other preventive services. However, by this time the practice, we hope, will have found that this approach to quality improvement works so well that it will establish other multidisciplinary teams to improve other processes of care (such as appointments, waiting time, test ordering, results reporting, or care for such clinical problems as urinary infections or back pain).

CONCLUSION Clearly, the above description is too brief to provide all of the information needed to make the best use of this new paradigm of CQI in medical practice. Each practice will have to learn much about efficient team function, statistical quality control measures, and how to understand better the needs and expectations of its patients and employees. Even before reaching that stage, however, it is likely that everyone associated with such a continuously improving practice will find it to be much more satisfying. Combining that satisfaction with the improved efficiency that is possible should result in a practice that is also thriving financially.

An important final question: What is going to make a clinical practice group want to go through changes like CQI, particularly for preventive services that may not be very profitable? The promise of thriving financially is not likely to be provable for at least a few more years. In the meantime, additional incentives will arise from some combination of the following:

- Idealism and the sense that preventive services are a medical responsibility of primary care practice;
- Patient expectations and competition for patients;

- Medical-legal risk management; for example, failure to diagnose breast cancer early enough is already a major legal problem and other prevention services are likely to follow soon; and

- Requirements from payers—government, employers, and insurance companies.

Each of these forces is likely to be stimulated by comparative data about the frequency with which preventive services are delivered in clinics. These data will surely soon be demanded, and they are easily obtainable from claims systems, in many cases. Although smoking cessation advice and assistance are more difficult to review than other preventive services, they are clearly important. Therefore, smoking intervention seems likely to be reviewed externally, perhaps through questions of patients on the satisfaction surveys that are being used increasingly to compare health plans and clinics.

At Blue Plus, we have already demonstrated to our satisfaction that it is possible to stimulate the development of traditional quality assurance systems in primary care clinics through a combination of requirements and assistance. Most of the 120 clinic groups with which we contract now have satisfactory or excellent quality assurance programs where none existed 5 years ago.

Moreover, many of those clinics are going well beyond our requirements in creative ways. An increasing number of clinics also are expressing interest in the concepts and techniques of quality improvement, and we are helping them to make that transition through conferences and on-site visits. We are convinced that many are now ready to use the above-described CQI approach to establishing systems for smoking cessation and other preventive services. Those that don't accept this challenge and opportunity will find themselves without long-term partnerships with us, and we shall know that through our use of audits from claims systems and satisfaction surveys.

Like quality improvement in other businesses, it is clear that the road to improved quality comes from two directions—from improving internal processes and from establishing close, long-term partnerships with those suppliers who are equally dedicated to that task. Working together, we must increasingly provide value (i.e., cost-effective health improvement) to our customers, and smoking cessation may be one of the most important tests of that commitment.

REFERENCES

Battista, R.N., Mickalide, A.D. Integration of preventive services into primary care: A conceptual framework for implementation. In: *Preventing Disease: Beyond the Rhetoric*, R.B. Goldbloom and R.S. Lawrence (Editors). New York: Springer-Verlag, 1990, pp. 466-473.

Belcher, D.W., Berg, A.O., Inui, T.S. Practical approaches to providing better preventive care: Are physicians a problem or a solution? In: *Implementing Preventive Services*, R.N. Battista and R.S. Lawrence (Editors). New York: Oxford, 1988, pp. 27-48.

Berwick, D.M. Continuous improvement as an ideal in health care. *New England Journal of Medicine* 320: 53-56, 1989.

Berwick, D.M., Godfrey, A.B., Roessner, J. *Curing Health Care.* San Francisco: Jossey-Bass, 1990.

Cohen, S.J., Kelly, S.A., Eason, A.A. Establishing smoking cessation programs in dental offices. *Journal of the American Dental Association* 20(Suppl.): 28S-31S, 1990.

Cummings, K.M., Giovino, G., Emont, S.L., Sciandra, R., Koenigsberg, M. Factors influencing success in counseling patients to stop smoking. *Patient Education and Counseling* 8: 189-200, 1986.

Deming, W.E. *Out of the Crisis.* Cambridge, MA: MIT-CAES, 1986.

Dietrich, A.J., O'Connor, G., Keller, A., Carney-Gersten, P., Levy, D., Nelson, E., Simmons, J., Barrett, J., Jr., Landgraf, J.M. Will community physicians participate in rigorous studies of cancer control? The methodology and recruitment in a randomized trial of physician practices. In: *Advances in Cancer Control: Screening and Prevention Research* (Progress in Clinical Biology Series, volume 339), P.F. Engstrom, B. Rimer, and L.E. Mortenson (Editors). New York: Wiley-Liss, 1990, pp. 373-381.

Glynn, T.J., Manley, M.W. *How To Help Your Patients Stop Smoking: A National Cancer Institute Manual for Physicians.* U.S. Department of Health and Human Services, Public Health Service, National Institutes of Health, National Cancer Institute. NIH Publication No. 90-3064, 1990.

Inui, T.S., Belcher, A.O., Carter, W.B. Implementing preventive care in clinical practice: I. Organizational issues and strategies. *Medical Care Review* 38: 129-154, 1981.

Juran, J.M. *Juran's Quality Control Handbook* (4th edition). New York: McGraw-Hill, 1988.

Kottke, T.E., Battista, R.N., DeFriese, G.H., Brekke, M.L. Attributes of successful smoking cessation interventions in medical practice: A meta-analysis of 39 controlled trials. *Journal of the American Medical Association* 259: 2882-2889, 1988.

McEachern, J.E., Neuhauser, D. The continuous improvement of quality at the Hospital Corporation of America. *Health Matrix* 7: 5-11, 1990.

Ockene, J.K. Physician-delivered interventions for smoking cessation: Strategies for increasing effectiveness. *Preventive Medicine* 16: 723-737, 1987.

Pommerenke, P.A., Weed, D.L. Physician compliance: Review and application to cancer detection and prevention. *American Family Physician* 43: 560-568, 1991.

Rogers, E.M. *Diffusion of Innovations* (3rd edition). New York: Free Press, 1983.

Solberg, L.I., Kottke, T.E. Smoking cessation strategies. In: *A Practical Guide for the Treatment of Substance Abuse,* M. Fleming and K. Barry (Editors). Chicago: Mosby-Yearbook, 1989, pp. 95-112.

Solberg, L.I., Maxwell, P.L., Kottke, T.E., Gepner, G.J., Brekke, M.L. A systematic primary care office-based smoking cessation program. *Journal of Family Practice* 30(6): 647-654, 1990.

Tornatsky, L.G., Fergus, E.O., Avellar, J.W., et al. *Innovation and Social Process: A National Experiment in Implementing Social Technology.* New York: Pergamon Press, 1980.

Walton, M. *The Deming Management Method.* New York: Putnam, 1986.

Computerized Reminder System To Aid Physicians in Assessment and Counseling of Patients Who Smoke[2]

Stephen J. McPhee, Joyce Adair Bird, Don Fordham,
Jonathan E. Rodnick, and Emilie H. Osborn

INTRODUCTION To overcome the barriers to physicians' performing smoking cessation counseling, reminder interventions of several types have been developed and tested (McPhee and Detmer, in press). Approaches during medical encounters, termed "inreach" interventions, have included medical record stickers, checklists and flowsheets, and computerized reminders.

In the past, reminder interventions have largely targeted physicians (often physicians in training) in university-based practices. The current project was directed to community-based physicians in solo or small group practices. The study was a randomized, controlled trial to test the efficacy of a computerized cancer prevention reminder system (CPRS) in promoting physicians' performance of several cancer prevention activities, including smoking assessment and counseling about smoking cessation (Fordham et al., 1990). The CPRS intervention was supplemented by professional and patient educational materials.

SUBJECTS The subjects of the study were primary care physicians who were members of the clinical faculty of the Department of Medicine and Department of Family and Community Medicine at the University of California, San Francisco. Such clinical faculty members have nonsalaried clinical appointments in recognition of their service as volunteer preceptors for medical students. Most have their practices in the San Francisco Bay area. Many of the physicians had expressed an interest in collaborative research (Osborn et al., 1991).

Physician Recruitment To recruit physicians for the study, we mailed each of the 307-member clinical faculty a letter describing the randomized, controlled trial and a self-addressed reply postcard, followed by a second mailing and telephone calls as needed.

Eligibility criteria for physician recruitment were as follows: (1) Each physician was in a full-time, private (fee-for-service) office practice of family medicine or general internal medicine; (2) each physician was in a solo or

[2] This work was supported by grant no. R01-CA46020-03 from the National Cancer Institute.

small group practice (sharing an office with no more than three other physicians); (3) the physician's office was located within reasonable distance (defined as 75 miles) of the university and research staff; (4) only one physician in a given office practice was eligible; and (5) each physician was willing to have a computerized CPRS installed and implemented in the office. Eligible physicians who agreed to participate were randomized into either the intervention or the control group.

Of the 307 physicians, 140 (46 percent) did not respond to the recruitment letters and telephone calls, 53 (17 percent) refused study participation, and 114 (37 percent) indicated their interest in the study. Among the last group, 39 did not meet the study enrollment criteria. Of the 75 eligible and interested physicians, 35 subsequently declined to participate, raising the total number of refusals to 88 (29 percent). The remaining 40 physicians were enrolled in the study.

The investigators met with potential subjects in their practice offices. Those meetings constituted the first of two essential steps toward gaining consent for study participation. The investigators described the study; discussed the benefits of the study to participants (e.g., the experimental group would receive computers, software, and educational materials; controls would receive software and educational materials at the end of the study); explained the contributions requested of participants (e.g., access to medical records, office staff time, questionnaire completion); investigated space, staff, and patient volume and demographics; and answered physicians' questions. All physicians were cooperative during the meetings; they approved of the study aims and indicated that they would like to take part. However, most were concerned that the CPRS requirements would overburden the office staff, and some were concerned about the space required for computer hardware. For many, those concerns led directly to refusal, whereas others waited to assess the reactions of their office staffs before making a decision.

Peer influence appeared to be an important factor in recruitment. During the meetings between the project physicians and the community physicians, the tone of the discussions was collegial, and discussions of medical issues usually related to prevention rather than research. In the few instances in which nonphysician investigators took part in recruitment, more time was devoted to the logistics of collecting the medical record data and implementing the intervention. In the latter discussions, the community physicians had greater opportunity to focus on the problems that might arise during the intervention; thus, the recruitment efforts by nonphysicians were less persuasive.

Medical Office Staff Recruitment

The second essential step toward gaining physicians' consent was acceptance of the intervention by the medical office staffs. Research staff members met with office staff members to describe the system and discuss their participation. In most cases, however, by the time these meetings took place, the physicians already had discussed the matter with their staff and decided whether to participate. Therefore, nearly all meetings with office staffs were held in practices of physicians who had decided to participate. In only one case was it clear that the physician had left the decision entirely in the hands of the office staff. In two cases, physicians made independent decisions to participate, choosing to operate the CPRS themselves rather than relying on their staffs.

Physician Characteristics

We enrolled 40 physicians in the study: 20 were assigned randomly to the cancer prevention reminders intervention and 20 to the control group. Three-quarters of the study physicians were male. The mean age of the physicians was 45 years, and the mean year of medical school graduation was 1971. Of the 40 physicians, 30 were family practitioners and 10 were general internists. Slightly more than half of the physicians (55 percent) were in solo practice. In general, physicians recruited for the study had a strong orientation toward preventive care (Osborn et al., 1991). For example, 80 percent believed it was their responsibility to urge patients to be screened for cancer, and 78 percent said they always advised their smoking patients to quit.

DESCRIPTION OF THE INTERVENTION

The CPRS is a software program developed by the investigators for MS-DOS-based microcomputers. The functions of the program are easily accessible through a branching menu design, and a user's manual takes the inexperienced user through the various features step by step. The program provides the physician with an up-to-date report of each patient's screening, assessment, and counseling status as a reminder to perform the maneuvers; also, the program provides a simplified version of the report for the physician to give to the patient. Additional features include the ability to generate summary reports of the percentage of patients in the data base who are overdue for a designated cancer prevention activity and listings of patients overdue for a designated activity. The patient listings with addresses may be printed on mailing labels and affixed to preprinted reminder postcards.

The printed reminder displays the list of appropriate assessment, counseling, and screening maneuvers (based on the patient's sex, age, and smoking status); the recommended assessment, counseling, or testing intervals; the last performance date; the due date for each next maneuver; and the patient's current "due" status (see Figure 6). The patient's smoking status is identified on each reminder report. If a patient's smoking status has not been assessed, the default identification is "smoker." The system reminds physicians to counsel smokers, to set a quit date, and to schedule a followup visit to discuss their progress. The physician is expected to indicate on the form whether or not each maneuver was performed or ordered, not applicable, or refused during the current visit. The annotated form then is used to update the computerized data base. The patient's copy of the reminder form includes space for physicians to write out specific recommendations as a prescription, such as "set a smoking quit date" (see Figure 7). This form also is intended to remind patients to schedule future appointments.

Figure 6
Physician cancer prevention reminder

Name: Andrews, Ms. Anne — Sex: F
Date of Birth: 03/03/33 — Age: 58
Today's date: Wednesday, March 27, 1991 — **SMOKER**

These reminders are based on the recommendations of the American Cancer Society for asymptomatic adults. The recommendations should be individualized depending on history and risk factors.

Procedure	**Date Last Done**	**Date Due**	**Overdue?**	**Done This Visit**	**Done by Others & Date**
Pap smear	11/12/90	11/12/91	NO	Y N NA R	_/_/_/_/
Mammography	05/05/89	05/05/90	YES-G	Y N NA R	_/_/_/_/
Smoking counseling	11/12/90	12/12/90	YES-H	Y N NA R	_/_/_/_/
Set smoking quit date		03/27/91	YES-I	Y N NA R	_/_/_/_/
Schedule smoking followup		03/27/91	YES-J	Y N NA R	_/_/_/_/

NA, Not Applicable; R, Refused.

Key to Overdue Notes:

G. For women over 50, every year.
H. All smokers.
I. All smokers.
J. All smokers.

J.Q. Public, M.D.
450 Sutter St., Suite 250
San Francisco, CA 94138-1111
(415) 555-9000

Figure 7
Patient cancer prevention reminder

Name: Ms. Anne Andrews — **SMOKER**
Today's date: Wednesday, March 27, 1991

According to the American Cancer Society, the following cancer prevention activities should be considered as part of your preventive care. If the tests or counseling have been done by another physician or clinic, please let your doctor know.

Procedure	**Date Last Done**	**Date Due**	**Overdue?**	**If Done Today, Next Due**
Pap smear	11/12/90	11/12/91	NO	03/27/92
Mammography	05/05/89	05/05/90	YES	03/27/92
Smoking counseling	11/12/90	12/12/90	YES	04/27/91
Set smoking quit date	03/27/91		YES	04/27/91
Schedule smoking followup	03/27/91		YES	04/27/91

Goals and Recommendations

J.Q. Public, M.D.
450 Sutter St., Suite 250
San Francisco, CA 94138-1111
(415) 555-9000

The authors currently are developing further refinements and plans for nonprofit distribution of the CPRS. In the meantime, readers who wish a copy of the software should contact the authors.

IMPLEMENTATION OF THE CPRS

System Initiation

We derived the initial data for the CPRS from preintervention review of a sample of medical records and from the medical records of patients aged 40 and older who were scheduled for visits during the first 2 or 3 weeks of the intervention period. At the beginning of the intervention period, the research staff installed computers and software, entered patient data, and oriented the intervention group physicians and their office staffs to the CPRS.

Office Staff Training

The appropriate staff members in each office were trained to use the CPRS. Usually, only one staff person was designated by the physician, but occasionally two were chosen for training. In each of three practices, the trainee was a high school student, hired by the physician to implement the CPRS after school hours. In a few instances, the physician also attended the training sessions.

Training was conducted in two 1-hour sessions. The first session covered basic features that would be used regularly: adding new patient names, editing names, adding data, printing reminders, and backing up data. The second session addressed special features that would be used occasionally, such as generating summary reports, deleting data and names, preparing mailing labels, indexing, and establishing individual patient exceptions. Thereafter, telephone and on-site consulting was provided as needed. Project staff members visited experimental group offices monthly to provide supplies, inquire about problems, and monitor implementation of the CPRS. Office staff members with no prior computer experience had some trouble with basic word processing skills, following the branching menus, and concepts such as saving new or edited data from the screen to the data base. However, most complaints about the CPRS by the office staffs were related to shortages of time and personnel.

We did not provide the office staff with directions or assistance in integrating the system into the general office procedures; each office had unique features, and therefore the staff for each practice determined its own method and procedures for handling the system. However, we did observe that offices with noticeably good office management and clear priorities handled these processes most easily and had fewer complaints about the amount of time the CPRS consumed.

Day-to-Day Operation

During the 12-month intervention period, the office staffs printed cancer prevention reminders prior to each appointment (for patients aged 40 or older). Usually, this work was done during regular office hours (eight cases), early in the morning before the first appointment (six cases), after hours (five cases), or during the lunch hour (one case). Among those who did the work during office hours, four had other duties to attend to at the same time.

After printing the physician and patient reminders, the staff person attached them to the medical records. The physician was encouraged to give the patient reminders to the patients during each visit. Typically, reminders were printed about four times per week, and the data base was updated about twice per week according to physicians' notations on the reminders.

Supplemental Intervention

Physicians in the experimental group were also given a rack of educational materials to assist them in counseling their patients. The patient education materials included the following:

- *Quit for Good* (National Cancer Institute);
- *Weight Control Guidance in Smoking Cessation* (American Heart Association);
- *Quit for Life* (University of California, San Francisco);
- *Getting Ready To Get Ready To Quit Smoking* (Kaiser Permanente);
- *Guia para Dejar de Fumar* (University of California, San Francisco; National Cancer Institute); and
- *Would You Give a Cigarette to Your Unborn Child?* (National Cancer Institute poster).

Two professional education publications were provided:

- *A Clinician's Guide to Helping Patients Change Behavior* (Martin and Coates, 1987); and
- *Smoking Cessation Programs in San Francisco County, Marin County, East Bay Counties, Sonoma County and Peninsula* (University of California, San Francisco).

Physicians were free to choose where the educational material was placed—in their offices, in the waiting room, or outside exam rooms. A few physicians reordered materials during the intervention period.

ANALYTICAL METHODS

To assess the impact of the intervention, we measured each physician's assessment and counseling performance during 12-month preintervention and intervention periods. To do so, we drew independent, random samples of about 60 patients from each physician's practice register at the end of the preintervention and intervention periods and audited the medical records of those patients. We calculated the percentage of patients each physician assessed for smoking status, the percentage of current smokers among patients who had been assessed, and the percentage of assessed smokers who had been counseled to quit smoking. We calculated performance rates for both preintervention and intervention periods and used *t*-tests and ordinary least squares multiple regression to test the significance of differences in mean rates between physicians in the intervention and control groups for each period.

At the end of the intervention period, we conducted brief interviews with the physicians and their office staffs to assess the acceptability of the system and to document any technical or logistical problems they experienced.

RESULTS

Preintervention performance rates did not differ significantly between intervention and control physicians for either smoking assessment or smoking cessation counseling. The mean percentage of patients whose smoking status physicians had assessed during the preintervention period was 30.1 percent, and the mean percentage of smokers whom physicians had counseled was 34.8 percent. The mean smoking rate among patients in the 40 practices (for patients whose smoking status appeared in the medical records) was 36 percent.

Table 1 shows the differences in mean postintervention performance scores between control and intervention group physicians. Performance rates of the intervention group were significantly higher than the control group for both smoking assessment and smoking counseling.

Results of multiple regression analyses provide stronger evidence of the intervention's impact on smoking assessment and smoking counseling performance (Table 2). When controlled for preintervention rates, estimated smoking assessment rates of intervention group physicians were 10.2 points higher than controls (p=0.02), and smoking counseling rates were 17.3 points higher than controls (p=0.03). A more detailed desciiption of the analytical methods and results is provided elsewhere (McPhee et al., 1991).

Physicians' verbal reports during the exit interviews corroborated these findings, dispelling any concern that observed differences between the experimental and the control group simply reflected better recordkeeping by physicians in the intervention group. Approximately two-thirds (13 of 20)

Table 1
Postintervention performance scores, by intervention group

	Mean (SD) Performance Score[a]		
	Control n=19	Cancer Prevention Reminders n=20	*t*-test,[b] p value
Smoking Assessment	32.4 (13.9)	45.0 (16.6)	0.014
Smoking Counseling	41.8 (22.2)	58.8 (23.0)	0.027

[a] *Percentage annual rates.*
[b] t*-test for differences between group means.*

Table 2
Regression results: effects of interventions on performance scores controlled by preintervention scores

	Constant[a]	Cancer Prevention Reminders
Smoking Assessment		
b[b]	15.0	10.2
p[c]	0.008	0.021
Smoking Counseling		
b[b]	39.7	17.3
p	0.000	0.027

[a] *Intercept.*
[b] *Unstandardized regression coefficient.*
[c] *p value.*

of the physicians in the intervention group said that they had done more counseling about smoking as a result of the reminders: 4 of 20 indicated they had done "slightly more" counseling, 6 had done "quite a bit more," and 3 had done "much more" counseling.

DISCUSSION The success of the CPRS is consistent with the results of other research studies demonstrating that physician reminders can be effective in promoting performance of smoking cessation counseling (Cohen et al., 1987 and 1989; Cummings et al., 1989a and 1989b).

Strengths Of the Intervention We designed the CPRS intervention specifically to address several barriers to performance of cancer screening activities, including physician forgetfulness and time constraints, identified in our previous research (McPhee and Bird, 1990; McPhee et al., 1986). The positive effects of the intervention in the present study strongly suggest that the same problems are implicated in physicians' limited performance of smoking assessment and counseling.

Compared with hard-copy flowsheets, the CPRS is more costly to initiate, because a 20 Mb personal computer and printer cost between $1,500 and $2,500; however, the CPRS has several distinct advantages when compared with other types of interventions. First, it is readily exportable to a variety of practice settings. Many physicians already have microcomputers in their offices for billing and other purposes (Schmittling, 1989); installing the CPRS software is done quite easily. It also can be built readily into in-place computerized ambulatory medical records systems, such as CO-STAR. Second, unlike other reminder systems (such as "smoker" stickers attached to medical records), the CPRS can be used to prompt the performance of a variety of periodic preventive care activities, including other assessment and counseling activities, screening tests, and immunizations (Fordham et al., 1990). Third, we have found that the CPRS, compared with other strategies, such as an audit-with-feedback intervention, is cost-effective (Bird et al., 1990). Furthermore, because the CPRS is able to target a variety of periodic health maintenance procedures, it will remain more cost-effective than interventions that target only one or two activities. Fourth, the CPRS software enables physicians to monitor their own performance of various activities. Finally, the due date intervals of the CPRS are easily adjusted to meet new recommendations (or the physician's preferred standards).

Acceptability Physicians (n=17) estimated that office staff spent a mean of 2.8 hours per week using the system. Although most physicians had been concerned about whether their office staff would have enough time to implement the system, at the end of the intervention period, only 3 of 20 physicians said the system had been "very burdensome" to their staff, 4 said it was "moderately burdensome," and 9 said it was either "only a little" or "not at all" burdensome. Office staff members (n=14) estimated that the mean time requirement to operate the system was 3.7 hours per week. When asked how difficult it was to find time to maintain the system, 3 of 14 office staff members said it was "not difficult," 7 said it was "somewhat difficult," and 4 said it was "very difficult." In spite of their perceptions of the difficulty involved, 9 of 14 said they thought the time devoted to using the system was "definitely worthwhile," 4 thought it was "probably worthwhile," and only 1 said it was "probably not worthwhile."

Weaknesses Of the Intervention Special features of the CPRS were used by less than one-half of the physicians. For example, only 6 of 20 physicians used the CPRS summary option to audit their own behavior; only 8 used the mailing label feature to mail appointment-reminder postcards to patients. At the end of the study, 3 of the 20 physicians commented that they "didn't know" about the features—2 in regard to the summary option and 1 in regard to the mailing labels. The office staffs, not the physicians, were the major users of the system and were more familiar with the range of options. However, our observations in the practices suggested that staff members used system features only at the request of the physicians. Thus, the degree to which the system was used depended to a great extent on the degree to which physicians pressed their staff to keep the system up to date. Physicians with the busiest practices seemed to have less time to devote to system maintenance and seemed to experience more difficulty in consistently implementing the system.

Eight of the twenty physicians "always" or "nearly always" offered patients the patient reminder; six did so "occasionally," and six "never" did so. Physician's comments regarding the patient reminder ranged from "patients who received it, liked it" to "patients might be confused [by it]" to "it's not helpful; it was mostly discarded." It is probable that some physicians were reluctant to share with their patients any data that reflected their own forgetfulness or deviation from compliance with established standards.

With respect to smoking reminders, a few of the physicians expressed annoyance that they received repeated reminders to counsel patients about smoking, set a quit date, and schedule followup appointments. This may have reflected doubts that their repeated counseling could be effective in helping patients to stop smoking or their annoyance with their patients' noncompliance. The presence of three reminder messages related to smoking cessation, rather than only one, also may have contributed to physicians' irritation.

Suggestions for Improvement

Although it is clear that the CPRS was successful in prompting physicians to counsel their patients about smoking cessation, anecdotal evidence indicates that more is needed to assure that physicians persist in those efforts. Our experience and findings suggest that bringing physicians and staffs into the early planning process and prefacing implementation of the CPRS with additional education-intervention components—one for physicians and one for their medical office staffs—would have enhanced the acceptability of the CPRS. In addition, it is clear that many physicians are not convinced of the importance of their role in patients' smoking cessation efforts. Such orientation, along with training in smoking counseling methods, would have facilitated physicians' acceptance of repeated reminders as a reflection of the difficulty many patients have in quitting smoking, rather than as comments on the physicians' ineffectiveness or the patients' noncompliance. Although physicians may disapprove of patients' smoking, their continued concern and repeated counseling are more likely to assist the smoker in quitting than are disapproval or annoyance. Indeed, such counseling may be more cost-effective than treating hypertension or hypercholesterolemia (Cummings et al., 1989c). The educational component for physicians also might include videotapes of physicians providing smoking cessation counseling to patients. For medical office staffs, additional education might include information about cancer risks and the importance of cancer prevention.

The planning component might bring physicians and office staff into the process of participation at an earlier stage. In turn, this might enhance participants' sense of investment in the study and proprietorship of the intervention. For example, we observed that, among the busiest medical office staffs, some were more interested in the intervention than others and that their higher level of interest and commitment appeared to motivate them to find time for the CPRS, regardless of their workload. Educational and planning components such as these undoubtedly would have strengthened the physician and staff commitment to implementing the system more fully and consistently.

In addition, it is worth considering whether the reminders to provide counseling would be more acceptable to physicians if there were only one reminder related to smoking behavior. Individual patient counseling packages containing quit-date prescription forms and followup appointment forms could then encourage the physician to take further steps whenever a counseling reminder appears.

The "audit-with-feedback" function of the summary report might have been more successful if we had asked physicians to make this report part of their office staffs' regular assignments. Included in the summary is a display of the percentage of smokers in the practice who have not been counseled by the physician. We would expect that routine, monthly inspection of the summary of their overall performance would have further stimulated physicians' performance of smoking assessment and counseling.

Study Limitations This study was conducted among family physicians and general internists in solo and small group practices. The voluntary nature of their participation may have biased the results. Also, the findings may not be generalizable to other specialties or settings. Still, these physicians are more typical of U.S. primary care physicians than are residents in teaching hospital settings.

The novelty of the computerized reminder system may have intensified its impact. Had the intervention period been longer, the substantial effects we observed may have declined over time (Green et al., 1986). Still, because of the continuity of automated updating, computerized reminder systems may have more durable effects than written flowsheets, audit-with-feedback interventions, or other interventions. As with any system, however, effectiveness depends on fairly consistent use. As would be expected, we found the level of use to vary among practices. At the end of the 12-month intervention period, 13 of 20 practices continued regular use of the system. The major reasons given by those who stopped using the CPRS were related to changes in the practice (they moved or took over another's patients), staff turnover, and shortage of staff. Two of the practices that discontinued use later indicated their interest in resuming use of the CPRS, and another had acquired an alternative system that combined computerized reminders with billing procedures.

CONCLUSIONS The authors conclude that computerized reminders can significantly increase physicians' performance of smoking assessment and counseling activities in the private office practice setting. The results of multiple regression analyses (controlled by preintervention rates) estimated the experimental group's rates of smoking assessment and smoking counseling to be significantly higher—both statistically and clinically—than those of the control group.

The effectiveness of the CPRS strategy suggests that physician forgetfulness is an important barrier to smoking assessment and counseling in clinical practice. Clearly, other barriers, such as physicians' perceptions of their effectiveness and their need for counseling skills, must be reduced to close the gap between recommended and actual performance levels.

Computerized reminders have been used and tested for a variety of preventive medicine activities, especially for secondary prevention such as cancer screening tests (McPhee and Detmer, in press). To our knowledge, this is the first report of success with a computerized reminder system in promoting physicians' smoking cessation counseling. Also, in this trial, smoking assessment and smoking cessation counseling were placed in the context of other cancer prevention activities. The success of this approach may help to establish smoking cessation counseling as an appropriate activity for the primary care physician.

REFERENCES

Bird, J.A., McPhee, S.J., Jenkins, C., Fordham, D. Three strategies to promote cancer screening: How feasible is wide-scale implementation? *Medical Care* 28: 1005-1012, 1990.

Cohen, S.J., Christen, A.G., Katz, B.P., Drook, C.A., Davis, B.J., Smith, D.M., Stookey, G.K. Counseling medical and dental patients about cigarette smoking: The impact of nicotine gum and chart reminders. *American Journal of Public Health* 77: 313-316, 1987.

Cohen, S.J., Stookey, G.K., Katz, B.P., Drook, C.A., Smith, D.M. Encouraging primary care physicians to help smokers quit: A randomized, controlled trial. *Annals of Internal Medicine* 110(8): 648-652, 1989.

Cummings, S.R., Coates, T.J., Richard, R.J., Hansen, B., Zahnd, E.G., Vander Martin, R., Duncan, C., Gerbert, B., Martin, A., Stein, M.J. Training physicians in counseling about smoking cessation: A randomized trial of the "Quit for Life" program. *Annals of Internal Medicine* 110(8): 640-647, 1989a.

Cummings, S.R., Richard, R.J., Duncan, C.L., Hansen, B., Vander Martin, R., Gerbert, B., Coates, T. Training physicians about smoking cessation: A controlled trial in private practice. *Journal of General Internal Medicine* 4(6): 482-489, 1989b.

Cummings, S.R., Rubin, S.M., Oster, G. The cost-effectiveness of counseling smokers to quit. *Journal of the American Medical Association* 261(1): 75-79, 1989c.

Fordham, D., McPhee, S.J., Bird, J.A., Rodnick, J.E., Detmer, W.M. The cancer prevention reminder system. *M.D. Computing* 7(5): 289-295, 1990.

Green, L.W., Wilson, A.L., Lovato, C.Y. What changes can health promotion achieve and how long do these changes last? The trade-offs between expediency and durability. *Preventive Medicine* 15: 508-521, 1986.

Martin, A.R., Coates, T.J. A clinician's guide to helping patients change behavior. *Western Journal of Medicine* 146: 751-753, 1987.

McPhee, S.J., Bird, J.A. Implementation of cancer prevention guidelines in clinical practice. *Journal of General Internal Medicine* 5(Suppl.): S116-S122, 1990.

McPhee, S.J., Bird, J.A., Fordham, D., Rodnick, J.E., Osborn, E.H. Promoting cancer prevention activities by primary care physicians: Results of a randomized, controlled trial. *Journal of the American Medical Association* 266: 538-544, 1991.

McPhee, S.J., Detmer, W.M. Office-based interventions to improve delivery of cancer prevention services by primary care physicians. *Cancer*, in press.

McPhee, S.J., Richard, R.J., Solkowitz, S.N. Performance of cancer screening in a university internal medicine practice: Comparison with the 1980 American Cancer Society guidelines. *Journal of General Internal Medicine* 1: 275-281, 1986.

Osborn, E.H., Bird, J.A., McPhee, S.J., Rodnick, J.E., Fordham, D. Cancer screening by primary care physicians: Can we explain the differences? *Journal of Family Practice* 32: 465-471, 1991.

Schmittling, G.T. Computer use by family physicians in the United States. *Journal of Family Practice* 29(2): 198-200, 1989.

Physicians' and Dentists' Roles in COMMIT—The Community Intervention Trial for Smoking Cessation

Elizabeth A. Lindsay, Judith K. Ockene, Larry Berger,
Norman Hymowitz, Paul Pomrehn, and Douglas M. Wilson

INTRODUCTION The National Cancer Institute's Division of Cancer Prevention and Control has initiated and supported more than 60 smoking cessation intervention trials in North America since 1980. A major goal of these trials is to test the efficacy of delivering antismoking interventions through diverse sectors or channels within a community, for example, worksites, health care providers, existing clinical programs, schools, and mass media.

In 1987, NCI embarked on its most extensive effort to help large numbers of smokers achieve smoking cessation. The Community Intervention Trial for Smoking Cessation task is to implement community-based interventions that have been demonstrated to help smokers, especially heavy smokers, achieve and maintain cessation. COMMIT involves 11 matched pairs of communities throughout North America. One community from each pair was randomly selected for a comprehensive tobacco-use intervention (COMMIT Research Group, 1991).

Building on the extensive experiences of past and ongoing smoking cessation studies supported by NCI, community-based heart disease prevention efforts, and other groups involved in smoking cessation, COMMIT has combined interventions into a comprehensive program designed to have an impact on the smoking patterns of an entire community. Through a community organization approach, citizens from the community with professional staff support assume the major role in planning, adapting, and implementing the interventions (Lichtenstein et al., 1990-91).

TRIAL GOALS Although the overall goal of COMMIT is to reduce community-wide smoking in general and heavy smoking in particular, the primary hypothesis tested in COMMIT is that implementation of a defined intervention protocol will result in at least 10 percent higher quit rates among heavy smokers in the intervention communities than among those in the comparison communities. There are a number of intermediate trial goals that include

- Increasing the priority of smoking cessation as a public health issue;
- Increasing the community capacity to modify the smoking behavior of its residents;

- Enhancing existing political and economic factors that discourage smoking within the community; and
- Increasing societal norms and values that support nonsmoking.

TRIAL DESIGN AND ENDPOINTS

After the initial selection of communities, three general periods of activity characterize the trial: planning and mobilization (phase I, January 1987 to December 1989), intervention (phase II, January 1990 to December 1992), and final assessment and analysis (phase III, January to December 1993) (COMMIT Research Group, 1991).

Evaluation Of the COMMIT Intervention

Cross-sectional and cohort surveys will assess the smoking status of community members in both experimental and control communities. In addition, there are a wide variety of surveys and other data collection activities that will measure impact, process, and cost of the COMMIT interventions (Lichtenstein et al., 1990-91; Mattson et al., 1990-91).

Selection of Communities

At the beginning of this project, NCI selected 11 matched pairs of communities for participation in COMMIT: 10 in the United States and 1 in Canada. A community was broadly defined and could include well-defined portions of major metropolitan areas or two small cities in a geographic region. Ideally, communities within pairs were to have some geographical separation to maintain independence of intervention activities and prevent contamination. Within a pair, communities were matched for general sociodemographic factors, including population size, demographic profile (e.g., proportion of females, age distribution, educational distribution), mobility and migration patterns, extent of urbanization, estimated smoking prevalence rates, and access to intervention channels (e.g., health care services, number of worksites, media resources, cessation services).

The populations in the communities vary from 52,493 to 166,824, with comparable means for pooled intervention and comparison communities. Overall, the intervention and comparison communities are well matched on general sociodemographic variables. Another characterization of the matching process involved cluster analysis and respective American and Canadian census data for eight demographic variables on which the pairs should demonstrate agreement: racial distribution, Hispanic ethnicity, gender by age, gender by marital status, general occupational category, educational attainment, family income, and years resident in the current household. This analysis verified the comparability of the households.

A baseline survey provided information on smoking prevalence and recent quit rates for the community pairs, and we found that the community pairs were also well matched on smoking prevalence and recent cessation behavior (COMMIT Research Group, 1991).

TRIAL ORGANIZATION AND INTERVENTION The communities deliver the COMMIT intervention through an organizational approach in which the community volunteers and staff are heavily involved in the entire project and have considerable input in decisionmaking (Thompson et al., 1990-91). The research institutes and the communities work in partnership to maintain trial integrity. It is necessary to find a balance between the research requirements for standardization of the intervention and community needs for participation and control. COMMIT provides a standard protocol to the communities that allows enough flexibility to accommodate local variations. There are 57 activities described in the protocol, and these are divided into four categories: worksites and other organizations, cessation resources and services, public education, and health care providers. We focus here on health care providers. For a complete description of all the activities, see Ockene et al. (1990-91); Pomrehn et al. (1990-91); Sorensen et al. (1990-91); and Wallack and Sciandra (1990-91).

GOALS FOR HEALTH CARE PROVIDERS Based on the understanding of how health care providers can influence smoking cessation, the following overall goals guide activities in this channel:

- Health care providers will be aware of, promote, and play an active role in smoking intervention efforts in the community;
- Health care providers will regard smoking cessation advice as the minimal standard of practice; some providers will go beyond providing advice;
- All health care facilities will adopt and effectively implement policies for a smoke-free environment; and
- Smoking patients will more actively seek assistance from the health care system to stop smoking.

INTERVENTION PROTOCOL To achieve these specific goals, we developed activities and established impact objectives and timelines. Figure 8 presents the impact objectives. COMMIT surveys (Mattson et al., 1990-91) measure progress in achieving such impact objectives, but these data are not yet available. Primary care physicians and dentists are the focus of the health care provider protocol because they see a large percentage of smokers each year and because they are generally receptive to doing preventive interventions. Targeted physician groups include the primary care specialties of internal and general medicine, family practice, obstetrics and gynecology, and osteopathy. Targeted dental offices are those practicing general dentistry.

The protocol requires activities that educate practicing physicians and dental health teams, involve them in promoting community-wide smoking control activities, and establish smoke-free offices and hospitals. Figure 9 presents the required activities for this channel. Whenever possible, we promote links among other channel activities in the protocol to reinforce the

Figure 8
Health Care Provider Task Force impact objectives for 1993

1. Among heavy smokers who have visited a physician or dentist in the past 12 months, increase the percentage who report having been told to stop smoking or asked to set a quit date by their physician or dentist.
   - Sixty percent of smokers will report having been told by a physician and 35 percent by a dentist to stop smoking;
   - Twenty-five percent of smokers will report having been asked by a physician and 20 percent by a dentist to set a date for stopping smoking.
2. Increase the percentage of physicians and dentists who report setting stop-smoking dates with patients most of the time.
   - Twenty-five percent of physicians and 20 percent of dentists will report setting stop-smoking dates with patients most of the time.
3. Increase the percentage of health care facilities (e.g., doctor and dentist offices, clinics, hospitals) that do not allow smoking by either patients or staff.
   - Ninety percent of physicians' and dentists' offices and other health care facilities will be smoke-free.

effects of the protocol. For example, the smokers' network and local cessation program guides, both of which are primarily cessation resource activities, are actively promoted through health care settings.

Some communities are finding that other health care professionals such as pharmacists and occupational and public health nurses are ready and able to reach smokers and have chosen to include them in COMMIT activities. For example, in Brantford, Ontario, chiropractors attended training events with family physicians, and physician leaders provided special events for public health nurses.

Approximately 30 physician and 30 dental offices were randomly selected in each community for a telephone survey in 1990. Office staff in these practices were asked about office smoking policies and available cessation resources (impact objectives 2 and 3 in Figure 8). Mailed surveys were sent to all primary care physicians and general practice dentists to determine their counseling cessation practices.

Physician and Dental Training

There are three levels of training activities provided for physicians and dental care teams designed to achieve the educational goals and facilitate regular counseling of all smokers following a standard protocol.

The *most advanced level of training* develops leadership and educational skills for medical and dental care teams within the intervention communities. This *train-the-trainers* approach uses national training seminars to build the

Figure 9
Health Care Provider Task Force intervention activities

1. Train leaders for basic and comprehensive continuing education sessions for physicians and dental health professionals.
2. Provide basic continuing education sessions for physicians.
3. Provide comprehensive continuing education sessions for physicians.
4. Provide basic continuing education sessions for dental health professionals.
5. Provide comprehensive continuing education sessions for dental health professionals.
6. Determine strategies for motivating and training office staff.
7. Promote smokers' network.
8. Influence training of physicians and dental health professionals.
9. Promote smoke-free policies in health care facilities.

capacity of medical and dental care teams within the communities to deliver the other two levels of training. The objectives of these training events are as follows:

- Developing the leadership skills of health care providers from the community to enable them to offer education to their colleagues regarding smoking cessation;
- Teaching the participants the recommended content and timing for basic and comprehensive educational events and providing resources that will help them to be effective educators in their home settings;
- Providing a variety of learning strategies that demonstrate how to develop smoking cessation intervention skills; and
- Providing ideas for the marketing of educational events in smoking cessation.

A central component of these train-the-trainers seminars is an actual demonstration of the comprehensive workshop for community physicians and oral health teams. In addition, the faculty makes suggestions for how to plan, market, and deliver the course. It is expected that these health care providers will work with COMMIT staff and often with local continuing education organizations to make the courses successful.

National experts in the clinical aspects of smoking cessation designed the materials for the train-the-trainers seminars and serve as the instructors. The seminars provide both information and practice in conducting comprehensive training workshops in the local communities. The leaders place particular emphasis on experiential techniques and providing feedback to participants. Intervention strategies are taught through lectures, demonstration, practice, and videotaped simulations. In addition to the events specifically for COMMIT leaders, NCI offers these advanced workshops in conjunction with regional and national professional meetings, to encourage participation by community health providers throughout the United States.

One or two physicians from each of the intervention communities attended a national training seminar in January 1989. They learned how to deliver both a 1-hour introductory type of session (*basic training*) as well as the longer skills-development workshop. These physicians have served as training resources in providing continuing medical education opportunities for physicians during the 1990 program year. Parallel training was also provided for oral health teams from each community during 1990.

Basic training is a 40- to 60-minute presentation by local health care providers who attend the national training and by invited guest speakers. These sessions motivate physicians and dentists to intervene with smokers and promote interest in more comprehensive, advanced training. Basic training emphasizes the following areas:

- The health benefits of smoking cessation;
- Importance and effectiveness of health care provider intervention;
- How to create an office environment and practice that supports smoking cessation and maintenance;
- A brief summary of intervention strategies;
- Factors that often interfere with maintaining cessation and how to address them; and
- Steps to further develop clinical skills in cessation counseling.

The presentations work well when they are incorporated into established networks for professional development and continuing education, such as grand rounds at local hospitals and regular meetings of professional organizations.

Comprehensive training offers more detailed instruction and demonstrations of how to create and deliver effective smoking cessation interventions in physicians' and dentists' offices. This training includes video demonstrations and opportunities to practice intervention skills and build on the content of the basic training. Attendees receive a manual instructing them in the physician-delivered smoking intervention steps.

Training for the oral health care team is similar to the physician training but has a greater emphasis on the role of the dental assistant or hygienist. There is also more content on prevention of smoking because dentists see teenagers more often than do physicians. Dentists and other members of the oral health team attend training in intervention procedures and planning office routines. They receive an instructional manual and other resource materials designed especially for the dental office.

There are a total of 909 primary care physicians altogether (the mean was 83 per community) and 731 general practice dentists (the mean was 66 per community) in the intervention communities. During the 4 years of intervention, a major goal is to attract 80 percent (727) of primary care physicians and 65 percent (475) of general care dentists to training events. All sites have conducted health care provider training and have achieved the process objectives expected at this stage of the trial (Ockene et al., 1990-91).

Influential Activities

Each community, through a community analysis, has identified influential health care professionals who are interested in smoking as a community health problem. In addition to their involvement in continuing medical and dental education, these "influentials" stimulate community change by promoting smoke-free health care facilities; supporting new regulations—and the enforcement of existing regulations—about the sale of tobacco to minors, and smoking in public places, schools, and worksites; and serving as spokespeople with the media, schools, and community groups. COMMIT staff members provide assistance to health care provider "influentials" in the form of a training manual with learning resources; materials from Doctors Ought to Care (a national physician group involved in innovative—and often humorous—antitobacco activities); and materials and training in media and legislative advocacy.

DISCUSSION AND CONCLUSIONS

Physicians, dentists, and other health care providers can serve as role models, advocate healthier environments, and encourage smokers to quit. Given that a large percentage of heavy smokers visit a physician and/or a dentist each year, the clinician's role in facilitating smoking cessation is important from both clinical and public health perspectives. The results of the COMMIT baseline evaluation survey confirm the importance of health care providers in the smoking cessation effort. Most smokers are aware that smoking is harmful to their health and say that they would try to stop smoking if told to do so by their physicians. The general public is very supportive of nonsmoking norms for health care facilities, and many smokers agree that smoking should at least be restricted in such settings.

Given these considerations, there is considerable logic to the COMMIT protocol, including the health care channel. Key goals are to train physicians, dentists, and other health care professionals to counsel or advise smokers to stop smoking; to set up their office practices to facilitate smoking intervention; and to advocate smoke-free health care facilities and smoking-related legislation.

Health care providers affect their colleagues' response and professional norms through their leadership roles as members of the COMMIT community board, in the Health Care Provider Task Force, and as representatives of their own professional societies and agencies. Not all health care providers are participating, and there are barriers to the integration into practice of systematic, effective smoking interventions. These barriers include time constraints, provider skepticism that they can "really make a difference" in getting smokers to quit, competing demands, and limited training in cessation counseling techniques. However, the educational events and materials provided to health care professionals not only build skills in working with smokers but also demonstrate how to integrate this work into regular office routines. Appendix A, at the end of this chapter, provides case studies to illustrate how three communities have implemented the COMMIT standardized protocol.

The COMMIT intervention is built on the premise that the interaction of many activities will magnify the impact of any one approach. Mobilization of the health care community will increase the chances of achieving the goals of COMMIT and of having a demonstrable impact on smoking cessation.

REFERENCES

COMMIT Research Group. Community Intervention Trial for Smoking Cessation (COMMIT): Summary of design and intervention. *Journal of the National Cancer Institute* 83: 1620-1628, 1991.

Deyo, R.A., Bass, J.E. Lifestyle and low-back pain: The influence of smoking and obesity. *Spine* 14: 501-506, 1989.

Lanier, D.C., Stockton, P. Clinical predictors of outcome of acute episodes of low back pain. *Journal of Family Practice* 27: 483-489, 1988.

Lichtenstein, E., Wallack L., Pechacek, T.F. Introduction to the Community Intervention Trial for Smoking Cessation (COMMIT). *International Quarterly of Community Health Education* 11(3): 173-185, 1990-91.

Mattson, M.D., Cummings, K.M., Lynn, W.R., Giffen, C., Corle, D., Pechacek, T. Evaluation plan for the Community Intervention Trial for Smoking Cessation (COMMIT). *International Quarterly of Community Health Education* 11(3): 271-290, 1990-91.

Ockene, J.K., Lindsay, E., Berger, L., Hymowitz, N. Health care providers as key change agents in the Community Intervention Trial for Smoking Cessation (COMMIT). *International Quarterly of Community Health Education* 11(3): 223-237, 1990-91.

Pomrehn, P., Sciandra, R., Shipley, R., Lynn, W., Lando, H. Enhancing resources for smoking cessation through community intervention: COMMIT as prototype. *International Quarterly of Community Health Education* 11(3): 259-269, 1990-91.

Sorensen, G., Glasgow, R.E., Corbett, K. Promoting smoking control through worksites in the Community Intervention Trial for Smoking Cessation (COMMIT). *International Quarterly of Community Health Education* 11(3): 239-257, 1990-91.

Thompson, B., Wallack, L., Lichtenstein, E., Pechacek, T. Principles of community organization and partnership for smoking cessation in the Community Intervention Trial for Smoking Cessation (COMMIT). *International Quarterly of Community Health Education* 11(3): 187-203, 1990-91.

Wallack, L., Sciandra, R. Media advocacy and public education in the Community Intervention Trial for Smoking Cessation (COMMIT). *International Quarterly of Community Health Education* 11(3): 205-222, 1990-91.

Dissemination of Physician-Based Smoking Cessation Interventions[3]

Michael G. Goldstein, Nancy A. MacDonald,
Raymond Niaura, and Catherine Dubé

INTRODUCTION Although the vast majority of physicians recognize the importance of smoking cessation as a disease-preventive measure, few physicians are confident of their ability to help patients stop smoking (Ockene et al., 1988a; Orleans et al., 1985; Schwartz, 1987; Valente et al., 1986; Wechsler et al., 1983; Wells et al., 1984). Several factors help explain the limited involvement of physicians in smoking interventions: limited knowledge of the effectiveness of their own counseling and advice; lack of counseling skills; little or no reimbursement for counseling; lack of organizational support in the office environment; and limited availability of materials to aid them and their patients in smoking cessation efforts (Battista et al., 1986; Kottke et al., 1987; Lewis et al., 1986; Ockene et al., 1988a; Orlandi, 1987; Orleans et al., 1985; Valente et al., 1986; Wechsler et al., 1983; Wells et al., 1984). Therefore, it appears that deficits in primary care physicians' knowledge, skills, and attitudes about smoking interventions, system and organizational barriers, and lack of incentives interact to limit the effective use of smoking cessation interventions in primary care settings.

Phase III studies, defined by the National Cancer Institute as controlled intervention trials (Greenwald, 1985; Greenwald and Cullen, 1984), have demonstrated that physician behavior can be changed through training (Lindsay et al., 1989; Ockene et al., 1988b; Strecher et al., 1991; Wilson et al., 1988), reminders on patients' charts (Cheney and Ramsdell, 1987; Cohen et al., 1987; McDonald et al., 1984), computer reminders (McPhee et al., 1989), and other techniques (Battista et al., 1986). Phase III trials have also demonstrated clearly the effectiveness of physician-delivered interventions to achieve smoking cessation (Cummings et al., 1989a; Kottke et al., 1988; Ockene, 1987; Ockene et al., 1991; Schwartz, 1987; Wilson et al., 1988). However, physicians who have participated in such research were volunteers, which limits the generalizability of the findings.

The percentage of eligible, practicing, primary care physicians who participated in NCI-funded phase III studies of community-based physicians ranged from 5 percent to 50 percent (Cummings et al., 1989b; Kottke et al., 1990; Wilson et al., 1988). Thus, it is unknown whether proven physician-

[3] Supported in part by the National Cancer Institute, Cancer Prevention Research Consortium, grant no. P01-CA50087, to James O. Prochaska, David B. Abrams, Wayne Velicer, and Michael G. Goldstein.

delivered smoking cessation strategies can be effectively disseminated within a representative sample of community-based physicians. Phase IV studies (Greenwald, 1985) that employ representative samples of community-based physicians are needed to test the effectiveness of physician-delivered smoking cessation interventions.

Investigators at the NCI-funded Cancer Prevention Research Consortium (University of Rhode Island, Miriam Hospital, and Brown University) are addressing the need for phase IV studies by testing a strategy to accelerate the adoption and implementation of smoking intervention protocols within a defined population of primary care physicians. The following sections discuss the models and strategies used in the Physicians Counseling Smokers Project, a phase IV study of physician-delivered smoking interventions.

DIFFUSION THEORY AND APPLICATION

Rogers (1983) and Orlandi (1987) have described models for the process by which innovations in health promotion, such as physician-delivered smoking cessation interventions, are diffused throughout medical care settings over time. The first phase, adoption of an innovation in the primary care setting, occurs when physicians accept the innovation and begin to put it to use (Rogers, 1983). The adoption of a new technique or technology generally encompasses several steps, beginning with awareness of the innovation and a personal interest in pursuing further knowledge. An evaluation and trial period follows as a physician weighs the advantages and disadvantages of the innovation against current practices. For example, in the case of smoking interventions, the physician attempts to foresee how additional interventions with smokers would fit with current practice and workflow. The final step of adoption is taken when the innovation is accepted and a decision is made to use it.

Active approaches to influencing and enhancing adoption of innovations are termed dissemination efforts. In the medical setting, dissemination efforts may include the use of influential physicians as change agents (Rogers, 1983). Such physicians may influence adoption if they express support and encouragement to other physicians and serve as role models in their own practices. Recently, Lomas and colleagues had considerable success in changing physician behavior by using local physician leaders to disseminate practice guidelines regarding cesarean sections (Lomas et al., 1991). Brief presentations to increase awareness of the innovation at hospital staff meetings, grand rounds, or in professional newsletters may also enhance the dissemination process.

The second phase in the diffusion process is implementation, which can be defined as the effective use of the innovation by physicians over time. It is obvious that the eventual success of an innovation depends on how well it is implemented by the targeted user group (Orlandi, 1987). Successful implementation is enhanced by the use of specific protocols and materials as well as other resources that enable physicians to integrate the innovation easily into their office practice system (Orlandi, 1987).

Orlandi (1987) described a "linkage" process to overcome obstacles to diffusion; a linkage system serves as a bridge between the technology of health promotion, its supporting resources, and the actual recipients of the interventions. In the diffusion of physician-delivered interventions to general medical care settings, a linkage system might include medical societies and other professional organizations, regional health departments, government agencies (e.g., NCI), hospitals, health maintenance organizations, medical schools, and voluntary organizations (e.g., American Cancer Society and American Lung Association). The ideal linkage system contains representatives from the resource group that developed or planned the innovation, the intermediary providers of the innovation (i.e., physicians providing smoking interventions and medical decisionmakers from the health care system), and the patients who are the targets of the innovation (Orlandi, 1987). Following a collaborative model, the linkage system works toward identifying the needs, capabilities, and concerns of each group within the system. "Change agents" or new organizational structures may be established to facilitate the linkage process (Orlandi, 1987).

Influential physicians in the community can play an important role in the diffusion process, especially if they are "early adopters" (Rogers, 1983). Early adopters may serve as role models for other physicians who may initially be less active and involved ("laggards") (Rogers, 1983). Adoption and implementation rates may be affected also by factors such as compatibility and complexity of an innovation in comparison to current practices, the relative advantage of an innovation over current behaviors, the ability to adopt the innovation on a trial basis, and the degree to which results of an adopted and implemented innovation are readily visible or measurable (Rogers, 1983).

These principles of diffusion theory can be used in the design of interventions to increase the dissemination and implementation of physician-delivered smoking cessation methods.

TRANSTHEORETICAL MODEL

The transtheoretical model of change provides a conceptual framework for understanding the process of individuals' behavior change (Prochaska and DiClemente, 1983 and 1986). This model is based on observations that individuals considering or undergoing behavioral change, such as stopping smoking, pass through a predictable sequence of stages (Prochaska and DiClemente, 1983 and 1986), as shown in Figure 10.

Individuals in the precontemplation stage are either unaware of the problem or deny it, and they are not motivated to make a behavior change in the foreseeable future. The contemplation stage is a stage of ambivalence, when pros and cons related to change are weighed without a definite commitment to action. Individuals in the preparation stage have taken steps to change their behavior but have not yet taken definitive action. Those who have reached the action stage have initiated behavior change. Maintenance is reached when an individual has successfully made a change for some time but continues to monitor behavior to prevent slips or relapses. Prochaska and

Figure 10
Stages of change

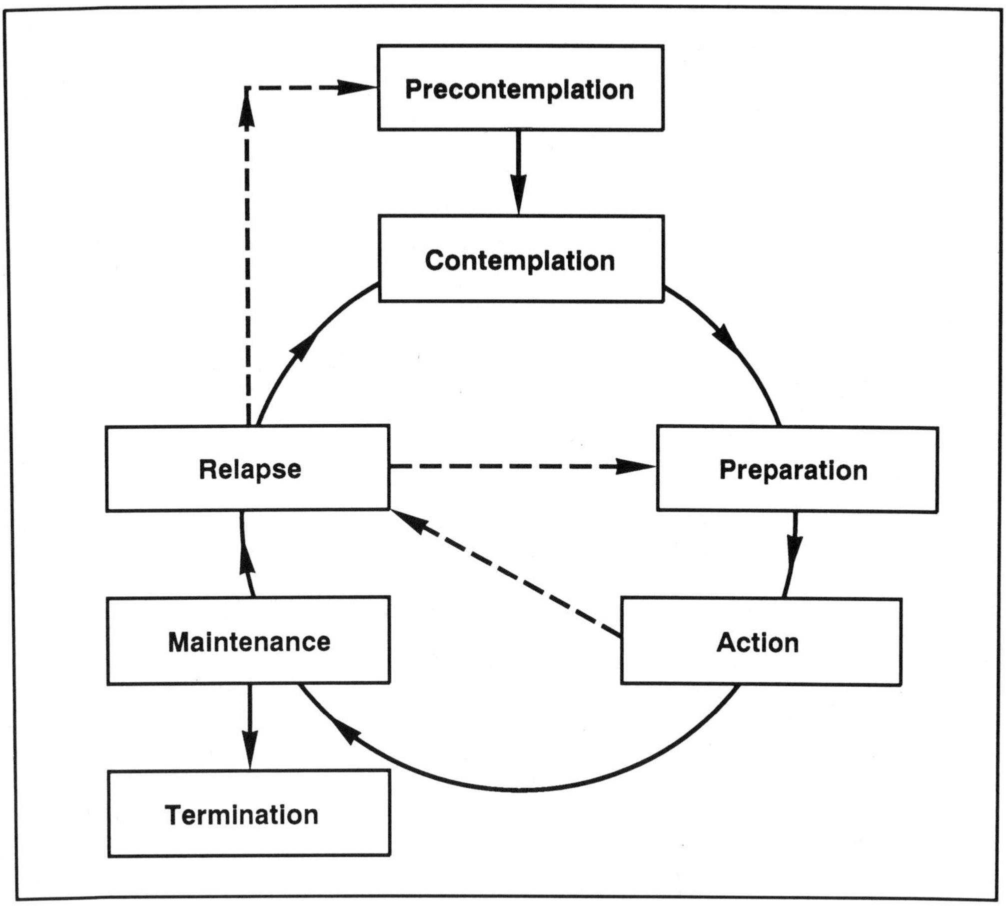

Source: Adapted from Prochaska and DiClemente, 1983.

DiClemente (1986) found that individual smokers may take several years to move through the stages of change, and moreover they may cycle repeatedly through the last four stages.

Prochaska and DiClemente (1983 and 1986) have also identified specific experiential, cognitive, and behavioral processes that facilitate movement through the stages of behavior change. Of great importance is their finding that the processes of change that are used by individuals vary across stages. For example, individuals in the precontemplation stage are more likely to use cognitive strategies, such as consciousness-raising, while individuals in the action stage are more likely to use behavioral strategies, such as stimulus control and counter-conditioning. On the basis of these findings, Prochaska and DiClemente have suggested that clinical interventions to facilitate behavioral change will be most successful if they are matched to the individual's stage of change (DiClemente et al., 1991; Prochaska and Goldstein, 1991) and have successfully tested this hypothesis in clinical smoking cessation trials (Prochaska et al., 1990). The transtheoretical model of change has now been successfully applied to behaviors other than smoking cessation, including behavior change that requires adoption of healthy behaviors (Marcus et al., 1992; Rakowski et al., 1992).

Physician behavior change, including the adoption and implementation of smoking cessation interventions, may also move through stages of change as described in the transtheoretical model. For example, physicians at the precontemplation stage have not yet accepted the idea of adopting smoking interventions into their office practices. Physicians in the contemplation stage are seriously considering providing smoking interventions but have not decided to take action, whereas physicians in the preparation stage have taken steps to implement protocols in their office (adoption) but have not used them regularly. Physicians in the action and maintenance stages are actively implementing smoking cessation protocols and systems.

This characterization of physician stage of change may assist those who attempt to influence the diffusion of physician-delivered interventions. Strategies that are matched to a physician's stage of change may be most effective in changing the physician's behavior and accelerating the rate of adoption and implementation of physician-delivered smoking cessation interventions. For example, physicians who express little or no interest in adopting smoking intervention strategies (precontemplators) might be more likely to respond if their awareness of the effectiveness of physician-delivered interventions were increased. Contemplators might respond to personal contact with a "consultant" who could assess their motivational barriers and offer potential solutions, resources, and support. Although these actions are not likely to lead to immediate adoption and implementation, physicians may move to an intermediate stage that will facilitate eventual adoption of the intervention practices. Physicians who are in the preparation or action stage are likely to be responsive to such intervention as the offer of counseling skills training or education in the use of smoker assessment questionnaires. Physicians in the maintenance stage may benefit from reminders to provide smoking counseling (e.g., chart stickers) or from reinforcement for their activity (e.g., from chart audits and/or feedback from patient satisfaction questionnaires).

PHYSICIANS COUNSELING SMOKERS

Diffusion theory and the transtheoretical model were used in the design of the Physicians Counseling Smokers Project, a component of the Rhode Island Cancer Prevention Research Consortium. The consortium was funded by NCI in September 1989. Physicians Counseling Smokers was designed to address the following specific aims:

- Assess the impact of a comprehensive, community-based intervention on the rates of adoption, implementation, and maintenance of physician-delivered smoking cessation interventions;

- Measure the impact of the comprehensive intervention on physicians' knowledge, attitudes, and practice behavior and on community smoking cessation outcomes; and
- Identify individual, system, and organizational factors that predict physicians' adoption, implementation, and maintenance of physician-delivered smoking cessation interventions.

The entire community of physicians providing primary care to the people of the State of Rhode Island is the target population for the study. All primary care physicians in one distinct Rhode Island geographic area received the experimental intervention for a period of 15 months. Physicians in two other geographic areas served as "untreated" controls. After 15 months, a crossover feature was implemented and a second area was targeted for intervention, while physicians in the third area remain "untreated" for the entire 3-year intervention period. The intervention began in the spring of 1991. Both physician outcomes (knowledge, attitudes, and behavior) and community and population smoking outcomes are to be measured. The population outcomes will be derived from a representative sample of approximately 4,200 Rhode Island smokers recruited for the Rhode Island Cancer Prevention Research Consortium projects.

Recruitment and Preparation

According to diffusion theory, adoption must precede implementation (Orlandi, 1987). For adoption to occur, physicians must become aware of the innovation and its potential usefulness. Thus, an important first step in the diffusion process is preparing members of the population to enhance their participation in the project. In a phase IV study (Greenwald, 1985; Greenwald and Cullen, 1984), the recruitment strategy must maximize participation among eligible physicians to create a representative sample and must avoid creating barriers to widespread participation. Care must be taken to avoid placing any additional burden on physicians by the requirements of participation in the research aspects of the study (e.g., measurement). Recruitment and enrollment of physicians into the study thus becomes a crucial first step in the overall strategy to increase diffusion of smoking interventions within this population.

Several avenues were used to enhance awareness of the project in an attempt to increase recruitment and hence participation. First, intermediary organizations were enlisted to help create a linkage system to aid in the recruitment of physicians (Orlandi, 1987). A physician advisory committee was formed, according to the principles of community activation (Bracht and Kingsbury, 1990), to generate ownership and demand for the intervention among the leaders in the physician community. Advisory committee members included local and state medical society leaders, hospital and health maintenance organization medical staff presidents, professional medical organization representatives, and voluntary agency board members. The project staff met with advisory committee members to familiarize them with the goals of the project and to solicit their input regarding the proposed recruitment and intervention process. Support was generated among advisory committee members for the intervention, and strategies to effectively reach and involve other physicians were discussed.

Committee members agreed to assist in the enrollment process through recruitment phone calls to colleagues. The demand on physician "recruiters" was kept minimal, in that each was asked to make only a brief phone call (2 minutes) to each person on a defined list of physicians (an average of 8 to 10 calls per physician). The recruiter was asked to state the goals of the project briefly, endorse the project, and encourage physicians to enroll when approached. Dietrich (1990), using a similar recruitment strategy, successfully recruited a large sample of community-based primary care physicians for an office-based cancer prevention project.

A targeted promotional campaign was also developed to increase awareness about the project. The campaign included items in hospital medical newsletters, mailings to eligible physicians from influential physicians (e.g., director of the State health department and president of the state medical society), and announcements about the project in the state medical society newsletters. Finally, grand rounds sessions were given in community hospitals during the recruitment period. In addition to providing an overview of the project and presenting compelling statistics about the importance of physician counseling for smoking cessation, each session included a short "trigger video" that was designed to increase physician awareness of patients' views about physician advice to quit smoking. Discussion points covered in the session included patient and physician expectations about recommendations to quit smoking and the positive impact physicians can have on patient decisions about health behaviors. The authors recognized the potential problem of contaminating the baseline survey by providing this session at grand rounds. When weighing the risk of influencing the physician baseline by providing this brief educational session versus the potential for increased enrollment, they decided that the grand rounds were needed to generate demand for the project and enhance recruitment. Grand rounds were provided in both the control and the intervention areas, decreasing the likelihood that the baseline would be affected differentially across conditions.

During the early phase of the recruitment process, the investigators learned several useful points. One was about the relative lack of interest in the scientific aspect of the project among eligible physicians. In Rhode Island, many physicians in community hospitals without university affiliations were not only reluctant but wary of being involved in a project that was designed primarily for research goals rather than service delivery. On the other hand, a factor that enhanced acceptance of the project (available only *because* the project is research-oriented) was the potential to provide physicians with feedback about their success in lowering smoking rates within their *own* communities. An overriding concern expressed by the advisory committee was that individual physicians might perceive that, by participating, they would have to do much more than they would do in typical interactions with patients. The investigators addressed this concern by emphasizing that physicians will be provided with the best available resources and strategies to allow smoking interventions to become a consistent, *more effective* part of their *usual* interaction with patients. It was emphasized that the research staff would also be working with office staff members to enhance their role in providing smoking interventions to patients, which could potentially decrease the current workload for physicians.

There were only two defined requirements for physician participation in the project: (1) completion of an annual questionnaire assessing physician knowledge, attitudes, and practices with respect to smoking cessation and interventions and (2) completion of an annual audit of each office practice to assess and document smoking cessation activities and resources that are currently in use. Physicians are able to select their level of participation in the intervention. They do not have to agree to use any of the protocols or resources that will be made available to them during the intervention period. Thus, the only requirements involved agreements to complete repeated assessment. Although surveys are often perceived as unpopular by physicians, the absence of a requirement to accept intervention protocols enhanced physician willingness to participate. We have succeeded in recruiting more than 80 percent of the eligible primary care physicians in the geographic areas selected for the study.

Delivery Of the Intervention

Delivery of the intervention to individual physicians is accomplished through the use of "office practice consultants," master's-level health care providers with health promotion training. Rather than using only the traditional CME format, an "academic detailing" approach will be used. This unique educational approach has been described by Soumerai and Avorn (1990); it extends the promotional practices used primarily by pharmaceutical sales representatives to university-based educational outreach. Characteristics of this approach include use of focus groups to understand the motivations of the targeted physicians, involving "opinion leaders," promoting active learner involvement, providing repetitive messages and reinforcement, using brief graphic materials, and training detailers to deal with resistant, indifferent, and less receptive physicians (Soumerai and Avorn, 1990).

Questionnaire data and informal interviews are used by office practice consultants to assess and "stage" individual physicians. As a result of the assessment, office practice consultants are able to personalize the intervention for each physician's practice. A physician-centered approach is used, in that each physician will have an intervention tailored to his or her expressed interest, current smoking cessation knowledge and attitudes, and baseline stage of adoption and implementation. Brief, intermittent "detail" visits and phone calls are scheduled with physicians to develop a plan of action for each physician, office, and staff. Printed materials developed by NCI and major voluntary agencies are distributed by the office practice consultants, when appropriate, to increase awareness, interest, knowledge, and activity. To facilitate the communication process, graphic flipcharts and brief handouts will be developed by the project staff. During four visits over a 1-year period, the office practice consultants can develop an ongoing relationship with physicians and office staff, negotiate plans for use of smoking cessation interventions, address barriers, and solve problems.

To increase the diffusion of available resources, the intervention will match individual physicians' interests and needs to their stage of adoption and implementation of smoking cessation protocols (Prochaska and DiClemente, 1986; Prochaska and Goldstein, 1991). For example, those physicians who have not yet made the decision to implement office systems to identify and track smokers (precontemplators or contemplators) are given information to increase their awareness of the effectiveness of such interventions without being asked for a commitment to implement them. During the course of the intervention, those physicians also are provided with a newsletter to inform them of the activity of their "early adopter" colleagues, who have already elected to implement aspects of the office-based smoking intervention program. Physicians in preparation and action stages who express a desire to implement smoking assessment and intervention systems are also provided with samples of resources and training on how to use them effectively.

Initial assessments by the office practice consultants are aided by new measures being developed by Prochaska and colleagues at the University of Rhode Island, which include the physician's stage of adoption and implementation of smoking cessation interventions. Our definition of stage of adoption was based on the NCI protocol for physicians that incorporates the four A's of patient counseling about smoking (Glynn and Manley, 1990):

- *Ask* (all patients about their smoking status);
- *Advise* (all smoking patients to quit);
- *Assist* (smoking patients with their smoking, regardless of their interest in quitting); and
- *Arrange* (followup visits with smokers).

The NCI counseling protocol was slightly modified, according to a patient-centered counseling approach (Grueninger et al., 1989), to include addressing the agenda (i.e., smoking) at each patient visit. "Ask" was changed to "assess" to cue the physician to assess the patient's stage of change as well as aspects of the patient's smoking history. Physicians who report that they routinely assist greater than 80 percent of their patients who smoke and arrange a followup specifically to discuss smoking are considered to be in the action stage.

Resources to be provided to the physician may include (1) educational materials about physician-delivered smoking interventions for physicians and their office staffs; (2) materials and systems for smoker identification, assessment, and tracking; (3) physician self-instruction manuals (i.e., Glynn and Manley, 1990); and (4) formal skill counseling workshops for physicians and staff members (see Table 3).

The education of physician participants, both during office practice consultant "detail" visits and at more traditional CME sessions, will include information on how to assess patients' smoking history, level of nicotine dependence, stage of change, reasons for smoking, pros and cons related to smoking, and ways to match interventions to individual smoking patients in light of these assessments (Goldstein et al., 1991; Prochaska and DiClemente, 1986; Prochaska and Goldstein, 1991). Training sessions for physicians in preparation or action stages will be voluntary and offered on site at community hospitals whenever feasible. These workshops will apply state-of-the-science educational techniques aimed at improving physicians counseling skills. Skill teaching will employ small-group methods, including role-play, video demonstration and review, and feedback techniques successful in the teaching of medical interviewing. In these sessions, physicians will be given the opportunity to learn more about smoking cessation counseling skills, practice applying these skills to simulated cases, and consider how these newly learned skills will be applied to their clinical practice. Other office personnel who provide primary care or patient education activities will be encouraged to

Table 3
Summary of intervention strategies for physicians

	Stage of Adoption/Implementation				
	Precontemplation	Contemplation	Preparation	Action	Maintenance
Office Practice Consultation	✔	✔	✔	✔	✔
Resource and Referral Lists	✔	✔	✔	✔	✔
NCI Office Manual	✔	✔	✔	✔	✔
Information About Reimbursement		✔	✔	✔	✔
Information About Physician Effectiveness	✔	✔	✔		
Materials for Patients			✔	✔	✔
Materials To Identify and Track Smokers			✔	✔	✔
Skill Training Workshop for Physician			✔	✔	✔
Training Workshop for Staff			✔	✔	✔

attend these sessions as well. Breakout groups will be employed for discussing the special concerns of each group of professionals attending the workshop.

Evaluation Of the Project

Efficacy of the physicians' intervention will be assessed through measured changes in (1) physician knowledge, attitudes, and behavior regarding smoking cessation interventions and (2) community smoking outcome measures. It is hypothesized that, after 3 years, physicians who receive the intervention will have increased their knowledge about smoking-related practices, developed more positive attitudes about smoking cessation, and increased their adoption and implementation of office-based smoking interventions. Moreover, this will result in a significantly smaller proportion of subjects who smoke in target intervention areas than in control areas. As noted previously, population-based outcomes will be derived from a representative sample of Rhode Island smokers recruited for the Rhode Island Cancer Prevention Research Consortium.

Presently, the investigators are in the final stages of developing the physician measures. They include

- An algorithm to categorize physician *stage of adoption and implementation;*
- A measure of *pros*, or benefits of the provision of smoking cessation interventions, and *cons*, or barriers to provision of smoking cessation intervention, adapted from a similar measure, the Decisional Balance Inventory, which was developed for smokers by Velicer and colleagues (Velicer et al., 1985);
- A *processes of change* measure, adapted from a measure derived from the transtheoretical model for smokers (Prochaska et al., 1988);
- *Smoking-related intervention practices* derived from Wells and colleagues (Wells et al., 1986);
- A *knowledge* questionnaire, derived from Ockene and colleagues (Ockene et al., 1988b); and
- A measure of physician *self-efficacy.*

As described previously, an annual audit of the office practice will be performed to assess and document smoking cessation activities and resources currently in use. The items to be assessed will include the presence of an office smoking policy, identification of an office smoking intervention coordinator, use of identification and tracking systems, use of patient education materials, use of a followup system, and presence of Physicians Counseling Smokers materials.

SUMMARY

The Physicians Counseling Smokers Project, a phase IV NCI-funded research project, was designed to assess the effectiveness of an intervention to disseminate physician-delivered smoking cessation protocols among a population of primary care physicians. In designing the intervention strategy, the investigators have incorporated principles of diffusion theory (Orlandi, 1987; Rogers, 1983), the transtheoretical model (Prochaska and DiClemente, 1983 and 1986; Prochaska and Goldstein, 1991); academic detailing (Soumerai and Avorn, 1990); and state-of-the-science physician educational strategies.

The population of physicians targeted for recruitment into the study is all primary care physicians serving adult smokers in Rhode Island. To recruit a representative sample of the physicians (more than 80 percent of eligible physicians in intervention areas), the authors had to develop a recruitment strategy that would maximize enrollment and participation. Thus, among the strategies used for recruitment are several that are derived from diffusion theory, including development of a "linkage system," and strategies to increase awareness of physician-delivered smoking interventions in the target population (Orlandi, 1987).

The intervention will disseminate the resources developed by NCI for physicians in office practice (Glynn and Manley, 1990) and will use academic detailers (Soumerai and Avorn, 1990), master's-level health care providers with experience in health promotion, to deliver much of the intervention. Physicians will be individually assessed, according to measures developed by the project team, and the intervention will be matched to each physician's stage of adoption and implementation, using the principles of the transtheoretical model developed by Prochaska and DiClemente (1983 and 1986).

If the intervention is effective in increasing the adoption and implementation of physician-delivered smoking cessation interventions, the investigators will be able to measure its effect on both physician behavior and patient smoking prevalence. Because the results should be generalizable to other community settings, a positive outcome will have much clinical and public health significance. Moreover, the intervention strategy could be easily adapted to diffuse other cancer prevention measures and, more generally, other health promotion innovations within the medical care community.

REFERENCES

Battista, R.N., Williams, J.I., MacFarlane, L.A. Determinants of primary medical practice in adult cancer prevention. *Medical Care* 24: 216-224, 1986.

Bracht, N., Kingsbury, L. Community organization principles in health promotion: A five-stage model. In: *Health Promotion at the Community Level*, N. Bracht (Editor). Newbury Park, CA: Sage Publications, 1990, pp. 66-86.

Cheney, C., Ramsdell, J.W. Effect of medical records checklists on implementation of periodic health measures. *American Journal of Medicine* 83: 129-136, 1987.

Cohen, S.J., Christen, A.G., Katz, B.P., Drook, C.A., Davis, B.J., Smith, D.M., Stookey, G.K. Counseling medical and dental patients about cigarette smoking: The impact of nicotine gum and chart reminders. *American Journal of Public Health* 77: 313-316, 1987.

Cummings, S.R., Coates, T.J., Richard, R.J., Hansen, B., Zahnd, E.G., Vander Martin, R., Duncan,C., Gerbert, B., Martin, A., Stein, M.J. Training physicians in counseling about smoking cessation: A randomized trial of the "Quit for Life" program. *Annals of Internal Medicine* 110(8): 640-647, 1989a.

Cummings, S.R., Richard, R.J., Duncan, C.L., Hansen, B., Vander Martin, R., Gerbert, B., Coates, T.J. Training physicians about smoking cessation: A controlled trial in private practice. *Journal of General Internal Medicine* 4(6): 482-489, 1989b.

DiClemente, C.C., Prochaska, J.O., Fairhurst, S.K., Velicer, W.F., Velasquez, M.M., Rossi, J.S. The process of smoking cessation: An analysis of precontemplation, contemplation and preparation stages of change. *Journal of Consulting and Clinical Psychology* 59: 295-304, 1991.

Dietrich, A.J., O'Connor, G., Keller, A., Carney-Gersten, P., Levy, D., Nelson, E., Simmons, J., Barrett, J., Jr., Landgraf, J.M. Will community physicians participate in rigorous studies of cancer control? The methodology and recruitment in a randomized trial of physician practices. In: *Advances in Cancer Control: Screening and Prevention Research* (Progress in Clinical Biology Series, volume 339), P.F. Engstrom, B. Rimer, and L.E. Mortenson (Editors). New York: Wiley-Liss, 1990, pp. 373-381.

Glynn, T.J., Manley, M.W. *How To Help Your Patients Stop Smoking: A National Cancer Institute Manual for Physicians.* U.S. Department of Health and Human Services, Public Health Service, National Institutes of Health, National Cancer Institute. NIH Publication No. 90-3064, 1990.

Goldstein, M.G., Guise, B.J., Ruggiero, L., Raciti, M.A., Abrams, D.B. Behavioral medicine strategies for medical patients. In: *Clinical Psychiatry for Medical Students*, A. Stoudemire (Editor). Philadelphia: J.B. Lippincott, 1990, pp. 609-628.

Goldstein, M.G., Niaura, R.S., Abrams, D.B. Pharmacologic and behavioral treatment of nicotine dependence: Nicotine as a drug of abuse. In: *Medical Psychiatric Practice* (volume 1), A. Stoudemire and B. Fogel (Editors). Washington, DC: American Psychiatric Press, 1991, pp. 541-596.

Greenwald, P. Prevention of cancer. In: *Principles and Practice of Preventive Oncology* (2nd edition), V.T. DeVita, Jr., S. Hellman, and S.A. Rosenberg (Editors). Philadelphia: J.B. Lippincott, 1985, pp. 197-214.

Greenwald, P., Cullen, J. The scientific approach to cancer control. *CA—A Cancer Journal for Clinicians* 34: 328-332, 1984.

Grueninger, U.J., Goldstein, M.G., Duffy, F.D. Patient education in hypertension: Five essential steps. *Journal of Hypertension* 7(Suppl. 3): S93-S98, 1989.

Kottke, T.E., Battista, R.N., DeFriese, G.H., Brekke, M.L. Attributes of successful smoking cessation interventions in medical practice: A meta-analysis of 39 controlled trials. *Journal of the American Medical Association* 259: 2882-2889, 1988.

Kottke, T.E., Blackburn, H., Brekke, M.L., Solberg, L.I. The systematic practice of preventive cardiology. *American Journal of Cardiology* 59: 690-694, 1987.

Kottke, T.E., Solberg, L.I., Conn, S., Maxwell, P., Thomasberg, M., Brekke, M.L., Brekke, M.J. A comparison of two methods to recruit physicians to deliver smoking cessation interventions. *Archives of Internal Medicine* 150: 1477-1481, 1990.

Lewis, C.E., Wells, K.B., Ware, J. A model for predicting the counseling practices of physicians. *Journal of General Internal Medicine* 1: 1-14, 1986.

Lindsay, E.A., Wilson, D.A., Best, J.A., Willms, D.G., Singer, J., Gilbert, J.R., Taylor, D.W., Hannah, W.J., Vayda, E. A randomized trial of physician training for smoking cessation. *American Journal of Health Promotion* 3: 11-18, 1989.

Lomas, J., Enkin, M., Anderson, G.M. Opinion leaders vs. audit and feedback to implement practice guidelines: Delivery after previous cesarean section. *Journal of the American Medical Association* 265: 2202-2207, 1991.

Marcus, B.H., Selby, V.C., Niaura, R.S., Rossi, J.S. Self-efficacy and the stages of exercise behavior change. *Research Quarterly for Exercise and Sports* 63(1): 60-66, 1992.

McDonald, C.J., Hui, S.L., Smith, D.M., Tierney, W.M., Cohen, S.J., Weinberger, M., McCabe, G.P. Reminders to physicians from an introspective computer medical record: A two-year randomized trial. *Annals of Internal Medicine* 100: 130-138, 1984.

McPhee, S.J., Bird, J.A., Jenkins, C.H., Fordham, D. Promoting cancer screening: A randomized, controlled trial of three interventions. *Archives of Internal Medicine* 149: 1866-1872, 1989.

Ockene, J.K. Physician-delivered interventions for smoking cessation: Strategies for increasing effectiveness. *Preventive Medicine* 16: 723-737, 1987.

Ockene, J.K., Aney, J., Goldberg, R.J., Klar, J.M., Williams, J.W. A survey of Massachusetts physicians' smoking intervention practices. *American Journal of Preventive Medicine* 4: 14-20, 1988a.

Ockene, J.K., Kristeller, J., Goldberg, R.J., et al. Increasing the efficacy of physician-delivered smoking interventions: A randomized clinical trial. *Journal of General Internal Medicine* 6: 1-8, 1991.

Ockene, J.K., Quirk, M.E., Goldberg, R.J., Kristeller, K.L., Donnelly, G., Kalan, K.L., Gould, B., Greene, H.L., Harrison-Atlas, R., Pease, J., Pickens, S., Williams, J.W. A residents' training program for the development of smoking intervention skills. *Archives of Internal Medicine* 148: 1039-1045, 1988b.

Orlandi, M.A. Promoting health and preventing disease in health care settings: An analysis of barriers. *Preventive Medicine* 16: 119-130, 1987.

Orleans, C.T., George, L.K., Houpt, J.L., Brodie, K.H. Health promotion in primary care: A survey of U.S. family practitioners. *Preventive Medicine* 14: 636-647, 1985.

Prochaska, J.O., DiClemente, C.C. Stages and processes of self-change of smoking: Toward an integrative model of change. *Journal of Consulting and Clinical Psychology* 51: 390-395, 1983.

Prochaska, J.O., DiClemente, C.C. Towards a comprehensive model of change. In: *Treating Addictive Disorders: Processes of Change,* W.R. Miller and N. Heather (Editors). New York: Plenum Press, 1986.

Prochaska, J.O., Goldstein, M.G. Processes of smoking cessation: Implications for clinicians. *Clinics in Chest Medicine* 12(4): 727-735, 1991.

Prochaska, J.O., Rossi, J.S., Velicer, W.F. A Comparison of Four Minimal Interventions for Smoking Cessation: An Outcome Evaluation. Paper presented at the Seventh World Congress on Tobacco and Health, Perth, Australia, 1990.

Prochaska, J.O., Velicer, W.F., DiClemente, C.C., Fava, J. Measuring processes of change: Applications to the cessation of smoking. *Journal of Consulting and Clinical Psychology* 56: 520-528, 1988.

Rakowski, W., Dubé, C., Marcus, B.H., Prochaska, J.O., Velicer, W.F., Abrams, D.B. Assessing elements of women's decisions about mammography. *Health Psychology* 11: 111-118, 1992.

Rogers, E.M. *Diffusion of Innovations* (3rd edition). New York: Free Press, 1983.

Schwartz, J.L. *Review and Evaluation of Smoking Cessation Methods: The United States and Canada, 1978-1985.* U.S. Department of Health and Human Services, Public Health Service, National Institutes of Health, National Cancer Institute, Division of Cancer Prevention and Control. NIH Publication No. 87-2940, 1987.

Soumerai, S.B., Avorn, J. Principles of educational outreach ("academic detailing") to improve clinical decisionmaking. *Journal of the American Medical Association* 263: 549-556, 1990.

Strecher, V.J., O'Malley, M.S., Villagra, V.G., et al. Can residents be trained to counsel patients about quitting smoking? Results from a randomized trial. *Journal of General Internal Medicine* 6: 9-17, 1991.

Valente, C.M., Sobal, J., Muncie, H.L., Levine, D.M., Antlitz, A.M. Health promotion: Physicians' beliefs, attitudes and practices. *American Journal of Preventive Medicine* 2: 82-88, 1986.

Velicer, W., DiClemente, C., Prochaska, J., Brandenburg, N. A decisional balance measure for predicting smoking cessation. *Journal of Personality and Social Psychology* 48: 1279-1289, 1985.

Wechsler, H., Levine, S., Idelson, R.K., Rohman, M., Taylor, J.O. The physician's role in health promotion: A survey of primary care practitioners. *New England Journal of Medicine* 308: 97-100, 1983.

Wells, K.B., Lewis, C.E., Leuke, B., Schleiter, M.K., Brook, P.H. The practices of general and subspecialty internists in counseling about smoking and exercise. *American Journal of Public Health* 76: 1009-1013, 1986.

Wells, K.B., Ware, J.E., Jr., Lewis, C.E. Physicians' attitudes in counseling patients about smoking. *Medical Care* 22(4): 360-365, 1984.

Wetzler, H.P., Cruess, D.F. Self-reported physical health practices and health care utilization: Findings from the National Health Interview Survey. *American Journal of Public Health* 75: 1329-1330, 1985.

Wilson, D.M., Taylor, D.W., Gilbert, J.R., Best, J.A., Lindsay, E.A., Willms, D.G., Singer, J. A randomized trial of a family physician intervention for smoking cessation. *Journal of the American Medical Association* 260: 1570-1574, 1988.

Clinical Interventions in Tobacco Control: A National Cancer Institute Training Program for Health Care Providers

Marc Manley, Roselyn P. Epps,
Robert Mecklenburg, and Corinne Husten

DISSEMINATING INTERVENTIONS

Other chapters in this monograph describe the clinical trials funded by NCI that examined the effect of health care professionals on smoking by patients. This section describes the training projects conducted by NCI to disseminate the research results after completion of the above trials.

Project Planning

At the time the five clinical trials were completed, there was very little information about mechanisms to disseminate behavioral interventions to practicing clinicians. Although the trials had demonstrated that physicians and dentists can change the smoking behavior of their patients, there was little in the literature about effective methods for rapid training of clinicians in the new techniques. One trial from the United Kingdom clearly demonstrated that mailing information on smoking cessation techniques to physicians resulted in very little change in physician knowledge and, presumably, very little change in physician behavior (Fowler et al., 1989). Given the volume of mail that most physicians receive and the demands on their time, such a result is not unexpected.

Experience from clinical trials in smoking cessation techniques indicated that physicians and dentists are willing and able to incorporate effective techniques into their practice after training in these skills. The trials showed that clinicians appreciate how tobacco use affects their patients' health and that health care professionals are willing to intervene with their smoking patients when provided with clinical techniques that are (1) effective and (2) easily incorporated into a busy practice.

Based on the concepts derived in the clinical trials, a decision was made to develop a training program that would provide clinicians throughout the United States with information about smoking cessation techniques and the skills to apply such techniques. A program for physicians and nurses began about 2 years before a similar effort was started for dentists and other oral health professionals.

Medical Materials Development

An early step in the development of the training project was the creation of effective training materials, which began prior to the completion of the clinical trials. A consensus on the development process for training materials was established while the major trials were in progress.

The investigators held regular meetings during the trials, and issues such as study design, comparability of data, intervention techniques, and validation were discussed in early meetings. At the end of the trials, extensive discussions focused on the principal findings, the results that were found in more than one trial, and the lessons that should be communicated to practicing clinicians.

Based on these discussions, a consensus document was written: *How To Help Your Patients Stop Smoking: A National Cancer Institute Manual for Physicians* (Glynn and Manley, 1990). The manual, designed for primary care physicians, nurses, and office staff members, was written as a "how to" guide, not as a scientific paper. It addresses two subjects: how to intervene with a smoking patient, and how to establish mechanisms in an office practice that result in systematic, routine treatment for all smoking patients.

Five steps are described for establishing and maintaining such an office system:

- Select a smoking cessation coordinator;
- Create a smoke-free office environment;
- Identify all smoking patients;
- Develop smoking cessation plans for patients; and
- Provide followup care.

These five steps establish a system that allows for the routine care of smoking patients. This office organization is planned to ensure that all patients who smoke are identified, monitored, and appropriately treated at every office visit. Because office practices differ, the exact procedures adopted will vary. However, it is important to involve as many members of an office staff as possible in smoking cessation. Involvement of the office staff results in more support for patients, increases the likelihood of patients' success, and reduces the amount of physician time required.

Within this framework of an office system, the NCI manual describes brief interventions that can be used by clinicians when they are face-to-face with a smoking patient. An intervention plan is presented and summarized with the four A's:

- *Ask* about smoking;
- *Advise* smokers to stop;
- *Assist* patients who want to stop; and
- *Arrange* followup care.

This intervention can be initiated at any office visit. The intervention typically lasts less than 3 minutes, but it may vary with each patient's needs and the clinician's skills. The recommended procedures are based both on data from the trials discussed above and on a meta-analysis of 39 controlled trials (Kottke et al., 1988), which showed that the most effective techniques used more than one modality (e.g., physician advice, self-help materials, nicotine gum), involved both physicians and other clinical staff, and involved more smoking messages over a longer period of time.

The next step in development of the training program was the creation of materials for teachers. The manual described above contained the basic information for a course, but experience from the clinical trials indicated that there were several different ways to teach this information. The development of teaching materials required extensive input from the trial investigators, as well as from experts in the design of training programs. The training materials design incorporated some new materials as well as ideas that had proved useful in the trials.

The training materials constituted a 3-hour course. Both longer and shorter training sessions had been used in the trials, and the 3-hour time was a compromise. A longer course would allow more time for skills development, which would be useful for physicians who received little formal training in behavioral change techniques. However, longer courses require more time commitment from the clinicians who attend. A shorter course, of 1 hour or less, is more typical in medical education and presents fewer logistical barriers; but a period shorter than 3 hours would allow little time for skills development exercises and could consist of only a lecture. A lecture can only transfer knowledge; it cannot teach skills.

The clinical trials indicated the value of conducting exercises that allow clinicians to practice techniques for smoking intervention. Most of the training in the trials included role-playing exercises. Another teaching technique frequently used was modeling of the intervention on videotape. The new training materials incorporated both techniques. Another exercise was designed that had small groups discuss typical smoking patients as an alternative to the role-playing exercise, because many of the course teachers would have had no experience with conducting a role-play. The small-group exercise was designed so that teachers with little experience in conducting exercises could lead a discussion of common intervention issues.

Other exercises in the training materials address issues of organizing the office and defining roles of staff members. Barriers to implementing an office system for smoking cessation also are discussed.

Finally, the order of topics covered during the course was considered. As mentioned above, the NCI manual included the intervention techniques (the four A's) within the framework of the office system approach, but this order was changed somewhat in the training materials. The training materials included an introduction that briefly addressed the importance of smoking cessation to patients' health. The introduction also discussed the crucial role of physicians and other clinicians in smoking cessation. Finally, the introduction reviewed the literature that demonstrated the impact of brief interventions on smoking among patients.

After the introduction, the course materials covered the four A's. Didactic material was followed by videotape demonstration of the techniques and then practice exercises. A short discussion of followup visits was then presented, including the importance of followup and the conduct of a typical followup visit. A videotaped demonstration of a followup visit was then shown. The final module of the course addressed the office system approach with didactic materials, slides, and exercises. A brief closing section reviewed the highlights of the course. The course materials, titled *How To Help Your Patients Stop Smoking: Trainer's Guide* (US DHHS, n.d.[a]), are contained in a three-ring binder that includes teaching notes, slides, handouts, and the videotape.

The final step was the design of materials to train the trainers. Courses for trainers were considered essential because few health professionals in this country had experience in smoking cessation techniques. A 1-day course for trainers was designed. A longer course might have been preferable, to produce trainers who can not only discuss the didactic information comfortably, but also conduct small-group and role-playing exercises; but, as with the course for clinicians, a longer course presents more logistical barriers and is likely to be attended by fewer health professionals.

The trainers' workshop demonstrated the 3-hour course to the participants and allowed them to discuss the teaching techniques used in the course. Approximately 6 hours of class time were allowed, so that questions about the didactic materials and the exercises could be addressed in detail. New materials were developed for the conclusion of the trainers' workshop, and issues relevant to implementing a course were discussed. The material was designed to involve the participants in a discussion of organizing and marketing a course to health professionals. That portion of the workshop was designed to help trainers develop a plan of action for conducting courses for their colleagues.

Training Activities As training materials were created, a plan was developed to reach clinicians with the training. An initial goal was to train 100,000 physicians within 3 years. (Subsequent goals were formulated for the training of other health professionals, as discussed below.) The goal was based on the number of practicing physicians in the United States and the proportion of primary care physicians among them.

A total of 50 workshops to train trainers are planned. With an average attendance of 40 trainers, 50 workshops will produce 2,000 trainers nationwide. Those trainers then conduct shorter courses (1 to 3 hours) for their colleagues. If each trainer can teach 50 other physicians, a total of 100,000 physicians will have been trained (see Figure 11).

This strategy does not require the development of a new training institution but seeks to incorporate the new course into established continuing medical education systems. To reduce the prevalence of smoking as rapidly as possible, initial efforts will be to train practicing clinicians rather than those still in internship and residency.

In order to reach clinicians throughout the country, NCI sought to collaborate with medical organizations (e.g., American Medical Association and American Cancer Society) that shared a commitment to cancer prevention and had a membership of practicing physicians or nurses. National associations initially approached were those that have state-level components, primary care specialties, and members likely to treat patients in high-risk populations. Through their members, interested organizations were encouraged to develop policies to sponsor, support, and promote training for clinicians in smoking cessation techniques.

Agreements with organizations committed to smoking intervention training were developed for implementing essential activities. Under those agreements, NCI provided expert faculty for trainers' workshops, as well as all training materials (trainer's guides and videotapes) for each workshop participant. Participants were also given as many copies of *How To Help Your Patients Stop Smoking* as needed for distribution to the clinicians they train.

The collaborating organizations were asked to promote the training to their members and make special efforts to ensure that the training reaches physicians who serve high-risk populations. The organizations also convened the trainers' workshops and, most importantly, recruited the trainers. Clinicians were sought who already had teaching responsibilities, so that this class could be easily incorporated into established teaching institutions.

These trainers not only were willing to attend the 1-day workshop, but also agreed to conduct classes for 50 of their colleagues. The trainers were also asked to use the NCI training manuals and to keep NCI informed of their progress in teaching.

Figure 11
Training 100,000 clinicians

Phase I—Training Trainers	Phase II—Training Clinicians
50	2,000
× 40	× 50
2,000	100,000

Source: National Cancer Institute, February 1990.

Discussions with the staff and leaders of professional and voluntary associations made clear that this kind of training strategy works for some associations but not all. The strategy requires staff time and commitment. To assure participation by members, association leaders and staff members must promote and organize the training efforts. In addition, the "train-the-trainers" model will not fit with every association's continuing education activities. Some groups already have activities that address the smoking issue, and some associations do not have continuing education programs in which to incorporate the NCI course.

Association Support Many medical associations and agencies, however, did adopt the NCI training into their activities. National associations that have done the most training have done so by encouraging the participation of their state affiliates. In particular, the American Cancer Society and the American Medical Association have formally encouraged their state divisions and component societies to adopt this project. Both organizations have staff members at the state level to work on the program, and both have local affiliates that can reach their members. Networks that allow programs to reach from national to state to local levels have proved invaluable in the dissemination of the training.

Several other associations have participated in this training effort. Several medical specialty organizations, even those with less extensive state and local organizations, conducted trainers' workshops at their national meetings. State health departments and large HMOs were also very active. Collaborators to date include the American Cancer Society, American Medical Association, Association of American Medical Colleges, American Medical Women's Association, Society of Teachers of Family Medicine, Association of Teachers of Preventive Medicine, American College of Preventive Medicine, National Medical Association, many state medical societies, and several large health maintenance organizations.

Typically, a trainers' workshop is sponsored by the state medical society and the state division of the American Cancer Society. After the workshop, the trainers conduct classes for their colleagues under the auspices of the sponsoring organizations. In many cases, a state medical society will encourage or assist local medical societies as they work with the trainers to conduct courses. The classes have been taught as special events, but usually they are incorporated into ongoing medical education systems. The 3-hour course can be taught in more than one session. A shorter version of the course also is taught, often to inform physicians of the need for training in smoking cessation and to identify those interested in more complete training.

NCI provides trainers with new teaching materials periodically. Among these materials are new publications that discuss interventions for preventing tobacco use among children and adolescents. The materials, developed by NCI with the collaboration of the American Academy of Pediatrics, discuss brief interventions for use by pediatricians and other physicians who care for children. Included in these materials are discussions of preventing exposure of children to environmental tobacco smoke, anticipatory guidance to prevent tobacco use, cessation by adolescents, and the role of physicians in schools and the community.

NCI reinforces the work of the trainers by providing periodic mailings to all health professionals they train. These mailings provide new information on smoking cessation and prevention techniques and augment the training with new materials and ideas. The NCI staff has also promoted the importance of smoking cessation training in articles in professional journals and through presentations at medical education conferences.

Clinical interventions in tobacco control are most effective when practiced by more than one health professional in an office and when the intervention is incorporated into routine office procedures. Accomplishing these tasks requires knowledge and skills on the part of physicians and nurses. For this reason, training in these techniques is most effective when entire office teams are trained, rather than just physicians. Whenever possible, trainers and sponsoring organizations are encouraged to recruit office teams to attend their classes. Nurses and others of the office staff can make the physician's intervention more efficient and effective, and they should receive training for this role. However, this is not always possible, and training of physicians alone is certainly valuable.

The training program has reached physicians and nurses in a variety of practices. The program has been adopted by HMOs, private practices, public health clinics in State and local health departments, family planning clinics, and specialty clinics. The trainers have also taught the course to residents, medical students, nursing students, and other health professionals in training. As of January 1, 1992, 34 trainers' workshops had been conducted, which produced more than 1,100 trainers. An estimated 40,000 health professionals have subsequently been trained by these trainers.

ORAL HEALTH TEAM RESEARCH

Design

As discussed above, the first efforts to train health care providers were directed at those professionals who work in primary care medical practices, especially physicians and nurses. In 1989, while the training of medical providers was under way, a similar program for dentists, dental hygienists, and dental assistants was planned. One study funded by NCI, as well as other trials, demonstrated that dentists can be as effective as physicians in influencing patients to quit smoking. Furthermore, it was recognized that oral health professionals, like medical professionals, see a large proportion of the smoking population every year. In addition, the oral health team routinely treats adolescents and young adults, who often have excellent health and therefore do not have frequent contact with physicians and nurses.

Tobacco use commonly produces or contributes to ill effects in the mouth (Mecklenburg et al., 1992). The dental care team can show patients their own oral health problems, thereby creating teachable moments, since tobacco-related conditions in tissues of the mouth often occur years before serious internal diseases become detectable. Tobacco use intervention is a reasonable complement to the preventive services common to dental practice.

The dental profession has concerned itself primarily with patients who use smokeless tobacco products. For example, moist snuff will produce leukoplakia in the oral mucosa in about half of users within 6 months after their beginning use. The oral effects of smoking are more diverse and less frequent. Without clear guidance about scientific methods to help smoking patients, and because of physicians' history of concern about smoking, fewer dentists than physicians have actively helped patients stop smoking.

Strategies

In 1989, an NCI program was organized to ensure that the oral health team and dental organizations are routinely involved in tobacco control activities. Eight strategies were identified to achieve this goal.

Some NCI dental program strategies included efforts to encourage dental professional organizations to play a more active role in tobacco control. Other activities were designed to train oral health care providers in tobacco control interventions.

Efforts to promote tobacco control as an appropriate function of oral health care providers were directed at the leaders and members of professional organizations. NCI convened meetings with organization leaders and committees to advise them of the Institute's interest in cooperating with the dental profession and to learn about any reciprocal interest. As a result, leaders from seven major dental organizations wrote to NCI, expressing support for NCI's tobacco control initiative and announcing their desire to work with the Institute to reduce the public's use of tobacco.

NCI recognized that dental clinicians would most readily adopt new tobacco intervention methods in their practices if their own professional organizations urged them to do so. Thus, several dental organization leaders were encouraged to introduce and seek approval of organizational policies and position statements that promoted tobacco control efforts by their members. Established policies were assessed and recommendations made for new policies.

To promote awareness about problems of tobacco use and methods of control, a series of symposia, panels, and special presentations were introduced into the annual meeting of several organizations, often using distinguished authorities in the field. Articles and news releases were prepared for dental organization media. Special announcements about the availability of NCI consultation and assistance were mailed to organization leaders through lists provided by dental organizations.

To promote communication and coordination among the organizations, NCI convened the National Dental Tobacco-Free Steering Committee, composed of representatives of 14 national organizations. Nearly all oral health clinicians in the United States are members of one or more of the organizations represented on the committee. The committee advises NCI about the most feasible and efficient means to advance tobacco control through the dental profession. The committee is a forum for organizational information exchange on tobacco control topics and it provides a means for recognizing previously isolated initiatives and coordinating dental profession activities with the larger community of tobacco control activities.

As was done for physicians, NCI assembled an *ad hoc* committee to propose methods for rapidly strengthening dental clinicians' knowledge, skills, and commitment with respect to control of tobacco use. Four basic differences from the medical development model emerged. First, the more generic term "tobacco" would be used instead of "smoking," because both smoking and smokeless tobacco are addictive, many users switch or use both types, and the involvement of dentists emerged primarily through their concern about the oral effects of smokeless tobacco.

Second, the term "oral health team" would be emphasized because research suggested that the clinical team approach led to more effective interventions than did individual efforts. Furthermore, the team approach promotes flexibility in developing clinical intervention systems.

Third, prevention services would be given attention equal to that for cessation services. About 75 percent of individuals aged 5 to 17 visit a dental office each year. Because more than 80 percent of tobacco users begin during their youth, the oral health team could intervene to persuade children and youth to avoid tobacco use. An intervention reinforced each year as adolescents grow to adults could help prevent psychological and physiological addiction.

Fourth, dental education institutions would be approached to encourage continuing education for graduate clinicians and the integration of tobacco intervention issues into the undergraduate curriculum. Toward this end, a special program was presented to faculty members of dental education institutions prior to specific followup with individual institutions. Dental institutions have been in transition because of changing patterns of disease. Thus, many schools have been open to concepts and methods that advance oral medicine and preventive practice services that had not been widely taught previously.

Training Methods Efforts to train oral health professionals in techniques to stop tobacco use, although modeled after the program to train medical professionals, were different. First, there are differences between the practices of medicine and dentistry that must be accommodated in a training program.

Second, the dental program was developed later and therefore benefited from experience gained in the medical program.

Two training publications were created for the oral health team. The first, *How To Help Your Patients Stop Using Tobacco: A National Cancer Institute Manual for the Oral Health Team* (Mecklenburg et al., 1990), was based on the manual for physicians and nurses but differed in several ways. The dental manual was organized into three parts with a chronology similar to the behavioral steps of stopping tobacco use:

- The first part, "Get Ready," addresses activities to create an office system to treat tobacco users.
- The second, "Help Patients," discusses the four A's. This discussion emphasizes treating patients who use smokeless tobacco. This section also includes a discussion about preventing the start of tobacco use among youth. Brief interventions for use with children and adolescents are described.
- The third part, "Follow Through," which discusses followup care of patients, includes a conceptual shift that goes beyond the processes of patient management. Follow Through asks the oral health team to work for tobacco control outside the office, that is, as citizens of their communities and in their personal behavior.

The second document developed was *How To Help Your Patients Stop Using Tobacco: Trainer's Guide* (US DHHS, n.d.[b]). As with the dental manual, case histories and other discussions of patients were modified from the medical model to reflect dental practice. An introductory section states the dental program goal, objectives, and strategy, and helps potential trainers with planning advice.

The trainers' workshop for the oral health team was also different from the physician training program. The physician's manual was organized such that course content and teaching methods were combined, so the course was truly a 1-day train-the-trainers program. The dental program equivalent taught the entire course content for clinicians during the first half-day. The first session thus served as a demonstration of the course as NCI recommends trainers teach it. The second session taught training methods, planning for training, background information about tobacco industry strategies, counter-strategies for clinicians, and NCI's Smoking and Tobacco Control Program. Because the two half-days are separate units, many individuals having an interest in applications in their own office environment attended the first half-day only. The second half-day included a high proportion of individuals who work in educational institutions, are affiliated with training programs, or have a specific interest in sharing tobacco use intervention information with professional colleagues.

Initial Observations Through work with professional organizations and the conduct of training programs, significant progress has been made in motivating oral health professionals to intervene in tobacco use. New tobacco control policies have now been adopted by professional organizations including the American Dental Association, National Dental Association, American Association of Dental Schools, American Dental Hygienist's Association, Academy of General Dentistry, and American Association of Public Health Dentistry. At one time, a few dental organization policies did little more than prohibit smoking during meetings. Now many organizations include comprehensive policies that address tobacco intervention services, intervention research, dental professional education, public education, organization administration, collaboration with nondental organizations, and advocacy. Many policies urge members to become trained in intervention methods and to assist their patients. Some organizations have joined coalitions of concerned citizens in the support of stronger public policy for tobacco control at community, state, and national levels.

Collaborative training programs have been conducted with national dental organizations. For example, the American Dental Association has a long record of supporting tobacco control through its professional development and public education programs. The American Dental Association developed new programs consistent with NCI tobacco intervention research results and increased the intensity of its promotion of clinician involvement in tobacco control issues. The Academy of General Dentistry has sponsored NCI training and has made the control of tobacco use a high-priority national initiative. This is significant because the Academy of General Dentistry is dedicated to professional excellence through continuing education. Most NCI training has been sponsored by state dental associations, state dental hygienist organizations, state health departments, state divisions of the American Cancer Society, and dental schools. California has conducted an independent training program through a special initiative. The State coordinates with NCI and uses NCI manuals and concepts in its dental courses.

As of January 1, 1992, 24 courses had been held in the United States, training 1,233 clinicians and 668 trainers. Data on the number of clinicians subsequently taught by the trainers are now being collected.

Dental assistants' interest in learning tobacco use intervention methods has accelerated as the program has progressed. Dental hygienists have been most responsive to the NCI training program and often may be the program coordinators for tobacco intervention in dentists' offices. Tobacco intervention methods are compatible with other preventive oral health services by hygienists. Tobacco use reduces the benefits of dental hygiene services, so there is a rationale for hygienists' involvement in intervention.

A few courses have had participants representing both medical and dental practices. If one profession is dominant, providing appropriate materials for the other has sufficed. If large numbers of both medical and dental participants attend, it has been necessary to change the order of presentation of dental materials. For improved flexibility, dental courses held in 1992 were planned to follow the presentation sequence used for medical training (i.e., "Introduction," "Help Patients," "Follow Through," and "Get Ready").

PROJECT EVALUATION The evaluation of the NCI training project will determine how effective the training program is in increasing the use of specific smoking cessation techniques by health care providers. The following questions will be answered by the evaluation:

- To what extent do the health care providers trained in NCI courses incorporate these techniques into their practices; and is there an increase in the use of these techniques that can be attributed to the training?
- Among trained health care providers, does the extent of technique adoption, both in total and in specific techniques, vary with professional characteristics, practice characteristics, training class characteristics, or time since training?
- How many health care providers have been trained through this project?
- What characteristics of trainers predict whether they will actively train their colleagues, and how have they used the NCI materials to conduct classes?

The first two questions will be answered by surveys of health professionals who have been trained. A sample of these professionals will be asked to complete written questionnaires prior to taking the course and 3 to 6 months after the course. In addition to asking about personal and professional characteristics, the questionnaire will ask about the use of smoking cessation techniques in their practices.

To answer the third and fourth questions, a telephone survey of all trainers who have participated in the project will be conducted. Trainers will be asked to provide details of all training they have conducted. Information about their own professional activities will also be sought.

CONCLUSIONS This project has attempted to take new information on tobacco control from clinical trials and rapidly disseminate it to practicing clinicians nationwide. To accomplish this, NCI has sought extensive help from professional organizations. Such organizations have willingly participated in the NCI health promotion project, recognizing its value to their clinician members and to patients.

Primary care professionals have expressed interest in the training program and have been willing to attend courses on this topic. The cost of this project—to both the Federal Government and participating organizations—is low.

The potential public health impact of this kind of program is enormous, especially in the context of other tobacco control efforts channeled through schools, worksites, mass media, and the community.

Future activities of the program will include formal efforts to incorporate this class into more training programs, especially medical and dental schools and residency programs in primary care. An expanded program directed to clinicians who care for children will also be implemented. Finally, efforts will be undertaken to make this information and training available to interested clinicians in other nations through collaboration with international organizations of health care providers.

REFERENCES

Fowler, G., Mant, D., Fuller, A., Jones, L. The "Help Your Patients Stop" initiative: Evaluation of smoking prevalence and dissemination of WHO/UICC guidelines in U.K. general practice. *Lancet* 1(8649): 1253-1255, 1989.

Glynn, T.J., Manley, M.W. *How To Help Your Patients Stop Smoking: A National Cancer Institute Manual for Physicians.* U.S. Department of Health and Human Services, Public Health Service, National Institutes of Health, National Cancer Institute. NIH Publication No. 90-3063, 1990.

Kottke, T.E., Battista, R.N., DeFriese, G.H., Brekke, M.L. Attributes of successful smoking cessation interventions in medical practice: A meta-analysis of 39 controlled trials. *Journal of the American Medical Association* 259: 2882-2889, 1988.

Mecklenburg, R.E., Christen, A.G., Gerbert, B., Gift, H.C., Glynn, T.J., Jones, R.B., Lindsay, E., Manley, M.W., Severson, H. *How To Help Your Patients Stop Using Tobacco: A National Cancer Institute Manual for the Oral Health Team.* U.S. Department of Health and Human Services, Public Health Service, National Institutes of Health, National Cancer Institute. NIH Publication No. 91-3191, 1990.

Mecklenburg, R.E., Greenspan, D., Kleinman, D.V., Manley, M.W., Niessen, L.C., Robertson, P.B., Winn, D.E. *Tobacco Effects in the Mouth: A National Cancer Institute and National Institute of Dental Research Guide for Health Professionals.* U.S. Department of Health and Human Services, Public Health Service, National Institutes of Health, National Cancer Institute/National Institute of Dental Research. NIH Publication No. 92-3330, 1992.

U.S. Department of Health and Human Services. *How To Help Your Patients Stop Smoking: Trainer's Guide.* U.S. Department of Health and Human Services, Public Health Service, National Institutes of Health, no date (a).

U.S. Department of Health and Human Services. *How To Help Your Patients Stop Using Tobacco: Trainer's Guide.* U.S. Department of Health and Human Services, Public Health Service, National Institutes of Health, no date (b).

APPENDIX A
Case Studies

The following case studies demonstrate how three communities have implemented the COMMIT standardized protocol. The protocol defines minimum criteria to ensure quality control, and the process objectives help all sites conform to the standardized quantity of intervention.

SANTA FE, NEW MEXICO

The Health Provider Task Force (HPTF) activities in Santa Fe reflected the unique personality of the city, an internationally recognized center for the arts and entertainment. Not surprisingly, the HPTF chose to produce a videotape on smoking cessation as its first major project. Physicians and dentists from the task force were filmed at their workplaces: a local health maintenance organization, the cardiac intensive care unit of the hospital, and a dental office. The chairman of the medical society and the hospital administrator also appeared. The videotape was distributed to all primary care physicians and dentists in Santa Fe. Physicians completing the accompanying evaluation form received 1 hour of CME credit and had their names listed in local newspaper advertisements encouraging smokers to "Ask-A-Doc" for help in quitting.

Santa Fe also was the site for the "Emphysema Slims" Tennis Tournament in 1990. This national antismoking event is sponsored by Doctors Ought to Care. The New Mexico President of DOC, a member of the HPTF, worked tirelessly to attract television personalities and other celebrities to help support the project, organize the city's first hot-air balloon event, and involve local and national media.

Santa Fe is unique also in supporting a spectrum of "alternative healers." The phone directory lists more than 40 acupuncturists, an equal number of chiropractors, and a number of hypnotists, naturopaths, and massage therapists. The chiropractors are the best organized, and their client population is from all socioeconomic strata. The opportunity to bring smoking cessation information to people who might not frequent allopathic physicians and the literature associating smoking with low back pain (Deyo and Bass, 1989; Lanier and Stockton, 1988) prompted the COMMIT staff in Santa Fe to organize a meeting with local chiropractors. The meeting outlined the goals and structure of COMMIT, the relationship of smoking and low back pain, options for patient intervention, establishing smoke-free offices, and opportunities for training in cessation counseling skills. As a result of the meeting, Santa Fe chiropractors have participated in each of the COMMIT task forces, and the chiropractic association is considering recruitment of a student from a chiropractic college to come to Santa Fe to prepare a teaching module on smoking and low back pain. By choosing to participate as individual members of established task forces, rather than organizing their own independent task force, the chiropractors have averted potential conflicts with physicians who might not want to be associated with a highly visible chiropractic initiative in the community.

The Santa Fe HPTF activities demonstrate the importance of individuals in creating opportunities for action. One physician member had a weekly radio program: Smoking-related issues figured even more prominently on his show after COMMIT began. After attending the American Medical Association's annual media training workshop, he took a lead role in producing the health provider videotape. A local pediatrician joined the HPTF, appeared in the video, became a speaker on pediatric aspects of smoking, and participated actively in developing a pediatrics initiative. The latter included T-shirts with relevant messages for pregnant women and newborns; a videotape on cessation for pregnant, low-income women; and cessation classes for women attending the WIC (women, infants, and children) nutrition program in Santa Fe. A family practice physician who had been leading smoking cessation classes in his own office for many years was able to win support for a cessation class at the Santa Fe hospital. The attendees were nurses, respiratory and physical therapists, and other hospital staff. The hospital administration was very supportive, arranging coverage for those employees attending the classes. The need for such an in-hospital program was not apparent until this trusted local physician offered his services.

Despite the enthusiasm of task force members, attracting other physicians and dentists in the community to attend advanced training workshops in smoking cessation was extraordinarily difficult. Providing continuing education credits, scheduling the workshops at convenient times and at attractive locations, and offering door prizes did not prompt sufficient interest to put on a workshop. It became clear that the health providers who joined the task force were not representative, with respect to recognizing the importance of smoking cessation, of the general medical and dental community. Most doctors and dentists were unwilling to give up 3 hours of their time for cessation training. Workshops were finally arranged through a contract with a physician to telephone health providers directly, inviting them to the workshop, scheduling the workshop in conjunction with a state medical meeting, and including outside speakers of national reputation. Another successful approach was to schedule training sessions over the lunch hour in providers' offices. When a task force physician or dentist was included in these extended lunch-hour sessions, the office physician or dentist would often join his or her staff (nurse, receptionist, dental hygienist) in learning about counseling skills, office procedures to promote cessation, and followup strategies. Further participation by physicians was encouraged through a newsletter. The first issue of the newsletter reviewed diagnostic codes that might be used to bill third-party payers for smoking cessation services.

The lessons learned from the activities of the Santa Fe HPTF include the importance of physician-to-physician contacts in providing information and promoting participation by community providers; the value of office-based educational approaches that include the entire office team in efforts to establish smoke-free policies and to identify, counsel, and support smokers' quit attempts; the need to have a broad representation of the health provider community, not just the "activist" members; and the desirability of designing initiatives around the skills and interests of individual task force members.

BRANTFORD, ONTARIO, CANADA

Brantford, Ontario, a city of 90,500, is surrounded by farmland and located on the edge of the most populated area in Canada. There are 72 primary care physicians and 35 dentists practicing in the city and 2 major health care facilities.

Several features of Canadian health care are important to understand, as they affect the implementation of the COMMIT protocol. Family medicine is a popular specialty and accounts for 80 percent of the total practicing physicians in Brantford. Most of the family physicians are in solo practice (87 percent), and not all physicians employ a nurse as a team member. Dentists also tend to be in solo practice, and most employ a dental assistant or hygienist.

Although all Ontario residents are covered by health insurance, smoking cessation counseling is not always a billable service. The COMMIT task force has taken action on this issue and through requests to the Ontario government has successfully convinced the health insurance policymakers to reimburse most tobacco-related visits.

During the early organization of the COMMIT board and task forces, the planning committee identified two physician leaders who have been central to the organizing and implementing of the health care provider protocol activities. The physician leaders have been key individuals in the creation of smoke-free environments in the city's hospitals, and one was known for his ability to give excellent presentations on smoking issues. These two physicians are from the mainstream of the practitioners in town; they are viewed as leaders but not extremists.

The HPTF has wide representation from the community, including physicians, public health nurses, occupational health nurses, pharmacists, chiropractors, dentists, and respiratory therapists. This group has met consistently and carried out the activities required. There have been many training events, and all process objectives regarding the number of professionals attending training have been met.

One of the comprehensive training workshops was attended by both physicians and chiropractors. This was a first in Brantford and has led to a clearer understanding of the roles of different professionals in the care of smoking patients. Referrals between physicians and chiropractors have become part of normal practice for those individuals who attended this joint training session.

Oral health team training is an innovation in Ontario. Although there is strong leadership from the team that was trained to conduct training events, it has been difficult to attract dentists and their staff to workshops. The COMMIT staff will try a new marketing strategy for the next event that will first attract the attention of the hygienists.

The Public Health Service in Canada operates differently from that in the United States. Through the Canadian Public Health Service, nurses access schools and homes to offer a variety of services that make them potential key players in the COMMIT interventions. Public Health Service nurses are able to work in neighborhoods and are working with COMMIT staff to develop neighborhood cessation programs. Neighborhood physicians will provide counseling as part of these programs.

In general, the task force has been concerned about the focus on physicians and oral health teams without requiring activities for other health care professionals. Therefore, from the beginning of the project they have been creative regarding the inclusion of activities for Public Health Service nurses, chiropractors (as mentioned above), and pharmacists.

There is strong support in Canada from the profession itself for pharmacies to stop selling tobacco. The task force has facilitated a community-wide letter-writing campaign in support of banning tobacco products in pharmacies. The pharmacist on the task force represented one of the first stores in Brantford to stop selling tobacco products.

Ensuring that offices are set up to support effective physician and dental interventions is a cornerstone of the health care provider interventions. This activity that motivates and helps receptionists and other staff to implement chart cueing, monitoring, and provision of self-help materials is one of the most challenging of the COMMIT activities. It is not enough to convey the importance of these procedures at the physician and dental training events. It is apparent that most offices do not get organized until a staff person from COMMIT visits the office and helps them establish their system of cueing, monitoring, and ordering resources. It will be important to build this function into the staff requirements in the dissemination stage of COMMIT activities for health care providers.

As one would expect in a volunteer committee, individuals make different contributions to the project. However, it is important that three or four key people have continued to be present and give their time and leadership. It is often difficult to find health care professionals who will give this level of support to a project, because time spent at meetings often means time lost from seeing patients and, therefore, a financial loss. Nevertheless, we have found that there are individuals who will make this contribution, and our perception is that without them the project would not succeed.

PATERSON, NEW JERSEY

Paterson, New Jersey, is an urban area with a predominantly poor minority population. The largely black and Hispanic citizenry is confronted by high rates of poverty, crime, drug abuse, poor housing, and high school dropouts. Despite this, the COMMIT protocol has been accepted by the community board, and virtually all of the mandated activities are being carried out with vigor and imagination. In many respects, the HPTF has led the way.

Three large hospitals and many health clinics that serve Paterson have representatives on the board and task forces. By year 2 of the trial, all of them are smoke-free, and they provide a variety of smoking cessation activities and services for their employees and the public. They have actively participated in the Great American Smokeout during each year of the trial to date, and they also participated in two major events (e.g., "Quit Month," "Cancer Education Month," "Blood Pressure Month," "Non-Dependence Day"). The hospitals and clinics work closely with COMMIT in sponsoring health screening, inviting speakers to symposia, and continuing education activities, all of which include the topic of cigarette smoking on the agenda.

Several Paterson physicians and dentists, as well as other health professionals, have stepped forward as influentials. To date, one Paterson hospital has sponsored grand rounds on smoking, and the HPTF has carried out three all-day symposia and workshops on smoking cessation for health professionals (comprehensive training).

Paterson physicians and dentists who attend the comprehensive training, as well as many others, received an office visit from a COMMIT community organizer who works under the direction of the HPTF. The organizer then carries out basic training for the physicians and dentists and their staffs and, in many cases, "Office Training and Activation of Office Staff." The content of these visits may vary, but certain features remain constant and provide necessary structure for the community organizer as well as the physicians or dentists and their staffs. Typically, the organizer will select a time when the office is relatively free. At lunch time, he will bring pizza or sandwiches and soda. We use the National Heart, Lung, and Blood Institute video, "Making A Difference," for training physicians in smoking counseling. The office staff member, physician, or dentist then is presented with a comprehensive smoking cessation program in the form of the American Heart Association's Heart Rx kit or the American Academy of Family Physicians smoking counseling kit. These kits provide guidelines and material for mobilizing the office, counseling patients, and followup.

After discussion of the film, the kits, and COMMIT, the organizer assists with setting up the waiting room area to reduce smoking. He supplies brochures, buttons, key chains, and posters. Wall racks and a plastic brochure holder are distributed to provide easy access to self-help stop-smoking and health material. Information on the Great American Smokeout and Quit and Win, as well as the COMMIT newsletters and other events of interest are routinely displayed and distributed.

It is not sufficient to visit busy offices on only one occasion and expect to have a major impact on office behavior. The community organizer serves as a "drug detail representative," returning to the office many times per year with refill material, new brochures, newsletters, and publicity. Events such as the Great American Smokeout (November), Heart Month (February), High Blood Pressure Month (May), Non-Dependence Day (July), and Quit and Win (Fall) provide occasions for the community organizer to return to the offices to reinforce and support the staff and doctors. A recent "Ask Your Doc" campaign provided still another occasion to keep in close contact with the health care community.

In inner-city urban environments, reaching out to the community may be more important than it is in more affluent, middle-class communities. This is accomplished in Paterson, under the leadership of the HPTF, by the COMMIT community organizer traveling with high blood pressure teams sponsored by the hospitals and the Paterson health department. Typically, these teams travel to churches, social service agencies, worksites, and community organizations to measure blood pressure and identify hypertensive individuals. We also measure expired air carbon monoxide of smokers, distribute self-help and related material, enroll smokers in the network, and inform them of smoking cessation activities in the community.

In summary, despite real social problems and competing issues, the COMMIT protocol for health care settings has proved applicable to Paterson. Health care facilities are smoke-free; physicians, dentists, and other health professionals are being trained and mobilized; and the health care community participates in many community events and activities. A cessation resource guide is distributed, and health care facilities are used to recruit smokers into the network and related smoking cessation activities. Despite this, there is concern that, in a 4-year intervention, physicians and dentists will lose their competitive edge and stop counseling smokers, flagging charts, and selecting quit dates. We try to counter this by returning to their offices and clinics periodically, by keeping in contact through the mails, and by providing certificates of appreciation for their involvement. Still, smoking counseling is a frustrating business with few rewards. It is hoped that the community-based nature of COMMIT and its comprehensive approach will yield success.

Index

abstinence from smoking 55, 71, 87, 99, 108, 160-161
- hospital patients 152
- long-term 6-7, 99, 108
- TRACC intervention, rates of 148-150
- (*see also* **quit rates, smoking**)

abstinence from smokeless tobacco 160-161
academic detailing 8, 10, 302, 349, 353
Academy of General Dentistry 366
adolescents, tobacco use
- and carbon monoxide testing 163-164
- and problem behaviors 164-165
- counseling by pediatricians 229-230, 232, 238-244
- followup to intervention 163-164
- initiation of smoking 4-5
- interventions 46, 162-166, 361-362, 364-365
- prevalence of smoking 232
- prevention of 340, 361, 364-365
- quit attempts 164-165
- ST cessation programs 157

Adult Use of Tobacco Survey (AUTS) 17-21
advertising
- cigarette 27, 29, 31
- of clinic smoking intervention 79, 81
- tobacco products 7, 232

advice to quit smoking
- algorithms for delivery of 262-264, 288-291
- alone, physician intervention 144-149, 189, 191, 194, 196, 199-202, 224
- booster sessions 262, 264-265, 269-270
- brief 92, 94-96, 145, 202, 240
- chemical workers 272-280
- clinical trial 92-98, 170
- confidence in 92, 95-96
- demographic factors 18-19, 21
- dental practice 157-161, 272, 274
- dysfunctional reactions to 279, 284
- effects of 21, 273-274
- experimental 262-263, 288-291
- head and neck cancer patients 262
- initial 262, 288-289
- institutionalization of 301
- negative reactions to 273, 279-280, 284
- parents' attitudes 236-238, 241
- patients' attitudes 24-25
- patients report receiving 3, 17-20, 117, 130
- pediatricians 230, 233-236, 241
- personalized 60, 66, 242, 260
- physician and dentist study groups 117, 130
- physicians 7-9, 21, 24-25, 50, 88-89, 117, 160, 272-280, 301-303
- physicians compared to team approach 145, 149
- physicians report giving 3, 20-21
- recommendations for giving 280
- reminder sheets 95, 175-177
- repeated 79, 260
- resident training 189, 191, 194, 196, 199
- role-play for delivery of 263
- samples of 196, 223-225, 288-297
- timing of 267
- training in 94-96, 278
- usual care 262-263, 288
- with nicotine gum 92, 95-99
- (*see also* **counseling, smoking intervention; smoking interventions**)

African Americans
- *see* **black smokers**

age
- of smokers 12-13, 19, 21
- of ST users 159

alcohol 98, 231, 265, 269
American Academy of Family Physicians, smoking counseling kit 75, 373
American Academy of Pediatrics 361
American Cancer Society 257, 344, 360-361, 366
- cancer prevention recommendations 324-325
- self-help materials 155-156, 282

American Dental Association 128, 135, 366
American Heart Association 257, 373
American Lung Association 146, 257, 344
- self-help materials 156, 282
- smoking cessation program 275

American Medical Association 25, 360-361
anticipatory guidance, pediatrician 240, 243-244
antismoking messages 34-35
Asians/Pacific Islanders 12-13, 111, 261
assessment of smoking status 13-14, 116, 130-131, 133-134, 139, 144, 146, 153, 155, 257, 321, 323, 328-329
associations
- dental, NCI collaboration 363-364, 366-367
- medical, training programs 360-362

attempts to quit smoking
- *see* **quit attempts**

attitude and practice questionnaire 115, 121, 129, 135
attitudes of parents
- about effects of their smoking on children 236-238
- about pediatrician counseling 230, 236-238, 241

attitudes of patient to provider intervention 24-25, 247

attitudes toward smoking intervention, physician 48, 52, 82, 87-88, 102, 109-110, 203, 254-255, 260, 263, 330-332, 342, 352
pediatricians 233-236, 239, 241
residents 199, 209-210, 213-215, 239-240, 266
audit-with-feedback interventions 330, 332
barriers
to effectiveness of office-based interventions 10, 254-255
to implementation of training programs 208, 220-221
to pediatrician intervention 233, 235, 238-241, 244
to physician smoking interventions 88-89, 143, 265-266, 303, 321, 329, 341-342, 352
to smoking cessation 7, 104, 151, 195, 211-212, 265-266, 281, 292
bedside counseling in hospital 154-155
behavior
change 24, 344-346, 352-353, 356, 358
counseling, smoking intervention 189, 192, 194, 196, 199-203
shaping 72, 87
skills training 229, 231
therapy and smoking cessation 98, 100
beta-naphthylamine, exposure to 275, 277
biochemical validation of smoking status 57, 102, 105-106, 110, 115-117, 123, 127, 131, 213, 247
carbon monoxide analysis 92, 96, 115-116, 127, 131, 146-148, 150, 163-165, 213, 215
cotinine analysis 57, 164-165, 247
black smokers 12-13, 19, 21, 111, 128, 261, 372
Blue Cross/Blue Shield of Minnesota 75-76
Blue Plus 75-78, 81, 304, 307-308, 319
booster sessions, smoking intervention 262, 264-265, 269-270
sample of 289-291
training sessions 204-205
California Tobacco Survey (1990) 12-14
Canada
COMMIT implementation 337, 371-372
smoking cessation interventions 45, 48, 53-67
cancer
bladder, chemical workers at risk of 229, 231, 272-284
cervix 26
esophagus 156-157
head and neck, interventions for 229, 259-270
larynx 156-157, 259, 261
lung 25-26, 259
oral 156-157, 259, 261
pharynx 259, 261
radiation therapy for 260, 267
squamous cell 259-261, 267
ST-associated 156-157, 259, 261
stomach 156-157
cancer prevention reminder system (CPRS) 321-333
Cancer Prevention Research Consortium 308, 343, 346-347
carbon monoxide testing
see **biochemical validation**
cardiovascular risk 16, 26
change, behavioral 24
stages of 344-346
techniques 356, 358
transtheoretical model of 344-346, 352-353
charts, patient 46, 54, 56, 62, 146
clinic review of 311-312
computerized CPRS 323, 326-327
flagging 13-14, 241-242, 264
labeling of 72-73, 304-305, 314
marking systems 116, 122, 125-126, 129, 136-138, 140
notes on smoking assessment 256-257
prompt 189, 207, 210
reminder system 207, 210
reminders 46, 116, 125-126, 129, 140, 264
smoking record card 314
chemical workers
bladder cancer risk and smoking 272, 274-275, 284
exposure to carcinogen 272, 274-275
medical/dental advice and counseling 229, 231, 272-276, 278-280
recruitment for intervention 274-278, 283
children
asthmatic 233-234
exposure to environmental tobacco smoke 29, 230, 362
parental smoking, effects of 220, 230, 232-234, 238
parents' attitudes about pediatrician counseling of 239
pediatrician smoking intervention 229-230, 232, 239-243
prevalence of smoking 232
prevention of tobacco use 229-230, 232, 239-240, 243, 361-362, 364-365
respiratory illness 232-234, 242
tobacco use intervention 361-362, 364-365
chiropractors 337, 369, 371-372
cigarettes
advertising 27, 29
and ST use 159-161
demarketing 29, 31
first of day 71, 217-218
initiation 4-5
marketing 31
clinic-based smoking interventions 7-9, 69-89, 305-313
Blue Cross/Blue Shield 75-76
Blue Plus 75-78, 81, 304, 307-308, 319

components of 72-73
cost-benefit adequacy 79, 81
Doctors Helping Smokers 69-89
Doctors Helping Smokers collaborations 75-89, 304-308, 314-315, 318
environment program 72-73, 79-81, 83, 89
feedback system 79, 81
HMO Midwest 75-76
level of implementation 82
marketing and advertising 79, 81
Nokomis Clinic 14-15, 72-75, 79-80, 304-305
orientation program 79-80
patient experience 84-85
patient surveys 84, 311-313
physician participation 78-80, 82-83, 87-89, 305-307
program evaluation 79, 81
recruitment for 70, 76-79, 81-82, 86-88
research environment 72-73
spirit-building component 79, 81, 83
stress of clinic 306-307
support staff 78-80, 82, 84, 89
supporting elements 74

clinic environment program 72-73, 79-81, 83, 89
clinic quality improvement 301, 303, 319
Clinical Interventions To Prevent Tobacco Use by Children and Adolescents 239-240
clinical trials, smoking intervention 158, 191, 342-343, 347, 352, 356-358, 362
design 213
phase III 145, 342
physician advice 92-98
Quit for Life 104-109
recruitment for 92-94, 193-194
resident smoking interventions 207, 213-221

CME
see **continuing medical education**
COMMIT
see **Community Intervention Trial for Smoking Cessation**
community
awareness and action 33-36
smoking outcome measures 347, 352

community-based physician interventions 45, 53, 302, 342-344, 346-348
Community Intervention Trial for Smoking Cessation (COMMIT) 51, 302, 334-341, 369-374
case studies 337, 369-374
community organizer 373-374
design and endpoints 335
goals 334-337
physician and dental training 337-340, 371-373
protocol 334, 336-337, 369, 371, 374
workshops 338-339, 370-371, 373

computerized reminder system 302, 321-333
consent form 93, 97, 115, 123, 128, 170
continuing dental education 338-339, 364, 370
continuing medical education (CME), smoking intervention
associations 361
methods 51
objectives 49-50
office-based 48-52, 54, 349-351
physician attitudes 52
physician counseling 103, 106, 108, 111
physicians 48-52, 54, 59, 62, 338-339, 349-351, 360
protocol for McMaster/Waterloo Project 53
workshops 59, 62, 94, 370
(*see also* **training programs, smoking intervention**)

continuity of care 10, 265-266
continuous quality improvement (CQI) 10, 309-311
system for smoking cessation 311-319

contract to quit smoking 32, 55, 67, 196-197, 260, 264-265
adolescent/child 243

cost-benefit adequacy of clinic intervention 79, 81
cotinine analysis 57, 164-165, 247
counseling, physician training 189-191, 194, 196-197, 199-200
advice alone 189, 191, 194, 196, 199
amount of time 203
counseling skills 269, 351
frequency of 190
maintenance of skills 199-200
patient-centered behavioral 194-197, 203-204
plus nicotine gum 189, 191, 194, 197, 199
prompts 189-190
research/questions to resolve 203-204
resident training 189-191, 194, 196, 199, 203
samples 196, 198, 223-226
tutorials 189-190

counseling, smoking intervention
attitudes, patients 24-25
behavioral 194, 199-202
clinical trials, residents 207, 213-221
content 213, 215-218, 220
cost-effectiveness 102, 110-111, 149
CPRS 321-333
dental patients 130
dentists 24-26, 143, 157
examples of 224-225
flowchart 210-212, 278
four A's 13-15, 240, 242-244, 350, 357-359, 365
frequency 213, 215-218, 220
in hospital 154
minimal contact 207-210
nature of 280-283

NCI protocol 350
nurse-assisted 46, 52, 109, 144-151, 166
of chemical workers 229, 231, 275-276
of children and adolescents 229, 232, 239, 241-243
of head and neck cancer patients 231, 259-270
of parents 229-230, 232
of pregnant women 229-230, 233, 246-258
of women 246-247
patient reports of 117, 214, 217
physician practices 25, 102-104, 109-111, 143-150, 214-216, 301-302
physician vs. patient reports 217-218
resident training 189, 192, 194, 196, 199, 203, 207-212, 220
self-efficacy 274, 276, 281-284, 295-297
special practice settings 229-244
steps in process 103-104
strategies for 30-33
team approach 143, 145, 149-151, 165-166
techniques 103-104, 213-214
training of nurses 251-254
training of physicians 103, 107-108, 246, 351
tutorial 207, 209-210, 213, 215-218
use of prompt 189-191, 207-210, 213, 215-218
(*see also* **advice to quit smoking; smoking interventions**)

counselors, smoking cessation 275-276, 281
training 276, 283-284

CPRS
see **cancer prevention reminder system**

CQI
see **continuous quality improvement**

demarketing of cigarettes 29, 31

demographics of smokers 12-13
and advice to quit 18-19, 21

dental associations 363-364, 366-367

dental education 337-340, 364-365, 370
(*see also* **training programs, smoking intervention**)

dental professionals, tobacco use intervention
differences from medical model 364
NCI training 362, 366-367
smokeless tobacco intervention 157-162
smoking intervention 14, 135, 340
training, COMMIT 340
training manuals 365
(*see also* **oral health team**)

dentists, smoking interventions 9, 13-15, 143, 157
advice to quit smoking, chemical workers 272-280
attitude and practice questionnaire 129, 135
barriers/problems 133-135, 139
compared to medical 113, 141
comparison of approaches 137-138
continuing education 337-340
counseling behavior 138-140
feedback reports 129
followup 159-161
maxillofacial prosthodontists 229, 231, 259-260, 266, 268-270
NCI program 362-367
NCI studies 113, 127-141, 362
of head and neck cancer patients 231, 259-270
office staff 27-28, 132-138, 140-141
patient reports of counseling by 130
patient visits per year 25, 364
provider acceptability/attitude 160
quit rates 131-132
receptivity of patients 157, 160
recruitment 45, 301-302
recruitment for studies 128, 133-135, 139
role in COMMIT 336-337, 340-341
role of 4, 9-10
success of intervention 160
surveys of practices 102, 109
training 45-46, 128-130, 135-137, 268-270, 301-302
training, COMMIT 337-340, 370, 373

dentists, tobacco use intervention 363-367
ST 46, 157-162, 363-365

determination of smoking status 13-14, 116, 130-131, 133-134, 139, 144, 146, 153, 155, 321, 323, 328-329

diffusion theory, smoking intervention 343-344, 346-347, 353

dissemination
of interventions 301-302, 342-353, 356, 367
of training 361
process 343

Division of Cancer Prevention and Control 334

Doctors Helping Smokers (DHS) 12, 45, 69-89, 304-308, 314-315, 318

Doctors Ought to Care (DOC) 27-28, 34-35, 340, 369

education
associations 361
continuing dental 364
level of patient and advice received 13, 19, 21
of physicians, use of nicotine gum 104, 110
(*see also* **continuing medical education; training programs, smoking intervention**)

educational materials
for dentists 365
for office staff 351
for patients
see **self-help materials, smoking cessation**
for physicians 75, 239-240, 257, 351, 357-360
on snuff 159

"Enough Snuff" 159

environment, clinic 72-73, 79-81, 83, 89
environmental stimuli 6-7
environmental tobacco smoke 29, 36, 230, 362
examples of physician interventions 196, 198, 223-226
exit interview 57, 64, 123, 138, 213-215, 217-218
experimental intervention 262-263, 288-291
face-to-face interaction 86, 260
Fagerstrom tolerance scale 95, 261
family practice physicians, smoking interventions 92-100, 120
- clinical trials 207, 213, 215, 220
- computerized reminder 321, 323, 332
- counseling 207, 229, 239, 332
- Quit for Life project 102-103
- recruitment for trial 92-94
- training 45-46, 48-50, 53, 193-194, 207, 210, 213, 239

Family Practice Smoking Cessation Project, McMaster/Waterloo 48, 53-67
fear arousal 279-280, 282, 284
feedback system 79, 81, 97, 330, 332
female smokers
- health risks 25-26
- lung cancer 25-26
- physician visits 12-13
- pregnant 26, 229-230, 233, 246-258, 370
- report receiving advice to quit 18, 21

flowcharts
- CQI system 314-317
- smoking counseling 210-212, 278

flowsheets 329, 332
- for patient office visit 55-56, 62

FOCUS-PDCA cycle 310-318
followup, dental ST intervention 159-161
followup, resident tutorial 190, 220
followup, smoking intervention
- 1-week 211
- 6-month 71-72, 92, 96, 184, 191, 198, 200-201, 214, 218-220
- 12-month 71-72, 191, 198, 201
- 18-month 191, 198
- 24-month 191, 198
- adolescents 163-164
- by nurses 252
- by pediatricians 242-243
- difficulty implementing 306
- head and neck cancer patients 262, 269-270
- hospital patients 154-156
- how to deal with 50-51
- interviews 70-71
- letters 197, 200
- long-term 49, 65-67, 191
- maximal 191, 197-198, 200
- minimal 191, 198, 200
- nurse-assisted, TRACC program 144-150
- office 33, 134, 357
- oral health team 365
- patient characteristics 67
- patient flowsheet 56
- patient reports and perceptions 64-65
- postcards 262, 264-265, 270
- questionnaires 95-96, 183-185
- Quit for Life 103-105, 107
- telephone 33, 46, 197-198, 200-201, 203, 269, 305
- training 63-64, 359
- use of nicotine gum 185
- videotape of 359
- visits, structuring and timing of 61-62, 66
- visits, supportive 54-55, 61
- (*see also* **quit rates, smoking**)

four A's of patient counseling 13-15, 350, 357-359, 365
- use by pediatricians 240, 242-244

generic reminder sheet 95, 175
grand rounds, smoking intervention 8-9, 115, 348, 373
Great American Smokeout 7, 373-374
gynecological patients 229-230, 246-247, 256-258
head and neck surgeons 229, 231, 259-260, 263, 266-270
Health Care Provider Task Force 337-338, 341
health care providers
- barriers to smoking intervention 341
- in COMMIT 336-337, 340-341
- training, COMMIT 337-340, 371

health effects
- of passive smoking 232-234, 237-239, 242
- of smoking 25-26, 229, 259, 272-275, 278, 280, 288
- of ST use 26, 156-159, 363-364

health maintenance organization (HMO) 304, 306-307
- adolescent smoking cessation intervention 162-166
- clinical trial recruitment 104, 106
- HMO Midwest 75-76
- intervention study 120, 122-123, 125
- office staff involvement 106-108
- pregnant smokers' intervention 248, 256
- smoking intervention training 46
- smoking intervention trials 102-111
- surveys of internists 109-110
- TRACC smoking intervention 143-151

Health Provider Task Force (HPTF) 369-371, 373-374
health risks, screening questionnaire 92-93, 169
health status, self-reported 12-14
Hispanics
- COMMIT 335, 372
- head and neck cancer patients in intervention 261

smokers, physician visits 12-13
smoking behavior 111
Hospital Corporation of America (HCA) 310-311
hospitals
activities, smoking cessation 373-374
patients, smoking intervention 46, 151-156
smoke-free 152-153, 371, 373
hotline, stop smoking 6, 146, 150, 163
How To Help Your Patients Stop Smoking 75, 239, 257, 357, 359-360
How To Help Your Patients Stop Using Tobacco 365
HPTF
see **Health Provider Task Force**
hygienist, dental
see **dental professionals, tobacco use intervention**
individualizing interventions 29-30
initial advice 262, 288-289
institutionalization of smoking intervention 8, 301
intention to quit 48, 57-58, 92, 95-97, 236, 238
internal medicine, smoking interventions
clinical trials 207, 213, 215, 220
CPRS intervention 321, 323, 332
HMO 102-107
NCI intervention study 113-114, 120
primary care trial 92-98
private practice 102-103, 105-107
recruitment for trials 92, 104-105
surveys of 102, 109-110
training 46, 193-194, 207, 210, 213, 215, 220, 239
intervention strategies for physicians, summary 351
interventions, smokeless tobacco
see **smokeless tobacco interventions**
interventions, smoking
see **smoking interventions**
Johns Hopkins Medical School, smoking prevalence 15-17
Johns Hopkins Precursors Study 15-16
Kaiser Permanente 46, 103-104, 106-107, 152
adolescent smoking cessation interventional 162-165
Dental Care Program 158
nurse-assisted smoking intervention 144-145, 147-148, 151
Latinos
see **Hispanics**
leadership, clinic smoking intervention 306-307
legislation, smoking-related 340
linkage system, diffusion of interventions 344, 347, 353
magazines
cigarette advertising 27
in waiting rooms 27-28
sticker for 28
without tobacco advertising 38-39
maintenance of smoking cessation 87, 262, 264-265, 270, 273
male smokers
lung cancer 25
physician visits 12-13
report receiving advice to quit 18, 21
marketing
of cigarettes 27, 29
of clinic smoking intervention 79, 81, 83
of educational events 52
McMaster/Waterloo Project 48, 53-67
media
and legislative advocacy, training in 340
campaigns 6-7
medical associations, training programs 360-362
medical materials development 356-359
medical records
computerized system 323, 326, 329
prompt on 189-190
(*see also* **charts, patient**)
medical screening form 93, 174
medical students, smoking prevalence 12, 15-17
meta-analysis of smoking cessation trials 71-72, 87, 240, 303, 358
minimal-contact smoking counseling 207-210
minimal followup to smoking cessation 191, 198, 200
Minnesota Heart Health Program 69-70
morbidity and mortality, smoking 25-26, 28, 35
motivation
and physician reinforcement 102, 104, 260
money 30-32
of health care providers, smoking intervention 8-9, 50, 97, 260, 301
to quit smoking 7, 28, 30-33, 102, 104, 111, 195, 209, 211, 214, 272, 274
National Cancer Institute (NCI)
associations, collaborative training programs 360-364, 366-367
Cancer Prevention Research Consortium 343, 346-347
clinical trials, smoking intervention 106, 334, 342-343, 347, 352, 356-358, 362
COMMIT 51, 302, 334-341, 369-374
counseling protocol 350
dental program strategies 363-364
dental team training programs 127-141
dentist manuals 365
Division of Cancer Prevention and Control 334

Doctors Helping Smokers 12, 69-71, 75-89, 304-308, 314-315, 318
elements of medical advice 272
four A's of patient counseling 13-15, 240, 242-244, 350, 357-359, 365
How To Help Your Patients Stop Smoking 75, 239, 257, 357, 359-360
How To Help Your Patients Stop Using Tobacco 365
medical and dental models compared 364-365
oral health team training 362, 364-366
patient materials 146, 155, 197, 327
phase III trials 342
phase IV studies 343, 347, 352
physician and dentist interventions, studies of 113-141
physician manuals 75, 239-240, 242-243, 257, 353, 357-360
physician smoking cessation trials 260
Physicians Counseling Smokers Project 343, 346, 352
"Quit for Good" pamphlet 115, 121, 129, 136, 197, 327
Smoking and Tobacco Control Program 365
smoking intervention 3, 12
Smoking, Tobacco, and Cancer Program 207, 209
training materials 356-360, 365
training programs 246, 256, 302, 356, 359-362, 366-367
training workshops 339, 359-360
National Health Interview Surveys 17-21
National Heart, Lung, and Blood Institute
counseling protocol for smokers 115, 129
preventive cardiology awards 16
video 373
National Institutes of Health 308
negative reactions to advice 273, 279-280, 284
nicotine addiction 4, 211, 274
nicotine gum 9, 98, 100, 209, 212, 214, 218, 274
and group therapy 98
black smokers 111
dentist training 130, 136-137
effects on smoking cessation 46, 55, 129
followup questionnaire on use 96, 185
instructions on prescribing 122, 137
NCI dentist intervention study groups 127-131, 136-137
NCI physician intervention study groups 113-114, 116-118, 121-123
patient instructions on use 55, 125, 280, 292
patient use 57-59, 67
physician training in use of 45, 50, 54, 60, 104, 110, 116, 121-122, 195
plus physician advice 92, 95-99
plus physician counseling, training 189, 191, 194, 197
plus reminder 113, 116-118, 127, 130-131
prescription of 110-111, 212, 214, 218, 279-281, 292
quit rates 116-118, 131-132
reminder sheet 176
trial group 92, 95-97
nicotine replacement therapies 7, 92, 94, 98, 100
patch 9, 87
(*see also* **nicotine gum**)
nicotine substitutes, patient instructions 125, 140
Nokomis Clinic (Minnesota) 14-15, 72-75, 79-80, 304-305
Nurses Guide 251-253
nurses, smoking interventions 14, 81, 109, 121, 123, 230, 240, 357
adolescents 162-164
burnout 254-255
COMMIT 337, 372
counseling 46, 52
CQI system 314
prenatal clinic 250-255
smoking status of 253, 255
TRACC 144-151, 166
training 145, 151, 240, 250-253, 255, 362
obstacles to smoking cessation
see **barriers**
obstetrical care practice
see **pregnancy**
office-based smoking interventions 3, 7-10, 301-319, 349-350, 357-358
barriers to 10, 254-255, 358
clinics 303-309
constraints on 249-250
cueing and monitoring system 62
dental 127-141
dissemination 301-302
examination 28-29
flowcharts 314-317
institutionalization 8, 301
interval between visits 250
medical 113-126
obstetrical 256-258
process of development 7-8
public prenatal care clinics 247-255
recall systems 134
reception area 27-28
recruitment 301-302
steps for 357
office staff, smoking interventions
clinic intervention 78-80, 82, 84, 89
components of successful system 46-47
CQI system 311-319
HMO 106-107
intervention study groups 123, 137-138
involvement in smoking intervention 45-46, 49, 52, 106-108

NCI intervention, dental 130, 132-138, 140-141
NCI intervention, physician 115, 119-126
nurse 46, 52
office practice consultants 349-351
private obstetrical 256-258
public prenatal care clinics 249-250
recruitment 45, 301-302, 322-323
role in smoking intervention 221, 357-358
staff coordinator 79-80, 95, 138, 357
support of 79-80, 89
TRACC program 145-146
training 10, 98, 301-302, 304, 326, 331, 349-351, 362
turnover 119, 122-126, 135, 139, 141

oral health
see **health effects**

oral health team
term defined 364
tobacco cessation 362
tobacco use prevention 362
trainers' workshop 365
training 135-137, 338-340, 363-365, 371-373
(*see also* **dental** entries; **dentists** entries)

parents
attitudes about pediatrician counseling 230, 238-239, 241, 244
attitudes about smoking 236-238
beliefs 234-235
effects of smoking on children 220, 230, 232-234, 238
pediatrician counseling/intervention 210, 220, 230, 232-238, 241-242
stage of change/readiness to quit 230, 238

passive smoking, effects of 232-234, 237-239, 242

patient-centered counseling 194-197, 202-204
cholesterol lowering 204
four A's of 350
physical exercise 204
smoking cessation 195-197, 202-203

patient-provider interaction 3, 73, 88, 191-192, 317

patients, smokers
adherence to intervention 266
assessment/determination of smoking status 13-14, 116, 130-131, 133-134, 139, 144, 153, 155, 321, 323, 328-329
attitudes 24-25, 247
cancer prevention reminders 324, 326-327
charts
see **charts, patient**
compliance 254
confidence in physician advice 92
consent form 115, 123, 128
demographics of 12-13, 18-19, 21
dentist visits per year 3, 25, 301, 364
exit interview 57, 64, 123, 138, 213-215, 217-218
experience in Doctors Helping Smokers 84-85
flowsheet for office visit 55-56, 62
health status, self-reported 12-14
hospitalized 151, 154
initial office visit 54-55
instruction on use of nicotine substitute 125
intake process 10, 210
motivation to quit smoking
see **motivation**
office visits, structure of 50
perceptions of physician intervention 64-66
physician visits per year 3, 12-14, 17, 25, 98, 102, 301
profile of 12-13
provider interaction flowchart 317
questionnaires 92-93, 95-97, 146, 149-150, 169-174, 179-182
race 12-13, 19, 21, 111, 335
recall of office visit 58
receptivity to interventions 157, 160, 166
recruitment for intervention 192-194, 202, 260-261
recruitment for NCI studies 115, 123, 128, 133-135, 139
report receiving advice to quit 3, 17-21, 25, 214, 217-218, 241
reports on physician and dental counseling 117, 130
screening of 28, 72-73, 115, 128, 304-305
self-efficacy counseling 274, 276, 281-284
self-help materials
see **self-help materials, smoking cessation**
smoking history 33, 55, 62
surveys 17-21, 84, 158, 160, 311-313
tracking of 10, 264
(*see also* **smokers**)

pediatricians, smoking interventions 229, 232-244
anticipatory guidance to prevent smoking 240, 243-244
attitudes and practices of 230, 233-235, 239, 241
attitudes of parents 230, 236-238, 241
barriers 233, 235, 239-241, 244
best opportunities to give advice 235-236
children and adolescents 229-230, 232, 239, 242-243, 361-362
clinical trials 207, 213, 215, 220
COMMIT 370
confidence in delivering advice 230, 233-235, 241
followup 242-243
four A's for counseling 240, 242-243
incorporating advice into office visits 241-243
NCI manuals for 239-240, 242-243, 361-362
office personnel 240
parents 229-230, 232-236, 238, 240-241
prevention 229-230, 232, 239-240, 243-244
publications for patients 287, 361-362
questionnaire 233-236
residents 207-210, 213, 215, 220, 239

surveys of 233-234, 241
training 207-210, 213, 230, 232, 236, 238-240
personalizing risks/benefits 211, 272, 278
pharmacists, COMMIT 337, 372
pharmacological therapies 92, 98-100
(*see also* **nicotine gum; nicotine replacement therapies**)
phase I studies 48, 53-61
phase II studies 48-49, 61-67
phase III clinical trials 145, 342
phase IV studies 343, 347, 352
physician coordinator 79-80
physician counseling
see **physicians, smoking interventions**
Physician-Delivered Smoking Intervention Project 194
physician-patient contact 54, 191-192
Physician Smoking Trials 207, 209
physicians
as trainers 208, 210
attitude and practice questionnaire 115, 121
attitudes to intervention 48, 52, 82, 87-88, 102, 109-110, 203, 254-255, 260, 263, 330-332, 342, 352
behavioral influence on 24
community activities 34
community-based 342-344, 346-347
continuing education
see **continuing medical education**
counseling behavior 24-25, 87-88
counseling practices 204, 213-218
focus groups 349
forgetfulness of 329-330, 332
intervention tasks 89
motivation of 8-9, 50, 97, 260, 301
patient visits per year 3, 12-14, 17, 25, 98, 102
peer influence 24, 322, 343-344, 370
recruitment 70, 76-79, 86, 114-115
reimbursement 8-9, 24-25, 52, 55, 110, 254, 371
reinforcing factors in counseling 24-25
reminders 72-73, 95, 175-177
report advising smokers to quit 3, 20-21, 214-218
smoking counseling rates 323, 328-329
stages of change 346, 350-351
tobacco use 12, 15-17, 25, 230, 255, 260, 307
(*see also* areas of specialty; e.g., **pediatricians**)
Physicians Counseling Smokers Project 343, 346, 352
physicians, smoking interventions
adoption and implementation of 343-344, 346-347, 350, 352-353
advantages and disadvantages 143
advice alone 144-149, 189, 191, 194, 196, 199, 200-202, 224
advice plus gum 92, 95-99
advice training 94-96, 278
cancer prevention reminder system 321-333
checklist for implementation 70
clinical trial on advice 92-98, 170
clinics 78-80, 82-83, 86-89, 305-307
communication grid 223
compared to dental 113, 141
compared to team approach 145, 149
comparison of approaches 199-203
compliance 53, 100
computerized reminder system 302, 321-333
confidence 24, 215, 342
content of 213, 215
counseling 57, 117, 143-149, 189, 191, 194, 196-197, 207-221, 224-225
counseling plus gum 189, 191, 194, 197
counseling skills training 351
CQI system 301
criteria 303
dissemination of 301-302, 342-353, 356, 367
educational materials 75, 239-240, 257, 351, 357-360
effectiveness of 342-343
examples of 196, 198, 223-226
for chemical workers 272-276, 278-280
four A's 13-15, 240, 242-244, 350, 357-359, 365
frequency of 213, 215
implementation of 343-344, 346-347, 350, 352-353
institutionalization 8, 301
McMaster/Waterloo project 48, 53-67
motivating patient
see **motivation**
NCI manuals for 75, 239-240, 242-243, 257, 353, 357-360
NCI studies 113-126, 260
NCI training 356, 359-362
nurse-assisted 46, 51-52, 144-151, 166
obstacles
see **barriers**
office practice consultant visits 349-351
office staff
see **office staff, smoking interventions**
patterns of advice 18
personalized 60, 66, 211, 242, 260, 272, 278
Quit for Life project 45, 102-110
recruitment for 45, 53, 301-302, 321-322, 347-349, 353
reminders 72-73, 302-303, 305
responses to patients' concerns 226
results of 199-203
role in COMMIT 336-337, 340-341
samples of 196, 198, 211-212, 223-226
summary of strategies 351
time constraints on 143
TRACC intervention 143-149
training
see **training programs, smoking intervention**
transtheoretical model of change 344-346, 352-353

willingness to intervene 191
(*see also* **advice to quit smoking; smoking interventions**; and areas of specialty)
postcards, smoking cessation maintenance 262, 264-265, 270
pregnancy
physician smoking intervention 229-230, 246-258
prenatal care 29, 247-258
smoking cessation 229, 247-248, 370
smoking during 26, 233
prevalence of smoking
adults 232
children and adolescents 232
medical students 12, 15-17
physicians 12, 15-16, 25
pregnant women 233
women 230, 233
prevention of tobacco use
by adolescents and children 229, 232, 238-240, 243-244, 361
by head and neck cancer patients 229, 231
by pregnant women 229, 233
clinic activities 318-319
computerized reminder system 332-333
dental office 9, 340, 364-365
(*see also* **smoking interventions**)
Preventive Cardiology studies 15, 17
primary care physicians, smoking interventions
brief advice 240
clinic-based 304-319
clinical trials 207, 213-221
COMMIT 336, 340
computerized reminder system 321-322, 332-333
Doctors Helping Smokers 45, 82-83
NCI dissemination studies 342-343, 347, 353
private practice 45-46, 102-103, 106-108
Quit for Life 102-105, 111
recruitment for trials 92-94, 97, 104-105, 321-322
TRACC program 143-151
training 207-208, 213, 220, 359-362
trials 46, 92-100, 113
prompt, smoking intervention 207-210, 213, 215-220
on medical records 189-191
provider attitudes and characteristics 254-255
provider-patient bond 260, 266
psychological treatment, smoking cessation 98, 100
public information 6-7
public prenatal clinics 247-255
quality assurance systems 10, 301, 308-309, 319
quality improvement paradigm 309-310, 319
questionnaires
dental intervention 159-160
for clinical trial 92-93, 95-97, 169-174, 179-185
on smoking 146, 149-150
parents' attitudes 236-237
pediatricians' attitudes and practices 233-235
Quit and Win 373-374
quit attempts 4-7, 22, 33, 89, 92, 212, 240, 281-282, 292
adolescents 165
log of 95-96
rates of 15, 71, 96, 148, 220
quit date
contracts 260, 262, 264
NCI study groups 117
physician verification form 95, 178
prescribing 209, 211, 213-214, 218
setting 14, 32, 55-56, 62, 104, 108, 117, 144-148, 150, 159, 209, 211, 213-214, 218, 242-243, 274, 279, 312
training for 50, 54, 67
"Quit for Good" pamphlet 115, 121, 129, 136, 197, 327
Quit for Life 327
Quit for Life project 45, 102-111
quit rates, smoking
1 year 49, 57, 59-61, 65-66, 74, 284
6 months 96, 189, 191, 200, 202, 218-219, 221
and level of physician intervention 200-202
and physician counseling 218-219, 221, 284
and physician training 57, 59-61, 65-66
cancer patients 259
dental intervention 160-161
expectations of 21, 30, 210, 240, 254
hospital patients 151, 155
long-term 49, 108, 191, 273-274
NCI intervention studies 116-118, 131-132
nurse-assisted counseling 149-150
pregnant smokers 247-248
reminder intervention 116-118, 130-131
short-term 59-60, 65
with brief advice 240
with gum use 55, 57, 59-61, 65-66, 96, 218
quit rates, ST 160-161
race, smokers 12-13, 19, 21, 111
radiation oncologists 260, 265-266
randomized factorial trial 210, 213-214
design of 213-214
randomized studies 106, 114, 153, 158
readiness to quit smoking 32, 150, 154-155, 229-230, 238, 251, 278-279
reception area 27-28
receptionist
clinical trial recruitment 93, 97
dental intervention 158, 160
patient screening 93
smoking intervention 14, 52-53, 132-133, 146, 150, 166

reimbursement 8-9, 24-25, 52, 55, 110, 254, 371
reinforcement of interventions 143, 145, 162-163, 257, 260, 303
reinforcing factors in physician counseling 24-25
relapse, smoking 22, 33, 50, 63, 71, 212, 251, 273, 279, 282-283, 289-290, 292
  abstinence violation effect (AVE) 289-290
  postpartum 248
  prevention counseling, training 205, 208
  prevention, hospitalized smokers 151, 155
  risk associated with alcohol 265
  stage of change 344-345
reminders
  computerized systems 302, 321-333
  for physicians 48-49, 72-73, 95, 175-177, 302-303, 305, 321-333
  intervention study groups 113, 116-118, 127, 129-131
  patient charts 116, 125-126, 129, 140, 207, 210
  plus nicotine polacrilex 113, 116-118, 127, 130-131
  quit rates with 116-118, 130-131
research assistants
  in dental studies 130, 132-134, 137-139
  in physician studies 115, 118-119, 122-124
residents, smoking interventions
  attitudes about 199, 209-210, 213-215, 239-240, 266
  clinical trials 213-221
  family practice 194, 207, 210, 213, 215, 220, 239
  integration of training 202
  internal medicine 46, 193-194, 207, 210, 213, 215, 220, 239
  maintenance of counseling skills 199-200
  pediatric 207, 210, 213, 215, 220, 232, 239-240
  posttraining data 199-201
  primary care 207-208, 213, 239
  prompt 207-210
  receptivity to 204
  recruitment for 190, 192-194, 204-205
  relapse prevention 205
  surgical 266
  training programs 8-9, 189-221, 223-226, 239
  tutorial 189, 207, 209-210
respiratory therapist 229, 275, 278
Rhode Island Cancer Prevention Research Consortium 343, 346-347, 352
risks of smoking 25-26, 229, 272-273, 280, 288
  and bladder cancer 272-275
  communication of 24, 279-280
role-playing in intervention training 95, 103-104, 263, 276, 351, 358
  nurses 253
  residents 195, 198, 200, 202
scare tactics 279-280, 282, 284
screening
  bladder cancer 274-278
  cancer prevention 329, 332
  clinical trial questionnaires 92-93, 97, 169, 174
  patients for NCI study 115, 128
  patients for tobacco use 28, 72-73, 304-305
self-efficacy counseling/intervention 272-274, 276, 281-284
  recommendations for 282-284
  sample 293-294
  transcript of 282, 295-297
self-help materials
  dental 159
  distributed by physician 104, 108, 209, 214, 218, 288-289, 305
  for children/adolescents 239-240, 242-243
  for head and neck cancer patients 264-265
  for nurses' intervention 251-252
  for patients 55, 144-148, 151, 155, 197, 257, 264-265, 270, 280, 282, 327, 373
  for smokers in public prenatal clinic 250-253
  for spouse/family 262, 265, 270, 288-291
  hospital patients 155-156
  Minnesota Heart Health Program 69-70
  NCI, for patients 146, 155, 197, 327
  ST cessation 159
  "Tip Sheets" 55
  videos 146-148, 150, 156, 373
seminar, training 121, 128, 141, 208
smoke-free health care facilities 337-338, 340, 374
  clinic/office 79-80, 83, 256-257, 305, 357
  hospitals 152-153, 371, 373
smokeless tobacco (ST)
  effects 26, 156-159, 363-364
  interventions 29, 46, 141, 156-162, 363-365
  users 156-157, 159-161
smokers
  African American
    see **black smokers**
  assessment of status 13-14, 116, 130-131, 133-134, 139, 144, 146, 153, 155, 321, 323, 328-329
  chemical workers 272, 274-278
  coping skills 274, 281
  demographics of 12-13, 18-19, 21
  dental visits per year 25, 301, 364
  desire to quit 71, 87, 89
  females 12-13, 18, 21, 25-26
  identification of 10, 28, 46, 72-73, 89, 133-134, 210, 351
  males 12-13, 18, 21, 25
  motivation to quit 7, 28, 30-31, 102, 104, 111, 195, 209, 211, 214, 272, 274
  physician visits per year 3, 12-14, 17, 25, 98, 102, 301
  physicians 12, 15-17, 25, 230, 307

pregnant
see **pregnancy**
profile of 12-13
providers of health care 230, 255
publications for spouse/family 262, 265, 270, 288-291
questionnaires 92-93, 95-97, 169, 171-174, 179-182
race 12-13, 19, 21, 111
readiness to quit 32, 149, 154-155, 229, 251, 278-279
report receiving advice 3, 17-20, 25, 241
resistance to advice 279
self-efficacy/ability to quit smoking 92, 95-97, 272-273, 281-284
self-help materials
see **self-help materials**
sex of 12-13, 18, 21
stages of change 149-151, 154, 251, 273-274, 277-279, 282
women, nonpregnant 246-247
(*see also* **patients, smokers**)
smoking
and anesthesia 267
and ST use 159-161
dependency 4-5, 211, 274
first cigarette in day 71, 217-218
health effects of 25-26, 229, 259, 272-275, 278, 280, 284, 288
initiation of 4-5
mortality from 25-26, 28, 35
oral health effects 26, 363
passive 232-234, 237-239, 242
physician attitudes about 110
prevalence 12, 15-17, 25, 230, 232-233
risks of 25-26, 229, 272-275, 278, 280, 288
social unacceptability 7, 36
Smoking and Tobacco Control Program (STCP) 365
smoking cessation
algorithms for delivery of advice 288-291
benefits of 25-26, 209, 229, 272, 278, 280, 288
biochemical validation
see **biochemical validation of smoking status**
cardiovascular patients 151
contract 32, 55, 67, 196-197, 243, 260, 264-265
hospital patients 151, 155-156
long-term 6-7, 99, 108, 191, 273-274
maintenance of 87, 262, 264-265, 273
motivation 7, 28, 30-31, 102, 104, 111, 195, 209, 211, 214, 272, 274
obstacles to/barriers 7, 104, 151, 195, 211-212, 281, 292
process of 4-7
progress toward 272-273, 279
reasons 7
rewards 30-33
scare tactics/fear arousal 279-280, 282, 284
self-help materials
see **self-help materials**
short-term 6-7, 59-60, 65, 273
stress of 282, 297
success 5-7, 30, 72
Surgeon General's report on 25, 233
transtheoretical model of change 344-346
weight gain 50, 63, 95, 211-212, 230, 253, 282, 292, 327
(*see also* **followup, smoking intervention; quit attempts; quit rates, smoking)**
Smoking Cessation and Reduction in Public Prenatal Clinics project 247, 249-251
training for 251-254
smoking cessation, stages of 22, 344-346
action 5-6, 150, 274, 277, 279-280
contemplation 5-7, 149-151, 154, 230, 251, 273-274, 277, 282
maintenance 87, 262, 264-265, 270, 273
parents 230, 238
precontemplation 5-7, 149-151, 229, 251, 273-274, 277, 284
pregnant women 229-230
readiness to quit 32, 150, 154-155, 229-230, 238, 251, 278-279
relapse
see **relapse, smoking**
smoking interventions
advice
see **advice to quit smoking**
approaches 189, 191, 194, 196-203, 248
audit-with-feedback 330, 332
barriers to effectiveness 254-255, 265-266
booster sessions 262, 264-265, 269-270
chemical workers 229, 231, 272-284
clinic-based 7-9, 69-89, 305-313
clinical trials
see **clinical trials, smoking intervention**
COMMIT 334-341, 369-374
comparisons 48-49, 113, 141, 199-203
computerized CPRS 321-333
cost-effectiveness of 102, 110-111, 149
counseling
see **counseling, smoking intervention**
criteria for effectiveness 303
dental assistant/hygienist 14, 135, 340, 362, 366, 372
dentists
see **dentists, smoking intervention**
dissemination of 301-302, 342-353, 356, 367
Doctors Helping Smokers 12, 45, 69-89, 304-308, 314-315, 318
dysfunctional reactions 279, 284 for adolescents
see **adolescents, tobacco use**

for pregnant smokers 246-250
for women 246-258
head and neck cancer patients 229, 259-261
HMO 144-151, 162-165
hospital patients 46, 151-156
individualizing 29-30
institutionalization 8, 301
McMaster/Waterloo Family Practice Smoking Cessation Project 48, 53-57
medical office 144-151
minimal-contact counseling 207-210
NCI studies 113-141
nicotine polacrilex study groups 113-114, 116-118, 121-122, 127-130
nicotine replacement 7, 92, 94, 98, 100
Nokomis Clinic 14-15, 72-75, 79-80, 304-305
nurse-assisted
see **nurses, smoking interventions**
office-based 3, 7-10, 301-319, 349-350, 357-358
office coordinator 79-80, 138, 357
office staff
see **office staff, smoking interventions**
oral health team 338-340, 362-368, 371-372
pharmacological therapies 92, 98-100
physicians
see **physicians, smoking interventions**
prompt 207-210, 213, 215-219
Quit for Life project 45, 102-111
reinforcement of 143, 145, 162-163, 257, 260, 303
reminder system study group 113, 116-118, 127, 129-131
reminder systems 302, 321-333
resident training 8-9, 189-221, 223-226, 239
samples of 196, 198, 223-226
self-help materials
see **self-help materials**
self-quit 146-149
software 323, 326, 329
spirit-building component 79, 81, 83
team approach 46, 52, 118, 120-121, 123-126, 135, 143-151, 165-166, 314, 364
TRACC program 46, 143-167
training
see **training programs, smoking intervention**
trials 104-109, 207, 213-221
trials, NCI 334, 342-343, 347, 352, 356-358, 362
tutorial 207, 209-210, 213, 215-219
use in smokeless tobacco interventions 157
worksites 275, 277
(*see also* **nicotine gum**)
smoking prevalence, U.S. 12, 15-17, 230, 232-233
smoking prevention
see **prevention of tobacco use**
smoking status
assessment of patient 13-14, 116, 130-131, 133-134, 139, 144, 146, 153, 155, 257, 321, 323, 328-329
of health care providers 230, 253, 255
of nurses 253
of physicians 15-17, 25, 230, 307
Smoking, Tobacco, and Cancer Program (STCP) 207, 209
Physician Smoking Trials 207, 209
social support materials 262, 265, 270, 288-291
software program, physician reminder system (CPRS) 323, 326, 329
ST
see **smokeless tobacco**
stages of behavior change
physicians 204, 346, 350-351
smokers
see **smoking cessation, stages of**
transtheoretical model of 344-346, 352-353
Stanford Cardiovascular Risk Reduction project 55
state-level intervention 360-361, 366
STCP
see **Smoking and Tobacco Control Program; Smoking, Tobacco, and Cancer Program**
stop-smoking contracts 32, 55, 67, 196-197, 243, 260, 264-265
(*see also* **quit date**)
success rates, NCI interventions 116-118, 131-132
Surgeon General's reports
see **U.S. Surgeon General**
surgeons, head and neck 229, 259-260, 263, 266-270
surveys
Adult Use of Tobacco Survey (AUTS) 17-21
California Tobacco Survey 12-14
cardiovascular risk of medical school students 16
Johns Hopkins Precursors Study 15-16
National Health Interview Survey 17-21
of health professionals' practices 102, 109-110, 233-234, 241
of patients 84, 241, 311-313
tobacco use 158, 160, 311-313
teachable moments 28-29, 143-146, 151, 167, 259, 363
dental care 157, 160, 162, 229, 231
teachers, materials for 358
team approach to tobacco interventions 46, 52, 314
compared to physician-centered 145, 149
CQI system 314
dental 135-141, 338-340, 362-365, 371-372
medical staff 118, 120-121, 123-126
TRACC 143, 145, 149-151, 165-166

teenagers
see **adolescents, tobacco use**
telephone
followup
see **followup, smoking intervention**
hotlines 7, 146, 150, 163
third-party payers 110, 370
tobacco and alcohol use 231, 269
tobacco control strategies 4-7, 33-35
dental 363-364
tobacco industry 31, 33, 36
advertising and promotion 7, 27, 29, 232
company sponsorship 33-34
Tobacco Reduction and Cancer Control (TRACC) program 46, 143-167
adolescent smoking intervention 162-165
hospital intervention 151-156
nurse-assisted counseling intervention 144-151
ST dental intervention 156-162
tobacco use
and alcohol 231, 269
by children 232
by physicians and office staff 307
cessation flowchart 316
health risks
see **risks of smoking**
identification of 28
prevention among children and adolescents 362, 365
prevention and cessation services, dental intervention 364-365
screening of patients 304-305
surveys of 17-21, 84, 158, 160, 311-313
(*see also* **smokeless tobacco; smoking**)
TRACC
see **Tobacco Reduction and Cancer Control program**
train-the-trainers approach 204, 207-208, 210, 220, 337-339, 361, 365
training materials 340
development of 356-359
for trainers 358-361
training programs, smoking intervention
advice only 189, 191, 194, 196, 199
and prompts 189-191, 208-210, 213, 215-216
approaches 189, 191, 194, 196-203
associations, medical 360-362
at practice site 94, 97
bedside counseling 155
behavioral skills 229, 231
booster sessions 204-205
brief advice 94-95
clinicians 359-360, 362
COMMIT 337-340, 370, 373
counseling 103-104, 145-146, 151, 189-191, 194, 196-197, 199-200, 203-204, 207-209, 223-226, 269, 351
counseling plus gum 189, 191, 194, 197, 199
counselors 275-276
dental staff 301-302, 338-340, 364-367
dentists 45-46, 128-130, 135-137, 268-270, 301-302
development of materials 356-359
educational methods used 194-195
family practice 45-46, 48-50, 53, 193-194, 207, 210, 213, 239
followup visits 63-64, 359
for Smoking Cessation and Reduction project 251-253
grand rounds 8-9, 115
incentives 195, 204
internal medicine 46, 193-194, 207, 210, 213, 215, 220, 239
maintenance of skills 199-200
materials for 199, 340, 358-360
McMaster/Waterloo Project 53-55, 61-63
medical office staff 301-302
methods of teaching 208-209
NCI dental intervention 128-130, 135-137, 141, 364-367
NCI materials 356-360
NCI physician intervention 115-116, 119, 121-122, 124, 256, 302, 356-362, 366-367
nicotine gum use 45, 50, 54, 60, 104, 110, 116, 121-122, 195, 280
nurse-assisted counseling 145-146, 151, 362
objectives 49-50
obstetrical office staff 256-258
office-based 301-302
office staff 10, 45, 119, 122-124, 126, 130, 135-137, 145-146, 351, 358, 362
office staff, CPRS 326, 331
pediatric 207-210, 213, 230, 232, 236, 238-240
physicians 45-46, 54, 62-63, 145, 189, 191-192, 204, 246, 278, 301-302, 304, 342, 351
posttraining data 199-200
practitioner 9-10
prenatal care nurses 250-255
primary care residents 207-208, 213, 220, 239
providers, head and neck cancer patients 263-264, 268-269
Quit for Life 103-104, 108-109
recommendations 49
recruitment to 190, 192-194, 204, 360
relapse prevention counseling 205, 208
residency curricula 8-9
residents 189-205, 207-210, 213, 223-226, 239
role-playing 95, 103-104, 195, 198, 200, 202, 253, 263-264, 276, 351, 358
self-efficacy counseling/intervention 276
self-training materials 204, 258
structure of sessions 205
trainers 358-362, 365
tutorials 189-190, 207, 209-210, 213, 215-216

videotapes
see **videotapes, smoking intervention for training programs**
workshops 50-51, 59, 62, 94, 305, 338-339, 351-352, 359-361, 365, 373
(*see also* **continuing medical education**)
training, tobacco use intervention, oral health professionals 364-365
differences from medical 364-365
NCI program 364-365
transdermal nicotine replacement 9, 87, 100, 110
transtheoretical model of change 344-346, 352-353
trial design, smoking counseling 213-214
trials, smoking intervention
see **clinical trials, smoking intervention**
tutorial
counseling group 207, 209-210, 215-220
plus prompt, counseling group 213, 215-219
resident smoking intervention 189-190
UCLA 259-260, 264, 268
University of North Carolina protocol 292
U.S. Surgeon General
report on health benefits of smoking cessation (1990) 25, 233
report on health consequences of smoking (1964) 15, 17
role of pediatrician (1985) 233
usual care group 262-263, 288
Veterans Administration patients 260, 266
videotapes, smoking intervention
by Health Provider Task Force 369-370
by National Heart, Lung, and Blood Institute 373
COMMIT 339
for adolescents 163
for hospital patients 154, 156
for physicians 54-55, 121, 136, 263-265, 339, 358-360, 373
for smokers 46
for training programs 195, 210, 276, 278, 358-360
impact on quit rates 150
interactive 166
physician recruitment for intervention 348
production and cost of 156
self-quit 146-148, 150
TRACC 46, 144-148, 150, 166
videotapes, ST intervention 159-160, 162
waiting room 27-28
weight gain 50, 230, 282
control of 63, 95, 253, 327
fear of 211-212, 292
white smokers 13, 19, 21, 111, 261
withdrawal
from nicotine 292
from smoking 50, 62, 282, 288, 297
women
attitudes to provider intervention 247
counseling by pediatricians 229, 233
in COMMIT 370
pregnant smokers 233, 246-250
risks from smoking 25-26
smoking intervention 246-258, 370
smoking rates 230
worker cohort recruitment 274-277, 283
workshops, intervention training 50-51, 59, 305, 351-352
clinical trial training 94
COMMIT training 338-339, 370-371, 373
Doctors Helping Smokers 78, 82
physician advice 94
trainers 359-362, 365
worksite smoking intervention 275, 277, 374